Neurology: A Clinical Handbook

# Neurology: A Clinical Handbook

Charles Clarke
*Honorary Consultant Neurologist, National Hospital for Neurology & Neurosurgery, University College London Hospitals NHS Foundation Trust, Queen Square, London, UK*

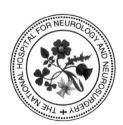

This Handbook is based on the Second Edition of *Neurology: A Queen Square Textbook*, which was co-edited by Dr Clarke.

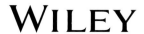

*Registered Offices*
John Wiley & Sons, Inc., 111 River Street, Hoboken, NJ 07030, USA
John Wiley & Sons Ltd, The Atrium, Southern Gate, Chichester, West Sussex, PO19 8SQ, UK

*Editorial Office*
9600 Garsington Road, Oxford, OX4 2DQ, UK

For details of our global editorial offices, customer services, and more information about Wiley products visit us at www.wiley.com.

Wiley also publishes its books in a variety of electronic formats and by print-on-demand. Some content that appears in standard print versions of this book may not be available in other formats.

*Library of Congress Cataloging-in-Publication Data*

Names: Clarke, Charles (Charles R. A.) author. | National Hospital for Neurology & Neurosurgery, Queen Square.
Title: Neurology: A Clinical Handbook / Charles Clarke.
Other titles: Neurology.
Description: Hoboken, NJ : Wiley, 2022. | Based on: Neurology : A Queen Square Textbook / edited by Charles Clarke, Robin Howard, Martin Rossor, Simon Shorvon. Second edition. Chichester, West Sussex, UK ; Hoboken, NJ : |b John Wiley & Sons, Inc., 2016. | Includes bibliographical references and index.
Identifiers: LCCN 2021054270 (print) | LCCN 2021054271 (ebook) | ISBN 9781119235729 (paperback) | ISBN 9781119235712 (adobe pdf) | ISBN 9781119235705 (epub)
Subjects: MESH: Nervous System Diseases | Neurology | Handbook
Classification: LCC RC346 (print) | LCC RC346 (ebook) | NLM WL 39 | DDC 616.8–dc23/eng/20211124
LC record available at https://lccn.loc.gov/2021054270
LC ebook record available at https://lccn.loc.gov/2021054271

Cover Design: Wiley
Cover Image: © Sergey Nivens/Shutterstock

Set in 9.5/12.5pt STIXTwoText by Straive, Pondicherry, India

Printed in Singapore
M064415_180522

# Contents

# Preface

In my training in the 1970s I was guided by many clinicians and also by books. Those large neurology tomes were useful, but it was the smaller texts that gave me insight into clinical practice. One by Dr Bryan Matthews, later Professor of Clinical Neurology at Oxford, was *Practical Neurology* published in 1963, when Matthews was a general neurologist in Derby. His was a book I could enjoy. Some comments are etched in my memory:

'There are many admirable textbooks of neurology but it is a matter of common observation that they are of more assistance in the passing of written examinations than in the management of practical problems'. Another, quoting Sir Geoffrey Jefferson, remarked ' . . . in life the tracts are not marked in red . . .'

And, from Matthews on dizziness: ' . . . there can be few physicians so dedicated to their art that they do not experience a slight decline in spirits on learning that their patient complains of giddiness.. . .'

There was thus some logic in taking *Neurology: A Queen Square Textbook*, Second Edition, the major reference work that I initiated and edited with colleagues, and turning it into this shorter, practical book. I hope this *Handbook* will serve two purposes. First, it is to be *read* – each chapter aims to give a brief overview of an area of neurology. Secondly, this book, a synopsis of our subject, provides a pointer to *Neurology: A Queen Square Textbook* in its forthcoming Third Edition, a completely separate project that has been fully updated and enhanced by Robin Howard, Dimitri M. Kullman, David Werring, and Michael Zandi. *Neurology: A Clinical Handbook* is based on the second edition of *Neurology: A Queen Square Textbook*. The editors and authors of *Neurology: A Queen Square Textbook* have not been involved in the development of this Handbook.

I struggled with several things. First: references. I decided, because one can source most references rapidly on a mobile phone, I would focus only on those references of personal interest. These are largely my own – but with one paper from my late wife Dr Ruth Seifert on *khat* and another from my father Professor Sir Cyril Astley Clarke on fatal methyl bromide poisoning – from the 1940s; both are in Chapter 19. Well, I thought . . . this is *my* book.

Secondly, with radiology: the internet is full of excellent neuroradiology (e.g. Radiopaedia *et al.*) that far surpasses printed images. Do please search for such sources – some are mentioned via the additional notes and references on my website:

https://www.drcharlesclarke.com.

My main experience for some 40 years, like that of Bryan Matthews, has been as a general neurologist in UK district general hospitals, largely the busy battleground of Whipps Cross, but always attached to a major neurology unit, initially St Bartholomew's and latterly Queen Square. I always found the variety within general neurology more attractive than its emerging specialties. I also broadened my experience by working further afield – during a meningococcal epidemic in Boston, in a leprosy clinic in Mysore, south India and elsewhere in India, Nepal and China, often in remote situations on mountaineering expeditions.

I thank many people. My parents Cyril and Féo Clarke were distinguished medical researchers, but I suspect they often despaired of me – their practical son who seemed focused on clinical practice and mountaineering, rather than research and publications. But they always gave me encouragement. Robin Coombs and Peter Lachmann grounded me in immunology at Cambridge. John Newsom-Davis and Angela Vincent took me into the world of myasthenia at the Royal Free, and my colleagues at Queen Square made *Neurology: A Queen Square Textbook* both a reality and the source of this book. They are acknowledged personally in each chapter. Wiley commisioned this book and Simon Shorvon suggested I write it.

Within the chapters, Dame Sally Davies and Dr Elizabeth Davies helped me with aspects of public health. Professor Peter Garrard guided me through cognition and dementia. Michael Hayle helped me with the nomenclature of recreational drugs. Professor Kailash Bhatia and Dr Eion Mulroy provided an excellent video of movement disorders (Chapter 7), hosted securely in my website. The new neuroanatomy illustrations were generously provided by Professor Thomas Champney, a fellow yachtsman, I soon discovered, of Miller School of Medicine, University of Miami, Florida – from his excellent book *Essential Clinical Neuroanatomy*, Wiley Blackwell 2016.

I also searched outside Queen Square, from our former alumni. I found willing and valued contributors, especially to neuroradiology – Professor Raymond Cheung in Hong Kong and Dr Patricio Paredes and Dr Pablo Soffia in Chile.

Why Chile? My partner, Professor Dame Marcela Contreras qualified in Santiago before emigrating to England, long long ago – and she has provided me with immeasurable support.

My daughters Rebecca and Naomi, who have carried their grandfather's 'Astley' into their successful business careers, have also helped, if distantly, by asking repeatedly *'Dad, when are you going finish this book?'*

My publishers Wiley have taken the project to its conclusion, smoothly and helpfully - in particular Mandy Collison, Managing Editor and Sophie Bradwell, Associate Editor for Clinical Medicine in the UK, Hari Sridharan and Sathishwaran P, Content Refinement Specialists in Chennai, South India.

Lastly, and to acknowledge the value of her expertise, Sallie Oxenham in Paris has worked tirelessly on my website design and its content. Also, two MacBook Air computers have been my constant companions – and I have retained not a page of paper. Both computers were stolen several years ago, but Dropbox provided backup without a word being lost – unlike T.E. Lawrence, who mislaid the manuscript of *The Seven Pillars of Wisdom* on Reading Station in 1919 and had to rewrite the entire book from memory.

In my study I have a portrait of Dr Thomas Sydenham, my distant grandparent, with a note from my 19th and 20th century Leicester grandfather Dr Astley Vavasour Clarke, whom also I never knew – a picture that Astley V. had left to my father. If genes have a role in these endeavours, they probably had a hand in this too.

*Charles Astley Clarke*
March 2022
https://www.drcharlesclarke.com

Matthews WB. *Practical Neurology*. Blackwell Scientific Publications, Oxford, 1963 and later editions.

## The National Brain Appeal

A proportion of the royalties from *Neurology: A Clinical Handbook* are donated to The National Brain Appeal. The charity raises funds to advance treatment and research at the National Hospital for Neurology & Neurosurgery and the UCL Institute of Neurology – *Queen Square*. Donations are used to improve outcome and quality of life for the one in six people affected by a neurological condition, by supporting pioneering research and helping to train tomorrow's clinicians.

UK Registered Charity Number: 290173

www.nationalbrainappeal.org

**The National Brain Appeal**
Funding advances
in neurology and
neurosurgery

# Foreword

As a medical specialty, neurology emerged in its modern guise in the second half of the nineteenth century, and it was then that the National Hospital at Queen Square opened its doors, the very first hospital in the world dedicated to neurological diseases. Since then, the stories of neurology and of the hospital have been intertwined. Throughout the twentieth and now the twenty-first centuries, *Queen Square* as it has become known has maintained its position at the cutting edge of neurology and remains one of the leading neurological institutions globally, both in terms of superlative clinical care and research. As neurology developed, the *Queen Square* clinical method evolved, a method that remains the standard approach to the diagnosis and treatment of neurological conditions.

Embedded in a knowledge of the anatomy, physiology and mechanisms of disease, this clinical method has at its core the taking of a detailed history, the performance of a systematised clinical examination, the judicious choice of well-focused investigation and a balanced approach to evidence-based treatment. The diagnostic approach is successful because it is a logical exploration of symptoms aligned to the principles of nervous system structure and function. Investigations, notably neuroimaging, neurophysiology and molecular biology, have also evolved enormously and assist this process. In terms of treatment, the parallel developments of surgical and medical therapies, also rooted in the modern neurosciences, have changed neurology from being what was essentially a diagnostic specialty to a therapeutic one. Again, *Queen Square* has been at the forefront. Linked to the science has been an emphasis on ensuring that the medical process is patient centred and responsive to patient needs. In view of these spectacular advances, neurology today would be hardly recognisable to its practitioners of long ago, yet this approach throughout the world remains the cornerstone for diagnosis and treatment. It also forms the backdrop to this book.

With advancing knowledge has come increasing subspecialisation. This has undoubtedly advanced the science of neurology but has had the drawback of narrowing of scope of individual medical practice. One solution is to incorporate the subspecialties within an integrated framework, and this has been a guiding principle at the hospital as it has evolved. The success of the strategy was demonstrated in the textbook *Neurology: A Queen Square Textbook,* that Charles Clarke initiated and propelled with many others to its completion. The *Textbook* comprised 26 chapters with contributions from over 90 physicians and surgeons. This present book, *Neurology: A Clinical Handbook,* is based on the second edition of the *Textbook*. It is Charles Clarke's distillation of practical knowledge and his wide experience. But it is more than this. This *Handbook* has the advantage of having been compiled and written by a single person, thus ensuring a seamless integration of knowledge from all the specialties. The result is a superb synopsis – a banner to herald our *Textbook* in its forthcoming Third Edition, edited by Robin Howard, Dimitri M. Kullman, David Werring and Michael Zandi.

Dr Charles Clarke is a senior neurologist who has maintained a wide-ranging general neurological practice and combined this with a knowledge of the advancing practice in the major specialist fields. Charles comes from a distinguished medical lineage and has demonstrated his skills in the production of this handbook, a consummate guide to neurological diagnosis and treatment, useful, up to date and practical, and one in which specialty knowledge has been integrated into a single framework. He has been able to bring together a text that is strikingly well balanced and authoritative. This is a crowning achievement, made possible not least because of the elegance and clarity of his writing. In the world of modern medicine, the ability to communicate clearly and precisely without savaging the beauty of the English language is a rare gift and one bestowed on Charles for all our benefit.

In all, this Handbook is a sparkling addition to the neurological library, a concise and clear guide to clinical practice in neurology, written in elegant prose, a tribute to *Queen Square* and to the contribution that both Hospital and Institute have made to neurology. It is the encapsulation of wisdom gained in a long career. For practitioners in the art of neurology, junior and senior, this is required reading.

Simon Shorvon
National Hospital for Neurology & Neurosurgery,
Queen Square, London

# 1

# Neurology Worldwide: Public Health and Essential Neuro-epidemiology

The world over, one-third of all serious illness is caused by brain disease and a tenth by other neurological conditions. I introduce here the epidemiology and burden of neurological illness. Public Health plays a minor role in neurology. It needs more attention.

## Basic Data

Incidence is new cases/100 000/year. Prevalence is the occurrence/1000 of the population, and lifetime prevalence the risk/1000 of acquiring a condition during life. These vary – between urban and rural settings and are linked to ethnicity, poverty, lifestyle/nutrition, vectors, war and sanitation. Data for specific age ranges are often more valuable than overall rates.

In the United Kingdom:
- For stroke, incidence overall is 190/100 000/year, but those over 65, 1100/100 000/year.
- For Parkinson's, incidence overall is 20/100 000/year and prevalence 2/1000. Over 65, incidence is 160/100 000/year and prevalence 10/1000.
- With epilepsy, the situation is shown in Figure 1.1.

A population's age structure impacts heavily: there are more children and young adults in poor than in rich countries (Figure 1.2). Degenerative age-related disease is increasing: the world's population over 65 is to double between 2020 and 2030. Doubling time depends upon mortality rates, on the number of offspring per mother, and on cultural, financial and religious pressure. Examples are in Table 1.1.

## Practical Neurology

Practical neurology is remarkably similar the world over – a neurologist in China, India or South America will be familiar with most conditions seen in Europe (Table 1.2). Variation between regions is determined largely by infections, such as malaria. Study of the full impact of Covid-19 is unknown and not discussed here.

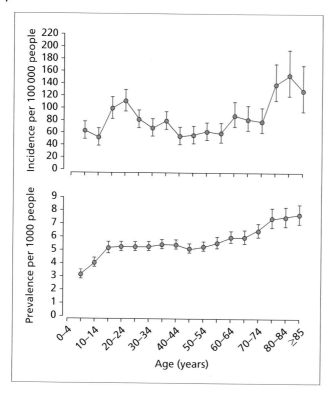

**Figure 1.1** Standardized prevalence and incidence rates of treated epilepsy in a population of 2 052 922 persons in England and Wales in 1995. (Bars indicate 95% CI.) Prevalence of treated epilepsy: overall 5.15/1000 people (95% confidence interval [CI] 5.05–5.25). *Source:* Wallace *et al.* 1998.

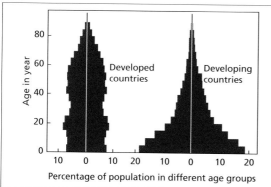

**Figure 1.2** Age structure in developed (Sweden) and developing (Costa Rica) countries. *Source:* Worldwatch Database, 1996, Worldwatch Institute.

## Causation

The cause of a neurological disease is rarely simple. A condition is either:

### Genetic

- Huntington's: a single gene disorder with high penetrance.
- Epilepsy: complex interactions between presumed susceptibility genes.
- Alzheimer's: genetic influences in 10%, but not in the majority.

### Genetic and Environmental

- Parkinson's disease: presumed genetic influences but susceptibility (curiously) reduced by smoking.

**Table 1.1**  Population size and doubling times.

| Country | Population (millions) | No. of births/mother | Doubling time (years) |
|---|---|---|---|
| Nigeria | 107 | 6.2 | 23 |
| India | 970 | 3.5 | 36 |
| China | 1236 | 1.8 | 67 |
| USA | 268 | 2.0 | 116 |
| Japan | 126 | 1.5 | 289 |
| UK | 60 | 1.7 | 433 |

*Source:* Data from The Population Reference Bureau, 2015

**Table 1.2**  Incidence and point prevalence.

| Disorder | Incidence (100 000/year) | Point prevalence /100 000 |
|---|---|---|
| Migraine | 370 | 12 100 |
| Acute stroke | 190 | 900 |
| Subarachnoid haemorrhage | 15 | |
| TIA | 30 | |
| Epilepsy | 50 | 710 |
| Dementia | 50 | 250 |
| Parkinson's disease | 20 | 200 |
| Chronic polyneuropathies | 40 | 24 |
| Bell's palsy | 25 | |
| Meningitis & infections | 15 | |
| Brain tumours | 10 | 10 |
| Trigeminal neuralgia | 4 | 1 |
| Multiple sclerosis | 4 | 90 |
| Motor neurone disease | 2 | 4 |
| Muscular dystrophies | 1 | 6 |

*Source:* Data from various WHO sources; excludes shingles.

- MS: genetic susceptibility and geographic location. MS is more common in latitudes around 50°N and S of the equator, and rare in the tropics (0°–23.5° N and S). Clusters of MS cases, for example on the W coast of Ireland.

### Evident and Preventable

- In traumatic brain injury, many severe brain injuries have been prevented by car seatbelts.
- Meningitis due to *Haemophilus influenza*, *Streptococcus pneumoniae* and *Meningococci*: immunisation.

Generally, where primary causes are poorly understood, causation can be divided into

- predisposing factors (e.g. age, gender, genetic susceptibility)
- enabling factors (e.g. hypertension, poor nutrition, inadequate medical care)

- precipitating factors (e.g. exposure to infectious or noxious agent)
- reinforcing factors (e.g. repeated or prolonged exposure).

Most neurological conditions are products of multifactorial influences, each of which alone would not cause the disease. It is thus helpful to study risk factors.

## Mortality, Life Expectancy and Quality of Life

Mortality rate: the number dying of a condition divided by the number in the population.
This information is of limited value without knowledge of the overall death rate.
Life expectancy (median survival age) is often lowered in neurological disease, but data are complex.
Taking epilepsy, one study followed over 500 cases for >10 years. The overall mortality ratio was 2.1. The hazard ratio (HR), or risk of death, for epilepsy overall, was 6.2. Life expectancy was reduced by some 2–10 years.

### Quality of Life

It is not enough to prolong survival. In high grade gliomas, radiotherapy is known to prolong life by about six months. Side effects are severe; the trade-off between survival and quality of life (QoL) is important. One study showed that how well a patient was before radiotherapy was a good indicator of disability-free life after it. For those already disabled, radiotherapy offered little gain.

### Other Important Measures

- *Birth rate*: number of live births/mid-year population;
- *Fertility rate*: number of live births/number of women aged 15–44 years (Figure 1.3);
- *Infant mortality rate*: number of infant (<1 year) deaths/number of live births;
- *Stillbirth rate*: number of intrauterine deaths after 28 weeks/total births;
- *Perinatal mortality rate*: number of stillbirths + deaths in first week of life/total number of births.

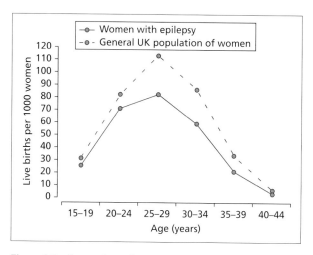

**Figure 1.3** Comparison of age-specific fertility rates in women with treated epilepsy and general UK population of women in 1993.

# Burden of Illness

This means all negative impacts, though the words are often used to define cost. Whilst cost studies produce fiscal measurements, it is absurd to measure QoL in cash. Utility measures such as quality-adjusted life years (QALYs) and disability-adjusted life years [DALYs] try to quantify this burden (Table 1.3).

## Cost of Illness Studies

The principal duty of a clinician is to provide individual care. However, doctors are now rightly involved in economic considerations. In any study of cost, analysis is of signal importance. Who was the study for, and who did it? The cost and burden for an individual have different parameters when compared with the effect on families, on health services and on society. Many studies are carried out from the point of view of society, with costs estimated in terms of lost employment, lost productivity and premature death, rather from the perspective of a patient, or their family.

- Direct costs mean any resource used – medical costs of primary care, out-patient and in-patient investigation, drugs, residential and community care, training and rehabilitation.
- Indirect costs are from lost economic production. They include premature mortality, dependency, unemployment and underemployment. The 'human capital' approach ascribes a monetary value to a person in terms of their potential productivity.

**Table 1.3** DALYs (Disability-Adjusted Life Year) for neurological and psychiatric conditions.

| Condition | DALYs × 10 | | | | |
| | Europe | Wealthy countries[a] | India | Sub-Saharan Africa | World |
| --- | --- | --- | --- | --- | --- |
| Neurological and psychiatric conditions (all)[b] | 53 009 | 24 682 | 23 949 | 15 788 | 165 082 |
| Cerebrovascular disease | 10 316 | 5166 | 5223 | 5487 | 45 770 |
| Unipolar depression | 4091 | 6721 | 10 064 | 6193 | 60 166 |
| Bipolar disease | 1541 | 1673 | 2867 | 1,785 | 16 722 |
| Schizophrenia | 1609 | 2151 | 2041 | 611 | 14 614 |
| Epilepsy | 633 | 427 | 848 | 526 | 4712 |
| Alcoholism | 4435 | 4611 | 1113 | 2387 | 18,973 |
| Dementia | 4531 | 3286 | 1192 | 453 | 10 135 |
| Parkinson's disease | 428 | 523 | 167 | 63 | 1278 |
| Multiple sclerosis | 303 | 222 | 253 | 140 | 1569 |

[a] Established market economies.
[b] This category excludes cerebrovascular disease.
Disability-adjusted life year is an indicator of the time lived with a disability and the time lost due to premature mortality. Reproduced with permission from the World Health Organization 1996b. The figures for Europe were separately calculated (Olesen and Leonardi 2003). *Source:* Modified from Olesen and Leonardi 2003.

Ethical and personal issues are intertwined with cost-effectiveness. Therapies that are neither cost-effective from the epidemiological nor from point of view of society can help an individual – such as the belief in homeopathic therapy, or travel to a centre for healing. Societal and evidence-based, clinical perspectives clash.

Social policy can greatly lessen the individual burden, for example by financial benefits and social support. It must be stressed that in the majority of countries, even those who pride themselves on wealth and power, there is either no or minimal support for those who are ill, either acutely or chronically.

### Stigma

Disease burden includes psychological, social, employment and legislative aspects. Some are rational, for example driving restrictions in epilepsy or stroke.

Stigma and discrimination deserve mention:

- enacted stigma – discrimination experience for example 'does he (the man in the wheel-chair) take sugar?'
- felt stigma – discrimination fear
- self-stigma – shame/withdrawal – response to discrimination perceived.

Complex interactions construct a stigma theory – to explain potential dangers people represent, either to others or to themselves. Whilst many no longer believe in witchcraft, in life after death, in the power of prayer or of the devil, some still do, and there remains a view that someone with a condition such as epilepsy, mental sub-normality or schizophrenia is in some way to blame.

Epilepsy is one example. To be regarded as *epileptic* can be more devastating than having *an occasional blackout*. Such beliefs are not restricted to poor societies. In Europe, with epilepsy, over 50% feel stigmatised. In the United States in some states until the 1950s, people with epilepsy were prohibited from marrying and could be sterilised; until the 1970s they could be excluded from restaurants and theatres.

Headache is another: people with headaches feel stigmatised at work. There is the well-known male attitude to women with headaches and menstrual discomfort.

Doctors and health professional should be aware, not only of such prejudices, but also of their own attitudes.

### Costs and Impact

Ill health imposes high costs, both on the patient and family everywhere. However, in poorer countries the proportion of family income spent on health is particularly high, not least as ill health results in unemployment.

- In the United Kingdom, any chronic illness (over one year) is likely to diminish the income of a family by >50%.

Even in countries where health services are free at the point of delivery, the cost of all illness is substantial.

Neurological illnesses because of their chronic nature are particularly onerous. The impact of a disease depends upon personal wealth, the healthcare system and social networks available.

### Treatment Gaps

Taking epilepsy again, a Treatment Gap is the percentage with seizures who do not receive anti-epileptic drugs (AEDs). In Pakistan, the Philippines and Ecuador there are epilepsy TGs of 80–95%, in India around 75%, but <5% in the United Kingdom, pre-COVID. Reasons include lack of health care, cost, drug availability, cultural factors, and stigma – and failure to grasp that AEDS are effective. Campaigns to narrow TGs are priorities.

## Improvements

Improvements in health delivery rest largely with governments, their knowledge and resources. Non-provision is largely due to policies. Success or failure to deliver provides stark contrasts, often unrelated to GDP. Most European countries have integrated care systems, that aim to improve the health of the populace. So does Cuba, despite its poverty. In the US, despite some of the world's finest medical institutions such a system remains in its infancy. Quite where we are heading in the United Kingdom and in Europe, from 2021, is known to no one.

## Acknowledgements

I am indebted to Professor Simon Shorvon who wrote the original chapter in *Neurology A Queen Square Textbook* Second Edition. Edited by Charles Clarke, Robin Howard, Martin Rossor & Simon Shorvon, Wiley Blackwell, 2016.

I am also most grateful to Dame Sally Davies, former Chief Medical of Health for England and to Dr Elizabeth Davies, Reader in Cancer & Public Health, King's College, London who reviewed and commented on my text.

## References

Olesen J, Leonardi M. The burden of brain disease in Europe. *Eur J Neurol* 2003; **10**: 471–477.
Wallace H, Shorvon SD, Tallis R. Age-specific incidence and prevalence rates of treated epilepsy in an unselected population of 2,052,922 and age-specific fertility rates of women with epilepsy. *Lancet* 1998; **26**: 1970–1973.

## Further Reading and Information

Shorvon S. Neurology worldwide: the epidemiology and burden of neurological disease. In *Neurology A Queen Square Textbook*, 2nd edn. Clarke C, Howard R, Rossor M, Shorvon S, eds. Wiley Blackwell, 2016. There are numerous references.
www.who.int/data/themes/mortality-and-global-health-estimates

http://www.healthdata.org/gbd

Davies E, Clarke C, Hopkins A. Malignant cerebral glioma. I: Survival, disability and morbidity after radiotherapy. *BMJ* 1996; **313**: 1507–1512.

Davies E, Clarke C, Hopkins A. Malignant cerebral glioma. II: Perspectives of patients and relatives on the value of radiotherapy. *BMJ* 1996; **313**: 1512–1516.

Please visit https://www.drcharlesclarke.com for free updated notes, potential links and other references. You will be asked to log in, in a secure fashion, with your name and institution.

# 2

# Movement, Sensation and The Silent Brain

Anatomical complexities of the nervous system became apparent in the late nineteenth century. Highlights were the pathways described by Santiago Ramón y Cajal in the 1890s and later the cortical mapping by Brodmann and the work of Alf Brodal. However, remarkably little neuroanatomy was required to practice sensibly and safely. To an extent this remains so. The neuroanatomy here is in excess of the needs of most general neurologists but further study is essential in many aspects of neuroscience.

First, here is an overview of the motor and sensory pathways of the brain and cord – the basic wiring that must be understood. I deal with this largely as illustrations. I also summarise what I call the Silent Brain, vital but less obvious – regions such as the thalamus. Cortical function is dealt with in Chapter 5. For neurones, nerves, glia and myelin see Chapter 10. Chapter 13 deals with the cranial nerves. Neuro-ophthalmology is in Chapter 14, Neuro-Otology in Chapter 15 and the autonomic nervous system in Chapter 24.

The overall anatomy of the brain is illustrated in Figure 2.1.

## ABC of Movement: Cortical, Extrapyramidal and Cerebellar Function

Movement – skilled, coordinated and fast – is highly developed in mammals. Rudimentary objectives are feeding, survival and reproduction and in Mankind, skilled use of tools, weapons and instruments of creative art.

A) Corticospinal (pyramidal) tracts originate in the motor cortex, somatosensory and limbic areas to reach cranial nerve nuclei and cord anterior horn cells. Dysfunction produces loss of skilled movement, weakness, spasticity and reflex change.
Pyramidal describes the triangular cross-section of the tract in the medulla. Pyramidal is used here interchangeably with corticospinal.
B) The striatal (a.k.a. extrapyramidal) system facilitates fast, fluid movement. Hallmarks of dysfunction are slowness (bradykinesia), stiffness (rigidity), rest tremor, all seen typically in Parkinson's and some movement disorders. Broadly, these are basal ganglia functions.
C) The cerebellum coordinates smooth movement, and balance. Ataxia and action tremor are features of dysfunction.

*Neurology: A Clinical Handbook*, First Edition. Charles Clarke.
© 2022 John Wiley & Sons Ltd. Published 2022 by John Wiley & Sons Ltd.

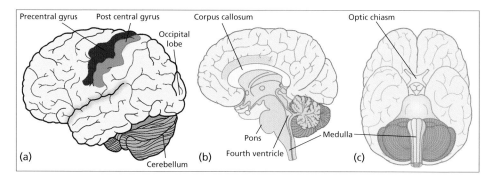

**Figure 2.1** Brain: overall anatomy (a) Lateral view (b) Midsagittal section (c) Ventral view. *Source*: Champney (2016).

## Cortex: Movement Force, Direction and Synergy

Movements are produced by neuronal groups in the motor cortex. These groups act synergistically to control force, direction and timing – and they communicate with sensation – to produce fine, skilled movements.

## Pyramidal System Anatomy

Figure 2.2 outlines the principal motor pathway from cortex to anterior horn cells.

Note:

- Pyramid: within rostral medulla
- Decussation of the pyramids: within caudal medulla
- Cortico-spinal axons synapse on cord anterior horn cells.

## Extrapyramidal System and Basal Ganglia Region

The word extrapyramidal is used in various ways. In neurology, extrapyramidal describes disorders such as Parkinson's disease – the slowing, stiffness and/or tremor. Extrapyramidal is also sometimes used to include dyskinesias, such as chorea, hemiballismus or dystonia. In neuroanatomy, as a more general term, extrapyramidal relates to the basal ganglia region (Figure 2.3), that is:

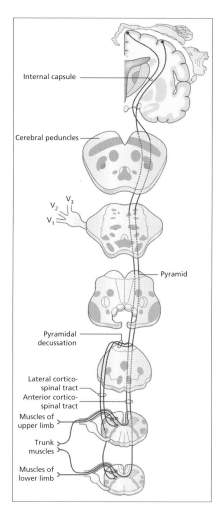

**Figure 2.2** Descending corticospinal pathways. *Source*: Champney (2016).

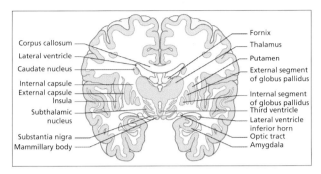

**Figure 2.3** Oblique coronal section: *putamen*, caudate, *globus pallidus,* subthalamic nucleus, *substantia nigra. Source*: Champney (2016).

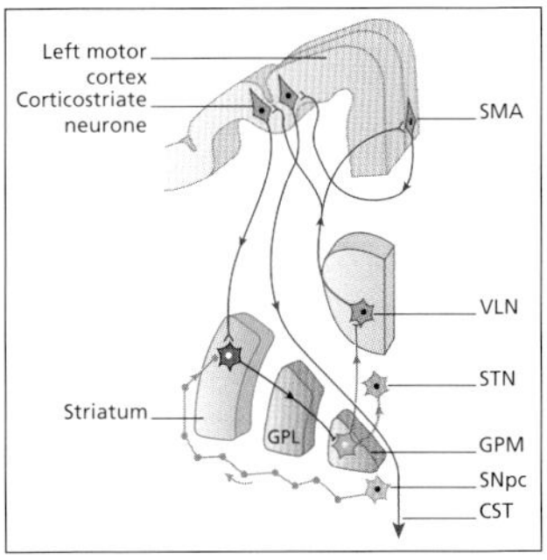

**Figure 2.4** A striatal motor loop. SMA - supplementary motor area, VLN - ventral lateral nucleus of thalamus, STN - subthalamic nucleus, GPL - *globus pallidus* (lateral), GPM - *globus pallidus* (medial), SNpc - *substantia nigra pars compacta,* CST- corticospinal tract. *Source*: Fitzgerald (2010).

- The *striatum* (caudate nucleus, *putamen* of lentiform nucleus, *nucleus accumbens*);
- *Globus pallidus* (GP) – lateral and medial parts. The GP extends into the *pars reticularis* of the *substantia nigra*;
- Subthalamic nucleus
- *Pars compacta* of the *substantia nigra.*

### Basal Ganglia Circuits

Neuronal servo-loops commence and end in the motor cortex. All pass through the striatum (*putamen* + caudate nucleus) and return via the thalamus, and within each loop there are two pathways: direct and indirect.

Transmission through each loop is controlled via the *pars compacta* of the *substantia nigra* to the lateral *globus pallidus*, where axons make two principal types of synapse, on excitatory $D_1$ (dopaminergic, direct pathway) and inhibitory $D_2$ (indirect pathway) receptors. Further receptors are now recognised in the D receptor series.

In normal subjects, the nigro-striatal tract is active, selecting preferentially the excitatory, direct pathway and thus leading, via the loop back to the cortex to activation of the supplementary motor area before a movement, and thence to a movement itself (Figure 2.4). This early activation of the cortex underlies the electrical readiness potential (*Bereitschaftspotential*).

Such servo-loops modulate, for example:

- Cognition/motor intention, contraction strength, suppression, speed control, storage of programmes
- Limbic (memory) loop: cortex→*nucleus accumbens*→ventral *pallidum*→thalamus→cortex.

## Cerebellar System

Zones of the cerebellum are illustrated in Figure 2.5.
The cerebellar peduncles and deep cerebellar nuclei are shown in Figure 2.6.
The essential cellular anatomy of the cerebellar cortex is shown in Figure 2.7.

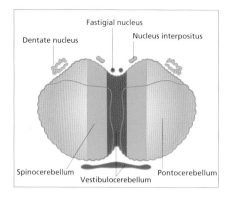

Figure 2.5  Zones of the cerebellum. *Source*: Fitzgerald (2010).

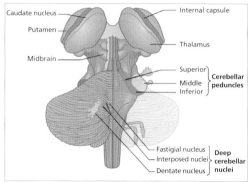

Figure 2.6  Cerebellar peduncles & nuclei: posterior view. *Source*: Champney (2016).

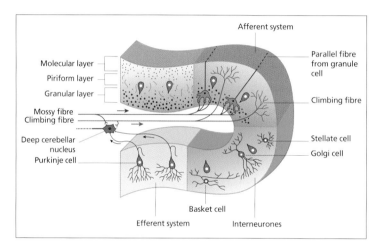

Figure 2.7  Cerebellum: cortical micro-anatomy. *Source*: Fitzgerald (2010).

### Afferent and Efferent Cerebellar Pathways

Afferent pathways include:

- Spino-cerebellar: posterior and anterior spino-cerebellar tracts – proprioceptive data from spinal cord.
- Ponto-cerebellar: originates in the cerebral cortex, and enters via middle cerebellar peduncle.
- Vestibulo-cerebellar: vestibular nuclei, enters via inferior peduncle.

Efferent pathways project to the vestibular system, to the cord, thalamus, motor cortex and to the red nucleus,.

The cerebellum and red nucleus in the midbrain tegmentum have a role in learned movement. The system modulates new motor activity:

- The red nucleus is a relay between cerebral cortex and the olive – the red nucleus is inhibitory, to the ipsilateral olive.
- When there is imbalance between movement intended (cerebral cortex) and movement already learned (cerebellum), the red nucleus is thought to modulate, to achieve harmony.
- A lesion of the red nucleus – a coarse tremor – is a breakdown of this harmonic, over-correcting each part of a movement.

In contrast to the anatomical complexity, signs of cerebellar disease are usually straightforward:

- A lateral lobe lesion – a tumour or an infarct – causes rebound and past pointing of the upper limb and similar lower limb signs.
- A vermis lesion – for example midline medulloblastoma – affects vestibular connection: truncal ataxia can be an early sign.
- Nystagmus – coarse, fast phase towards the side of a lesion, sometimes dramatic – is an inconstant feature.

## Sensory Pathways

Neurologists deal with the special senses – vision, hearing/balance, olfaction and taste – and the main five sensory modalities: touch, nociception, temperature, joint position, vibration and two-point position. Neuroscientists use an alternative vocabulary: sensation is either conscious or non-conscious and either afferent proprioceptive – from a limb, or enteroceptive – from gut, or heart.

### Sensory Pathways in the Cord and Brain

Two major pathways deliver sensory information to the thalamus and thence to the cortex (Figure 2.8):

- Spinothalamic pathways (nociceptive – pain, temperature);
- Posterior columns → medial lemnisci (touch, position, movement, vibration).

Each system consists of three orders of neurones.

- First order neurones are in the posterior root (dorsal root) ganglia;
- Second order neurones decussate before reaching the thalamus;
- Third order neurones project from thalamus to cortex;

There is somatotopic organisation throughout, and transmission can be controlled (inhibited/enhanced) at various stages (see Gate Control & Chapter 23).

### Dorsal Root Ganglia

The complexity of the laminae within the posterior horn and the cord pathways are illustrated in Figure 2.9, the detail of which is hard to remember. A single nerve root ganglion can contain around 100,000 neurones, each enshrouded by a modified Schwann cell. Two

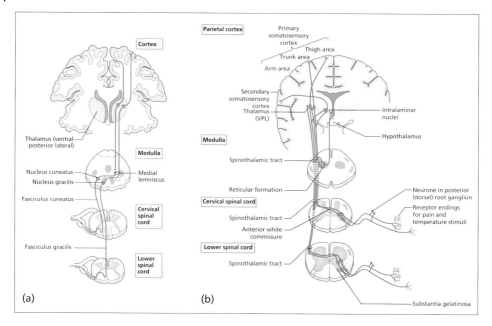

**Figure 2.8** Sensory pathways to the cortex. (a) Posterior columns, (b) Spinothalamic tracts. *Source*: Champney (2016).

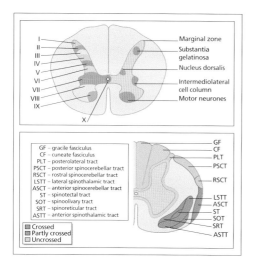

**Figure 2.9** Cord cross-section: dorsal horn laminae, ascending & descending tracts. *Source*: Fitzgerald 2010.

streams of axons, medial and lateral – the dorsal root afferents – synapse in various specific areas of the cord, to form the two main sensory pathways.

### Posterior Column→Medial Lemniscus Pathway

The cord posterior columns are formed partly by axons of posterior root ganglia and partly by axons of second order neurones in the dorsal horn of the spinal grey matter. These axons all project to the gracile and cuneate nuclei in the brainstem. Axons then decussate in the medulla to form each medial lemniscus (meniscus means a ribbon) that terminates in the ventral posterior nucleus of the thalamus. Thalamic neurones then project to the somatic sensory cortex.

### Spinothalamic Pathway

The anterior and lateral spinothalamic tracts pass from the posterior grey horn to the opposite thalamus. The two tracts merge in the brainstem to form the spinal lemniscus, enter the ventral posterior nucleus of the thalamus and project to the somatic sensory cortex.

Additional sensory pathways are concerned with non-conscious proprioception, reflex arc excitability, balance between agonists and antagonists, trunk and head orientation, arousal & motor learning:

- Posterior spino-cerebellar tract, cuneo-cerebellar tract, anterior spino-cerebellar tract, rostral spino-cerebellar tract
- Spino-tectal tract, spino-olivary tract, spino-reticular fibres.

We cannot recognise lesions of these pathways clinically – they are part of the wider framework of motor and sensory modulation.

## The Silent Brain

This section summarises the functional anatomy of the brainstem, reticular formation, limbic system and hippocampus, thalamus, hypothalamus, pituitary, and the little known circumventricular organs – regions I call The Silent Brain.

### Brainstem

I find that four points of reference simplify this region:

- Each cranial nerve nucleus denotes a different level in the rostral–caudal plane.
- Motor pathways lie ventrally.
- Sensory pathways lie dorsally.
- Reticular formation (RF) nuclei: most lie laterally, but the magnus raphe & median raphe nuclei are midline.

In our invertebrate ancestors, the brainstem was almost the entire forebrain. Olfaction and other sensations were connected, via the brainstem reticular formation (RF) to various movements – and thus to alertness, feeding and survival. With the evolution of the cerebral cortex, the brainstem became, in addition, a conduit connecting cranial nerve nuclei, cortex, cerebellum and cord, but remained the site of the RF and its connections – hence its complexity. What is needed is a general grasp of the levels of these brainstem nuclei (Figure 2.10).

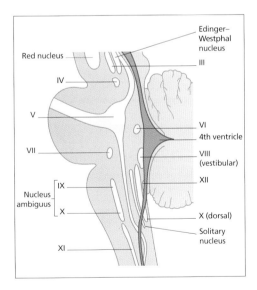

**Figure 2.10** Brainstem: lateral view – cranial nerve nuclei. *Source*: Hopkins (1993).

The way in which the nuclear arrangements arose is explained by a brief embryological perspective. Seven nuclear columns develop into cranial nerve nuclei.

Motor cranial nerve nuclei:

- III, IV, VI and XII arise from a paramedian nuclear mass – known as the general somatic efferent (GSE) column.
- V (motor), VII, IX and X (nucleus ambiguus) and XI (spinal accessory nucleus) arise from ventro-lateral cells – the special visceral efferent (SVE) and general visceral efferent (GVE) columns.

Afferent columns (general & special somatic and visceral afferents – GSA, SSA, SVA, GVA) develop into:

- Vth nerve nuclei
- Vestibular nuclei
- Tractus solitarius nucleus (taste).

## Reticular Formation

The RF has no single overriding function – and no single condition becomes apparent when it is damaged. It is a control centre, a polysynaptic network within the thalamus, hypothalamus, brainstem and cord involved in:

- Respiratory and cardiovascular control
- Sleep, wakefulness, arousal and mood
- Pattern generation – reflex activities, for example chewing, swallowing, conjugate gaze
- Micturition, bowel and sexual function
- Sensory modulation (see Gate control below, and Chapter 23)
- Autonomic and reflex activity (Chapter 24).

Essential anatomy and neurotransmitters: Figure 2.11 The raphe nuclei (pronounced 'raffay' = a seam in Greek) are the major source of serotoninergic neurones in the neuraxis.

### Gate Control: Sensory Modulation

Gating (also Chapter 23) means control of synaptic transmission between one set of neurones and the next. The RF has a role in gating sensory stimuli.

- Tactile sensation is gated at the posterior column nuclei. Nociceptive transmission from the trunk and limbs is gated in the posterior grey horn of the cord, and from the head in the spinal V nucleus. One crucial cord structure is the *substantia gelatinosa,* rich in excitatory glutaminergic neurones and inhibitory GABAergic and enkephalinergic neurones.
- Unmyelinated C fibres mediate dull, intense, prolonged, poorly localised pain. Short, sharp, well-localized pain is mediated by finely myelinated Aδ fibres. These synapse directly on relay neurones of the lateral spinothalamic tract.
- Large A (mechano-receptor) afferents from hair follicles and skin synapse on anterior spinothalamic cells and send collaterals to inhibitory (GABAergic) gelatinosa cells. These then synapse on lateral spinothalamic tract relay cells.
- Enhancement of RF inhibition from the magnus raphe nucleus, by rubbing, TENS, implanted stimulators, sleep and pain-modulating drugs reduces – that is, gates – C fibre activity.

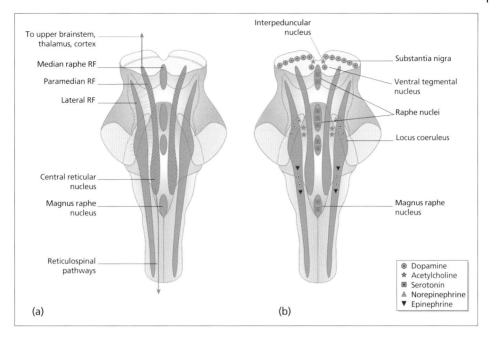

**Figure 2.11**   Reticular formation: (a) Nuclei (b) Principal neurotransmitter cell groups. *Source:* Fitzgerald (2010).

## Limbic System and Hippocampus

The limbic system includes:

- Hippocampi, mamillary bodies and septal area
- Insulae, cingulate and parahippocampal gyri
- Amygdala – subcortical nuclear masses adjacent to each temporal pole.

Other regions nearby are the *nucleus accumbens*, medial dorsal nucleus of the thalamus, hypothalamus and part of the RF. Orbital cortex, temporal pole, *corpus callosum*, choroid plexus and lateral ventricle are also nearby (Figure 2.12).

This region is involved in memory, arousal and mood – and in epilepsy (see hippocampal sclerosis, Chapter 7).

### Insula and Cingulate Cortex

The insula is involved in pain, and in language:

- Anterior: a cortical centre for pain perception
- Posterior: pain – emotional responses to/memories of
- Central: language – emotional responses.

The cingulate cortex has six zones:

- Executive: connected to dorso-lateral prefrontal cortex and SMA
- Nociceptive: afferents from thalamus (medial dorsal nucleus)

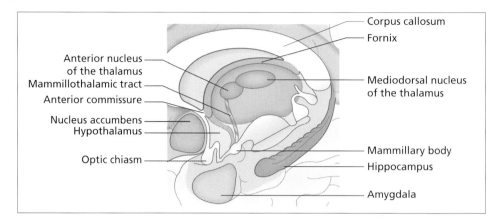

**Figure 2.12**   Limbic system: brain midline sagittal section. *Source*: Champney 2016.

- Emotional: happy thoughts light this area on fMRI
- Micturition: activity seen on bladder filling
- Vocalisation: active during decisions about construction of a sentence - changes in activation and reduced blood flow can occur in stammering
- Autonomic: respiratory and cardiac – responses to emotion, sweating and blushing.

### Amygdala and Kindling
Fear and anxiety are mediated via the amygdala, and there are widespread autonomic connections that provide potential explanations for everyday experiences, such as freezing with fear, hypertension with severe pain, and feeling nauseated, hypotensive and sweaty at the sight of blood. Kindling is a term used, often conjecturally for seizure activity developing in an area of brain contralateral to or distant from an epileptic focus. This phenomenon is as far as is known confined to the amygdala and hippocampus.

### *Nucleus Accumbens*, Septal Region and Basal Forebrain
Stimulation of areas of the ventral striatum (*nucleus accumbens*, ventral olfactory tubercle, ventral caudate and *putamen*) can lead to a sense of well-being akin to a shot of heroin, attributed to excessive dopamine release.

   Stimulation of the septal region in man produces pleasurable sexual sensations and/or orgasm. In animals, destructive lesions cause extreme anger – known as septal rage.

   The basal forebrain lies between the olfactory tracts and the amygdala. The magnocellular basal nucleus of Meynert and its cholinergic neurones extend throughout the cortex. These magnocellular basal nuclei, septal nuclei and neurones, and an area known as the diagonal band of Broca are also called basal forebrain nuclei. These nuclei exert tonic cholinergic activity within the cortex, and thus maintain wakefulness.

### Thalamus

The paired conjoined halves of each thalamus are large nuclear masses. Divisions and connections are shown in Figure 2.13.

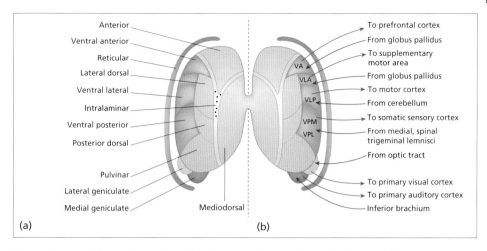

**Figure 2.13**   Thalamus (from above): (a) nuclei (b) connections of relay nuclei.
*Source*: Fitzgerald (2010).

Note the large 'Y' of thalamic white matter – the internal medullary lamina – that divides the nuclei into three cell groups:

- Anterior (within the 'Y')
- Medial dorsal
- Lateral nuclei.

Lateral nuclei are divided into ventral and dorsal tiers. The medial and lateral geniculate bodies lie posteriorly. The reticular nucleus surrounds each thalamus laterally, separated by an external medullary lamina traversed by thalamo-cortical fibres. The three groups of thalamic nuclei, somewhat uninformatively named are:

- Relay (specific) nuclei
- Association nuclei
- Non-specific nuclei.

Thalamic nuclei connect to most areas of the cortex, cerebellum and cord. The neurology of thalamic damage is confined largely to central post-stroke pain, a.k.a. thalamic pain, and sensory loss (Chapters 6 and 23).

## Hypothalamus and Pituitary

### Hypothalamic Region
The multiple paired nuclei of each hypothalamus lie each side of the third ventricle (Figure 2.14).

The hypothalamus is a central neural effector of basic survival, with roles in:

- Temperature homeostasis, regulation of food and water intake;
- Defence, arousal and sleep–wake cycles, sexual, endocrine and autonomic activity.

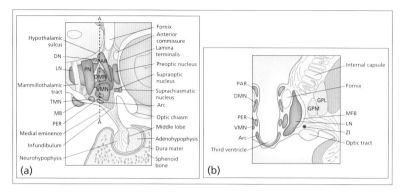

**Figure 2.14** (a) Hypothalamic & pituitary region: sagittal – from right (b) Partial coronal section through A-A. DN – dorsal nucleus; PN – posterior nucleus; LN – lateral nucleus; TMN – tuberomamillary nucleus; MB – mamillary body; PAR – paraventricular nucleus; DMN – dorsomedial nucleus; VMN – ventromedial nucleus; PER – periventricular nucleus; Arc – arcuate nucleus; GPL – globus pallidus lateral; GPM – globus pallidus medial; MFB – medial forebrain bundle; ZI – zona incerta. *Source*: Fitzgerald (2010).

For an area so intimately involved in essential activities, lesions of the hypothalamus are unusual. One reason is simple – bilateral destruction is necessary to produce clinical effects.

### Neuroendocrine Cells

These neurones, specific to the region, both conduct action potentials and also liberate into the bloodstream peptide and other hormones, the latter having been synthesised in the endoplasmic reticulum and stored in Golgi complexes. The peptides are attached to long-chain polypeptides – neurophysins. Cell bodies lie in the region of the preoptic nuclei and *tuber cinereum*. The principal nuclei that contribute to this system are the supraoptic, para-ventricular, ventromedial and arcuate nuclei.

Small neurone (parvocellular) axons in the tubero-infundibular tract reach the median eminence, where releasing and inhibiting hormones are liberated. Large neurone (magno-cellular) axons form the hypothalamo-hypophysial tract→ posterior pituitary.

### Sympathetic and Parasympathetic Hypothalamic Activity (See Chapter 24)
### Water Intake, Thirst, Appetite and Satiety

*Zona incerta* cells beside each lateral nucleus of the hypothalamus control thirst. Lesions lead to neglect of drinking. Other mechanisms contribute to osmotic homeostasis, for example serum sodium and glucose levels, and renal function.

Balance between lateral and ventromedial hypothalamic nuclei constitutes a satiety control system.

- Lateral hypothalamic (feeding centre) stimulation leads to overeating
- Lateral hypothalamic destruction leads to lack of interest in food
- Ventromedial hypothalamic (satiety centre) stimulation inhibits eating
- Ventromedial hypothalamic destruction (bilateral) leads to gross obesity.

Serotonin down-regulates appetite. Selective serotonin reuptake inhibitors (SSRIs) and most antidepressants tend to increase appetite.

### Mood, Sexual Arousal, Wakefulness and Memory

Aggression or docility are features of lateral/ventromedial hypothalamic imbalance. Obese animals with ventromedial lesions become aggressive. Underweight, ventromedially stimulated animals are docile. Hunger stimulates arousal. Maybe this explains why some people become grumpy when they are not fed at the time they expect to be.

Sexual arousal: specific neurones (INAH3 cells) in each preoptic nucleus are more numerous in males than in females. This is an area rich in androgen receptors, activated by testosterone and induces male sexual activity. In females, neurones rich in oestrogen receptors are found in the ventromedial nucleus: stimulation induces sexual arousal.

Sleep–wake cycles are set by the suprachiasmatic nucleus via pineal gland connections. Arousal is mediated via richly histaminergic neurones in the posterior hypothalamus (the tuberomammillary nucleus). These project widely (medial forebrain bundle, cortex, brainstem, cord). Hypersomnolence in Man is seen when the posterior hypothalamus is damaged bilaterally.

Memory: the mammillary bodies are stations on Papez's circuit (fornix → mammillary bodies → mammillothalamic tract → anterior nucleus of thalamus, Chapter 22). Mammillary body destruction produces a dramatic amnestic syndrome.

### Anterior/Posterior Pituitary Axes and Circumventricular Organs

These are mentioned briefly. In the anterior pituitary, ACTH (corticotrophin), FSH/LH, GH, prolactin and thyrotropin have peptide releasing hormones. GH and prolactin also have inhibiting hormones – prolactin IH is dopamine.

For the posterior pituitary, the hypothalamo-hypophyseal tracts pass from large (magnocellular) neurones of the supraoptic nucleus and paraventricular nucleus. There are also contributions from periventricular neurones (opiate and peptide neurotransmission) and brainstem (aminergic) neurones. Vasopressin (antidiuretic hormone) and oxytocin are secreted by the supraoptic and paraventricular nuclei – hormones are housed in axonal secretory granules (Herring bodies) before release into the capillary system within the posterior pituitary.

The circumventricular organs are neurones and glia adjacent to the ventricular system, each with an intimate relation to fenestrated capillaries:

- Neurohypophysis – ADH secretion
- Median eminence – anterior pituitary hormone release and inhibition
- VOLT (Vascular Organ of Lamina Terminalis) – feedback loop: low blood volume→renin→angiotensin II→VOLT/SFO→ADH
- SFO (SubFornical Organ)
- Area postrema – emetic centre, obex of 4th ventricle
- Pineal gland – melatonin, sleep-wake cycles.

## Acknowledgements

I am most grateful to Professor Roger Lemon, UCL Institute of Neurology for his contribution to our neuroanatomy chapter in *Neurology A Queen Square Textbook* Second Edition upon which part of this text is based.

Professor Thomas Champney, Miller School of Medicine, University of Miami, Florida, USA was most helpful in providing new illustrations, from Champney, TH. *Essential Clinical Neuroanatomy. Wiley Blackwell 2016.*

The late Professor MJ Turlough Fitzgerald, Emeritus Professor of Anatomy, National University of Ireland, Galway most generously provided all the neuroanatomy illustrations for *Neurology a Queen Square Textbook* Second & First Editions.

## Further Reading and Information

Clarke C, Lemon R. Nervous system structure & function. In *Neurology A Queen Square Textbook,* 2nd edn. Clarke C, Howard R, Rossor M, Shorvon S, eds. John Wiley & Sons, 2016. There are numerous references.

Champney TH. *Essential Clinical Neuroanatomy,* 1st edn. Wiley Blackwell, 2016.

*Fitzgerald's Clinical Neuroanatomy and Neuroscience,* 8th Edition. Mtui E, Gruener G, Dockerty P. Elsevier, 2020.

Hopkins AP, *Clinical Neurology: A Modern Approach.* Oxford Medical Publications, 1993.

Also, please visit https://www.drcharlesclarke.com for free updated notes, potential links and references. You will be asked to log in, in a secure fashion, with your name and institution.

# 3

# Aetiologies and Mechanisms: Genetics, Immunology and Ion Channels

Many neurological diseases have aetiologies that require an understanding of genetics, immune mechanisms and the way neuronal cell membranes – and thus ion channels – react. This chapter considers these briefly.

## Genetics

I have approached this in two ways. The first is to trace the embryological development of parts of the CNS – and here I have selected the spine and spinal cord, where genes have been identified that deal with either longitudinal or axial spinal development. The second is to illustrate how mutations and other abnormalities translate into neurological diseases. The basic genetics are summarised here, but picked up in the third section of this chapter – in channelopathies. I assume an understanding of Mendelian and mitochondrial inheritance, DNA, RNA, and chromosomes.

Despite the major advances, genetics plays little part in the day-to-day neurology of headache, seizures and even conditions such as malignant neoplasms, MS and most cases of Parkinson's. This may change in years to come.

### Essential Embryology of the Spine

The adult spine is divided into the cranio-cervical junction, cervical, thoracic, lumbar and sacro-coccygeal spine. In early foetal life the ectodermal germ layer forms the primitive neural tube that gives rise to the entire nervous system. This tube closes by the end of the fourth intrauterine week; failure of this primary neurulation results in fusion defects such as anencephaly or spina bifida. By this time the brain vesicles are present – the forebrain, midbrain and hindbrain. By the end of the fifth intrauterine week mesoderm that lies around the neural tube completes segmentation into somite pairs, from the occiput to the coccyx. Epithelioid cells of these somite pairs transform rapidly and migrate towards the notochord where they differentiate into three cell lines: sclerotomes – connective tissue, cartilage and bone, myotomes – segmental muscle and dermatomes. In the sclerotomes, chondrification leads on to ossification – anterior and posterior centres for each vertebral body and two for each arch. This is largely complete by the 12th week of foetal life.

Disruption during these stages accounts for many anomalies. After the third month the vertebral column and dura lengthen more rapidly than the cord. By term, the cord tip typically lies at the L2–3 interspace. The spine can be identified on ultrasound at 12 weeks and its integrity determined by 20 weeks.

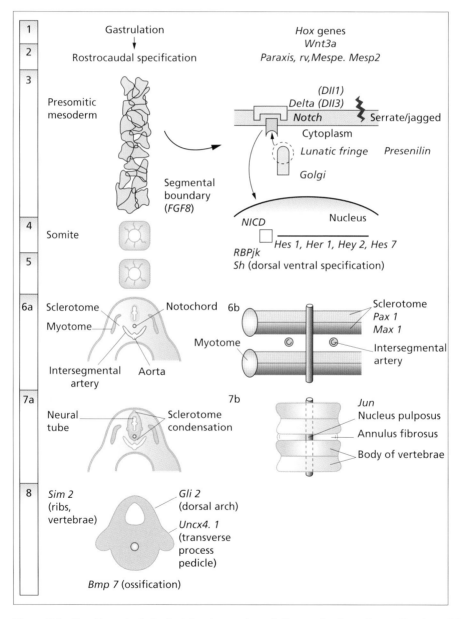

**Figure 3.1** Genetic control of spinal development – putative mechanisms. *Source:* Courtesy of Dr Simon Farmer.

**Genetic Control of Spinal Development**

The notochord provides the template for spinal development – its remnants persist as the nucleus pulposus of the discs (Figure 3.1). The notochord orchestrates production of numerous signalling molecules. One is initiated by the protein product of a notochord gene *Sonic Hedgehog*. Mesoderm becomes segmented into 44 somite pairs (4 occipital, 8 cervical, 12 thoracic, 5 lumbar, 5 sacral and 10 coccygeal) by the end of the fifth week. The driver for this presomitic mesoderm segmentation involves an intrinsic molecular oscillator, a.k.a the segmentation clock. There is rhythmic production of mRNA from genes within the *Notch* gene-signalling pathway. *Notch*-related genes include *Lunatic Fringe (LFNG)*, *Delta-like (DLL)*, *Presenilin* and *Mesoderm Posterior 2 (MESP2)*. Failure of oscillatory signalling leads to failure of segmentation in a rostral–caudal direction. The first, caudal somites are formed normally but then there is loss of segmentation, because of failure of this rhythmicity. Mutations cause skeletal and spinal abnormalities.

  *Notch* genes are involved in longitudinal segmentation. A second group of genes, the *Hox* (homeobox) family, specifies axial development and defines vertebral shape. In man there are four families of *Hox* genes (*Hox* A-D). Abnormal expression has been demonstrated in mice: for example, mutation of HOXB4 results in duplication of the atlas – a second atlas replaces the axis vertebra. Large *Hox* mutations produce a severely disrupted body habitus incompatible with intrauterine life. From analysis of mouse and human malformations, many genes have been identified: HOXB4, Notch, PAX1, PAX2, MEOX1, Gli2, Uncx4.1, BMP-7 and Jun.

## Chromosomal Abnormalities, Repeat Expansions and Mutations

These are usually categorised by their mode of inheritance:

- autosomal dominant (AD)
- autosomal recessive (AR)
- X-linked
- mitochondrial inheritance.

  Mechanisms typically comprise:

- Mutations or other gene defects that affect a protein or an ion channel
- Nucleotide repeat expansions such as in Huntington's disease
- Abnormalities in chromosomes, such as trisomy 21 (Down's)
- Digenic (two-locus) inheritance, such as in some familial Parkinson's cases

  Conditions where genes and environment appear to interact, in an unproven way, such as in MS are less clear.

**Autosomal Dominant Inheritance**

Huntington's disease, neurofibromatosis type 1, tuberous sclerosis and myotonic dystrophy are typical examples. There is usually a family pedigree.

**Autosomal Recessive Inheritance**

Most recessive traits are rare and typically follow consanguinity.

  AR cerebellar ataxias (Chapter 17), neuropathies (Chapter 10), hearing loss (Chapter 15) and progressive external ophthalmoplegia (Chapter 14) are examples.

Individuals who are heterozygous are usually phenotypically normal. However, when a population has a high gene frequency, heterozygote testing can identify high risk individuals and thus assist genetic advice. One example is Tay–Sachs disease.

### X-Linked Inheritance

Transmission is via an unaffected female carrier. Examples are Duchenne muscular dystrophy and Kennedy's disease. If the disease does not affect fertility because it allows survival into the reproductive period, such as in Fabry's disease and Becker-type muscular dystrophy transmission can be via female carriers and affected males. X-linked adrenoleucodystrophy, ataxia syndromes and forms of Charcot–Marie–Tooth disease are other examples.

### Mitochondrial Disorders

More than 70 different polypeptides interact to form the mitochondrial respiratory chain. Thirteen essential subunits are encoded by the 16.5 kb mitochondrial genomic DNA (mtDNA).

Mitochondrial diseases caused either by mutations in mtDNA or in mitochondrial genes are transmitted via maternal inheritance.

Examples are disorders such as myoclonic epilepsy and ragged red fibres (MERRF), mitochondrial myopathy, encephalopathy, lactic acidosis and stroke (MELAS) and Leber's hereditary optic neuropathy (LHON). Chronic progressive external ophthalmoplegia (CPEO) is usually the result of a large deletion. A single mitochondrial disorder can present with variable features. For instance, the m.3243A>G point mutation may cause either MELAS, CPEO, diabetes mellitus or deafness.

### Expanded Repeat Disorders

The majority of simple nucleotide repeats that occur frequently throughout the genome are not associated with disease. However, some are of great importance.

In 1991, an expansion in a trinucleotide (CAG) repeat in the androgen receptor gene was identified in X-linked spinal and bulbar muscular atrophy a.k.a. Kennedy's disease. The repeat normally 13–30 CAGs, lengthens to 40 or more CAGs in this condition.

Huntington's disease (see Chapter 7 for detail) and spinocerebellar ataxias – SCA1-3, Friedreich's ataxia are others. An expanded hexanucleotide repeat occurs in familial amyotrophic lateral sclerosis with fronto-temporal dementia.

Disorders can exhibit anticipation – severity worsens in successive generations. This correlates with the increased number of repeats.

### *Practical and Ethical Considerations*

When considering genetic testing it is important to understand the practicalities, cost and the advertising pressures placed upon patients and their families.

A three-tier approach is usual:

- Initial low cost screening for common defects
- Screening of rarer genes using a gene panel approach
- Diagnostic exome sequencing.

Predictive genetic testing is frequently offered to individuals at risk, such as in late-onset autosomal dominant inherited conditions. Most experience of predictive testing comes from Huntington's disease.

Important considerations:

- Do all involved understand the implications – work, insurance, plans, disclosure and confidentiality issues? In the past there has been a tendency to suggest that those potentially at risk have a duty to be tested. This pressure is now less common - and there are situations where individuals prefer not to be tested.
- Does the individual – rather than another family member – really wish to be tested and give informed consent?

## Immune Mechanisms: Concepts and Components

The immune system is dynamic and reactive. It is a system that distinguishes self from non-self and deletes, inactivates or supresses foreign invaders and distinguishes irreparable or altered tissue from normal, to maintain homeostasis. Where effective surveillance fails, infection or neoplasia can develop. Where active components become misdirected, autoimmune disease can follow. It is assumed that the reader has a basic understanding of the immune system and its components, the cytokine network and their interactions.

### Blood–Brain and Blood–Nerve Barriers

The blood–brain barrier (BBB) is a concept – that divides the systemic compartment from the CNS and across which fluids, solutes and cells can pass selectively. This gives CNS machinery relative resistance to immune attack but it also provides an environment in which unique autoimmune processes can occur, that either limit or cause damage. The blood–nerve barrier (BNB) is less well understood – the endoneurial space of the peripheral nerve. The BNB is more permeable than the BBB, but it undoubtedly modifies immune responses that would occur if nerves were not shielded. See Chapter 10.

### Cerebrospinal Fluid

The invasive nature of lumbar puncture and the normal CSF label of 'gin clear' tended to diminish its diagnostic value. Advances have shown that CSF is a useful fluid in which biomarkers can be identified.

#### CSF Solutes

In health, the CSF is maintained as a protein-poor solvent in which are dissolved proteins derived mainly from brain tissue. The normal levels of CSF antibodies, amyloid beta, tau and phosphotau proteins are a baseline from which change indicates disease.

When there is a dysfunctional BBB, CSF total protein contains contributions from both CNS and systemic compartments, but this is non-specific. Analysis of specific proteins is more useful.

- Albumin: no albumin is produced in the normal CNS. Any CSF albumin is present either via direct transport or leakage through a dysfunctional BBB.
- IgG: in health, all the CSF IgG is actively transported across the BBB. A raised CSF IgG in comparison to the serum (raised $CSF_{IgG}$ : $serum_{IgG}$) or the IgG quotient ($Q_{IgG}$) can indicate disease.
- Other solutes such as a-beta amyloid proteins, tau, neurofilament proteins, S-100 β and 14-3-3 protein can also be measured. Their profiles can provide biomarker support for the diagnosis of Alzheimer's disease versus frontotemporal dementia and other degenerative diseases (Chapter 5).

*CSF Cells and Other Constituents*

CSF is essentially acellular. Few cells are found in normal CSF: most laboratories quote <5 white cells/mm$^3$ as normal, but any cells should provoke suspicion. Cells are typically lymphocytes: macrophages or neutrophils are almost certainly disease-related. Red blood cells are always abnormal, though the commonest cause is a traumatic tap. Cytology/flow cytometry may be needed, for example in malignant meningitis and haematological malignancy.

Bacteria and fungi can be isolated by culture and seen on microscopy. Viruses: PCRs are specific but variably sensitive. Whole genome and next generation sequencing techniques are available. Oligoclonal banding pattern can identify the relative production of monoclonal or oligoclonal responses, useful in inflammatory diseases. The antigenic target in MS of oligoclonal bands remains a mystery.

## Immune Nervous System Diseases

While immunology, like genetics and ion channels, is a part of every chapter in this book, it is often difficult to make dogmatic statements. Here are examples where immune pathogenesis is truly relevant.

## Antibody-Mediated Diseases

Antibody-mediated diseases can be divided either into those where the antibody defines the disease and is responsible for its pathogenesis, or diseases where antibodies are simply markers.

### Neurological Disease with Pathogenic Autoantibodies

Myasthenia gravis (MG), Guillain–Barré syndrome, Lambert–Eaton myasthenic syndrome (LEMS), some autoimmune encephalitides and probably stiff person syndromes are examples of B-cell mediated diseases in which antibodies cause the clinical picture.

In MG, antibodies to the post-synaptic acetylcholine receptor (AchR) cause a complement-dependent disruption of the post-synaptic neuromuscular junction and fatigable weakness. The unsolved question remains: what initiates anti-AchR antibody production?

GBS: in the acute motor axonal neuropathy (AMAN) GBS variant, initiation of the antibody response is better understood. Some strains of *Campylobacter jejuni* have ganglioside-like epitopes on their lipo-oligosaccharide coat. Infection in individuals who have impaired self-tolerance and in whom sufficient adjuvant stimulation exists, make antibodies to their own peripheral nerve gangliosides. These antibodies have complement-dependent mechanisms that alter membrane characteristics at nodes of Ranvier and elsewhere, and thus damage both axons and myelin.

Similar mechanisms presumably exist in the common demyelinating Guillain–Barré syndrome.

Some CNS diseases also appear to be directly antibody mediated:

- Antibodies form to the voltage-gated potassium channel complex to two of its components: LGI1 and Caspr2. Antibodies to LGI1 cause a form of limbic encephalitis. Antibodies to Caspr2 produce Morvan's syndrome – peripheral nerve hyperexcitability, psychiatric features and sleep disturbance.

- Antibodies to *N*-methyl-D-aspartate (NMDA) receptors cause an encephalitis, mainly in women, associated with antibodies against NR1 or NR2 NMDA subunits.
- Antibodies to aquaporin-4, the water channel protein, and possibly to myelin oligodendrocyte glycoprotein (MOG), are associated with Devic's disease (Chapter 11).

### Neurological Disease with Systemic Disorders and Autoantibodies

Several diseases have antibodies that may have both systemic effects and effects on the nervous system. In others, antibodies are central to diagnosis but of questionable relevance to pathogenesis.

Anti-neutrophil cytoplasmic antibodies (ANCA) are associated with some vasculitides. Although antibodies may attack neutrophils, for example in granulomatosis with polyangiitis (GPA), they are not essential to the pathogenesis.

Antibodies to extractable nuclear antigens (ENA) are associated with primary and secondary Sjögren's syndrome – that causes a sensory neuronopathy.

Antibodies to phospholipid and cardiolipin are associated with the antiphospholipid syndrome – that may cause a disorder of coagulation, or in some cases an MS-like condition.

In paraneoplastic conditions there is overlap between humoral and T-cell mediated disease, but the antibody tends to define the syndrome.

Anti-Hu, anti-Yo and anti-Ri, associated with disorders such as sensory ganglionopathies, limbic encephalitis and the opsoclonus-myoclonus syndrome are also associated with tumour types such as small cell cancers, breast and ovarian tumours.

### T-Cell-Mediated Neurological Disease

T-cell-mediated disease is difficult to define, and targets of T-cell receptors hard to isolate. These conditions are less reversible than B-cell-mediated disease:

- In paraneoplastic diseases there are T-cytotoxic mechanisms of cell injury, such as with anti-Hu, anti-Yo and anti-Ri.
- Cerebral and peripheral nerve vasculitis: the final path to tissue damage involves T-cell infiltration.
- MS is the best-described T-cell disorder, but among the most mysterious. Whether the process of myelin and axonal destruction is a neurodegeneration, primarily autoimmune, and/or driven by some viral pathogen remains unknown.
- CIDP (Chronic Inflammatory Demyelinating Polyneuropathy) is an example of T-cell-mediated PNS disease. There are deficiencies in the autoimmune regulator protein AIRE, reduced T-regulatory mechanisms, failure of Fas-Fas ligand lymphocyte down-regulation and mixed Th1 and Th2 cytokine profile up-regulation, both in serum and endoneurium. B-cell-mediated pathways are also involved.

### Cytokine-Driven Processes

Primary cytokine-driven processes are also far from clearly defined. One example occurs in POEMS (polyneuropathy, organomegaly, endocrinopathy, M-protein and skin changes). It appears that central processes driving the disease are unregulated vascular endothelial growth factor (VEGF) and IL-6 production, possibly exacerbated by hypoxia-induced factor 1α (HIF-1α). This unregulated cytokine drive causes proliferation and maturation of B cells and increased cytokine production.

## Immunomodulation, Immunosuppression and Replacement Therapy

- Intravenous immunoglobulin (IVIg) acts by multiple mechanisms, by non-specific removal of soluble immune factors and possibly interferons. Interference with B- and T-cell interactions, macrophages and complement is important.
- Plasma exchange removes low molecular weight solutes including cytokines and antibodies, especially IgG – quick and effective in GBS, systemic vasculitides and antibody-mediated encephalitides.
- Interferons act at least in part via modulation of the cytokine network.
- Steroids, oral azathioprine, methotrexate, mycophenolate, and ciclosporin and IV cyclophosphamide immunosuppress non-selectively.
- IVIg is a replacement therapy in hypogammaglobulinaemias.

  Discussion related to therapies in MS: see Chapter 11.

## Targeted Ablative Therapies

Anti-CD20 and anti-CD52 monoclonal antibodies are increasingly used, sometimes in combination with other immunosuppressants such as rituximab or methotrexate. Idiosyncratic rare complications are limiting factors. For example, PML (progressive multifocal leukoencephalopathy) is a known, usually fatal complication of rituximab, natalizumab and others. When death or severe disability is not an outcome of the primary disease, these medications are ethically questionable.

## Specifically Targeted Molecules

Anti-TNF, anti-VEGF and anti-IL-6: some of these are targeted therapies, such as etanercept, widely used in rheumatoid. Others are antibodies with anticytokine activity such as bevacizumab which acts as an anti-VEGF agent, or tocilizumab which is anti-IL-6.

# Ion Channels and Inherited Mutations

Changes in ion channels can explain clinical features. Monogenic channelopathies provide insights into disease mechanisms and whilst they are rare, they frequently have features seen in common sporadic disorders such as epilepsy and migraine. The study of channelopathies can identify signalling pathways in many diseases. One feature is that many channelopathies cause discrete paroxysms; function returns to normal between attacks. Most channelopathies are AD inherited but this may simply reflect that AR disorders are hard to identify.

Channelopathies can present in all areas of neurology. The broad groups are summarised here.

## Migraine, Epilepsy, Movement Disorders and Ataxias

In AD familial hemiplegic migraine two genes identified encode ion channels.

In epilepsy, ion channel mutations can cause benign neonatal convulsions and early-onset epileptic encephalopathies. In families with generalised epilepsy with febrile seizures plus (GEFS+), seizures may persist beyond early childhood. Mutations of at least four ion channel genes cause GEFS+. Other ion channel mutations have been described, such as malignant migrating partial seizures of infancy.

Paroxysmal dyskinesia, ataxia and hyperekplexia (exaggerated startle reaction) can be caused by channelopathies.

## Nerve, Muscle and Neuromuscular Junction Diseases

Mutations of one sodium channel gene can cause either paroxysmal pain or congenital insensitivity to pain. Some potassium channel mutations lead to neuromyotonia. CMT X (an X-linked hereditary neuropathy) is caused by mutations of connexin32. Connexins make up gap junction proteins.

Channelopathies can cause congenital myasthenic syndromes, periodic paralysis or myotonia. Myotonic dystrophy may have a similar mechanism – DMPK gene mutations alter mRNA processing that encodes the muscle chloride channel.

## Disease Causation

To understand a channelopathy requires knowledge of the normal role of the ion channel, both in neurone or muscle excitability, action potential propagation and synaptic transmission and expression of the mutated ion channel. Mutations can have multiple effects – on channel genesis and operation.

Examples are:

- Premature stop codons – the message to create a protein is incomplete.
- Splice site mutations – alteration in the DNA sequence between an exon and an intron.

Other mutations can give rise to non-functional subunits that fail to assemble normally, alter trafficking and voltage-dependent or ligand-dependent gating. Deletions and duplications of entire exons or genes also occur.

### Voltage-Gated Potassium Channels

Voltage-gated potassium channels are the largest family. They are composed of four homologous pore-forming subunits, and four intracellular beta subunits. They contribute to regulation of excitability and termination of action potentials. Each subunit of a voltage-gated potassium channel typically contains six transmembrane $\alpha$-helices, of which the S4 segment acts as a voltage sensor. Such channels open in variable ways upon membrane depolarisation.

By contrast, the pore-forming subunits of inward-rectifying potassium channels lack the voltage-sensing module S4. These channels conduct potassium ions preferentially at negative potentials and have an important role: they stabilise membrane potentials at rest.

Dominantly inherited loss-of-function mutations of *KCNA1*, that encodes the Kv1.1 potassium channel, cause episodic ataxia type 1, characterised by paroxysms of dyskinesia and neuromyotonia.

Some gain-of-function mutations of a calcium gated potassium channel (*KCNMA1*) and a sodium-gated potassium channel (*KCNT1*) cause epilepsy.

### Transient Receptor Potential Channels

Transient receptor potential (TRP) channels are related to voltage-gated potassium channels. Several members are sensitive to temperature and chemical ligands and have a role in sensory transduction. Mutations of *TRPV4* can cause abnormalities of peripheral nerve development and function. Mutations of *TRPA1* – an ion channel best known as a sensor for pain and itch – can cause a paroxysmal pain disorder. Acquired changes may also explain some aspects of neuropathic pain.

### Sodium Channels

Sodium channels open rapidly in response to depolarisation; influx of sodium underlies the upstroke of the action potential. They are structurally similar to voltage-gated potassium channels. An important feature is that most close rapidly upon sustained depolarisation.

Impairment of such fast inactivation occurs in gain-of-function mutations that affect the muscle sodium channel NaV1.4 (encoded by *SCN4A*). Depending on severity, muscle fibres are either prone to repetitive firing (myotonia) or they enter a persistent depolarised state, with hyperkalaemia (hyperkalaemic periodic paralysis, Chapter 10).

Paradoxically, loss-of-function mutations of the *SCN1A* gene are an important cause of monogenic epilepsy. An explanation is that the α subunit of Nav1.1 is preferentially expressed in cortical interneurones. Impaired excitability of these interneurones predisposes to seizures. Other mutations of *SCN1A* are associated with familial hemiplegic migraine.

*SCN9A, SCN10A* and *SCN11A* encode different sodium channels expressed in peripheral nerves. Mutations that impair inactivation cause paroxysmal pain disorders. Recessive loss-of-function mutations can cause congenital insensitivity to pain.

### Calcium Channels

Calcium channels are structurally similar to sodium channels, though with slower kinetics. There are three groups:

- CaV1.1, one of the L-type channels has a central role in excitation–contraction coupling in skeletal muscle.
- P/Q type channels contribute to triggering neurotransmitter release at presynaptic terminals and are also expressed in the cerebellar cortex.
- Transiently activating T-type, low threshold channels have a role in burst-firing of thalamic neurones.

Hypokalaemic periodic paralysis (Chapter 10) is caused by mutations of *CACNA1S*, which encodes the muscle calcium channel. However, mutations of the sodium channel gene *SCN4A* can give the same phenotype, and most mutations of either channel causing hypokalaemic paralysis affect arginine residues in the S4 voltage sensor. These are positively charged residues and sense the transmembrane potential gradient. Although loss of an arginine residue might be expected to alter voltage activation, hypokalaemic periodic paralysis is actually thought to result from an abnormal cation pathway through a cavity lining the S4 segment, arising from substitution of an arginine residue by a smaller amino acid side chain. The association of paralysis with hypokalaemia may reflect failure of inward-rectifying potassium channels to stabilise the membrane potential, because these channels fail to conduct when the extracellular potassium concentration is low.

Loss-of-function mutations of *CACNA1A*, which encodes the pore-forming subunit of the CNS calcium channel CaV2.1, cause episodic ataxia type 2, while gain-of-function mutations cause familial hemiplegic migraine.

### Chloride and Ligand-Gated Ion Channels

In skeletal muscle, dimeric ClC-2 channels have an important role in setting the resting membrane potential. They activate further upon depolarisation. Loss-of-function mutations destabilise the membrane potential and predispose to repetitive discharges. Both dominantly inherited and recessive mutations occur – Thomsen and Becker myotonia.

Ligand-gated ion channels mediate fast neurotransmission. Many mutations have been identified.

### Acetylcholine Receptors

At the neuromuscular junction ACh opens nicotinic receptors made up of α1, β1, δ and ε subunits, encoded by *CHRNA1, CHRNB1, CHRND* and *CHRNE*. Mutations of these subunits can cause a congenital myasthenic syndrome.

Of the receptor subunits expressed in the CNS, mutations have been identified in *CHRNA4, CHRNA2* and *CHRNB2* (encoding the α4, α2 and β2 subunits, respectively) in autosomal dominant nocturnal frontal lobe epilepsy. CNS nicotinic receptors mediate fast excitatory transmission to a subset of cortical interneurones. How mutations give rise to epilepsy remains unclear.

### GABA$_A$, Glycine and Glutamate Receptors

GABA$_A$ receptors are structurally homologous to nicotinic receptors but are permeable to chloride ions instead of sodium and potassium. They mediate fast inhibitory transmission and are the sites of action of benzodiazepines and other anti-epileptic, and anxiolytic drugs. Loss-of-function mutations have been reported in epilepsy.

Glycine receptors also homologous to GABA$_A$ mediate fast inhibition in the spinal cord and brainstem. AD or AR loss-of-function mutations of *GLRA1* cause familial hyperekplexia.

Glutamate receptors mutations have been described in schizophrenia, and in rolandic epilepsy.

### Acquired Channelopathies

Several autoimmune disorders affect ion channels. Antibodies recognise extracellular epitopes, for example AChRs, P/Q-type calcium channels, glycine and NMDA receptors. Aquaporin 4 (see antibodies in Devic's, Chapter 11) is a transmembrane protein that permits the flow of water between glial cells. The way that an ion channel is affected is similar in both an acquired and hereditary channelopathy – as one might expect because each ion channel has a limited repertoire. More antibody-channel interactions are likely to be discovered and to be of significance.

## Acknowledgements

I am most grateful to Dimitri Kullmann, Henry Houlden & Michael Lunn for their contribution to *Neurology A Queen Square Textbook* Second Edition on which this chapter was based. I am also indebted to Simon Farmer & David Choi who wrote in Chapter 16 about spinal embryology in *Neurology A Queen Square Textbook* Second Edition.

## Further Reading

Kullman D, Houlden H, Lunn M. Mechanisms of neurological disease: genetics, autoimmunity and ion channels. In *Neurology A Queen Square Textbook*, 2nd edn. Clarke C, Howard R, Rossor M, Shorvon S, eds. John Wiley & Sons, 2016. There are numerous references.

Also, please visit https://www.drcharlesclarke.com for free updated notes, potential links and references as these become available. You will be asked to log in, in a secure fashion, with your name and institution.

# 4

# Examination, Diagnosis and the Language of Neurology

My purpose here is to outline how I approach day-to-day neurology:

- To provide a framework for examination, diagnosis and investigation
- To introduce terminology – the language and vocabulary we use.

There is some distance between anatomy, science, diagnosis and the words we use to communicate clinical features. I try to fill these gaps. Our first purpose is to answer one question: is there a recognisable disease? In no other speciality are clinical patterns more important, nor are they more reliable. Despite advances in imaging, neurogenetics and neuropathology, we follow a traditional approach:

- Assemble clinical observations – history, symptoms and physical signs, and assess investigations.
- Recognise, by sifting these, the site of the problem, and if possible a disease.

Good neurology is about getting this right. Failure to follow this approach can lead to over-investigation or missing a serious disease.

## Elements of Diagnosis

Diagnosis is the product of the history and examination. Many find neurology hard, both because of this interplay and also because of its breadth. In some conditions, such as migraine, a faint or a seizure, we rely on narratives. There are typically no physical signs. In others, examination is pivotal, for example signs of a spastic paraparesis. However, despite its sophistication the nervous system has a relatively limited repertoire. For example, a headache can be similar whether the problem is benign or sinister.

Try to answer:

- Do the history and signs point to the site of the lesion, or lesions or to a system?
- Do the time course and character of the findings point to a recognisable disease?

*Neurology: A Clinical Handbook*, First Edition. Charles Clarke.
© 2022 John Wiley & Sons Ltd. Published 2022 by John Wiley & Sons Ltd.

## History

The narrative, from the patient, and witnesses provides vital data. How to take a present, past and family history is assumed. Pitfalls occur in three areas:

First, vividness comes from a *verbatim* account. Abbreviations are rife. 'Fitted on way to A&E – bitten tongue. . ..' is familiar medical shorthand. The inference is a generalised tonic–clonic seizure, but it does not indicate what was actually said:

> I was standing on the 73 bus near King's Cross first thing taking mum to hospital. I felt all dizzy . . .. my eyes went all funny, my legs went weak and out I went. I came to on the floor, in a pool of blood. Mum says I fainted. But then the ambulance came and they said I was shaking. I'd bitten my lip. . ..I was right as rain in a minute but they said they thought I'd had a fit.

Syncope, a simple faint, is obvious.

Secondly, identify temporal patterns:

- Intermittent events with recovery. Common: epilepsy, migraine, syncope and TIAs. Rarer: paroxysmal dyskinesias.
- Intermittent, with relapses and remissions: MS is the typical example.
- Progressive, chronic: neurodegenerative and neoplastic disorders.
- Acute or subacute and progressive: usually infective, vascular or inflammatory.
- Acute onset, single insult, with some recovery. Stroke is the prime example. Guillain–Barré and traumatic brain injury are others.

The long time scale can sometimes be forgotten – prolonged febrile convulsions in infancy or a head injury long ago can be of relevance to later seizures. Family history may be relevant.

Thirdly, one's own attitude – the balance between critical appraisal and sympathy. Judgmental approaches interfere with diagnosis, and lead to complaints. Our principal purpose is to help.

Many patients find unfamiliar questions difficult. There is no such thing as a 'hopeless historian' – it's the neurologist's fault. Patients today are well-informed, but the unsympathetic neurologist remains well described. Patients do actually suffer from their complaints. That first visit carries a burden – a serious diagnosis is often in mind. Patients and relatives hang upon single comments. Depression and anxiety are common.

## Nature of Symptoms

Foundations of neurology emphasised distinctions between positive and negative or primary and secondary phenomena, though these are not rigid. Many brain, cord, root and nerve lesions are destructive, that is with negative, primary effects such as paralysis. Destructive lesions may also cause positive, secondary phenomena, typically release of neuronal inhibition, such as exaggerated tendon reflexes. Positive also describes irritative phenomena, such as seizures.

Symptoms can thus be of two types:

Primary (direct) abnormalities, often negative: one part fails to work. Primary abnormalities can also be positive (irritative) – focal seizures from a glioma, or pain in the distribution of a trapped median nerve.

Secondary (indirect) abnormalities, usually positive, indicate typically over-activity from release of inhibition, such as spasticity.

# Neurological Examination: Preliminary Assessment

Gordon Holmes wrote in 1946: 'More can often be learned of a patient's disabilities by observing his ordinary actions, as dressing and undressing, walking when apparently unobserved, than by specific tests'. We rely on this approach intuitively – it is the way we form impressions and gauge people. Refine these skills. Think about:

- Greeting, manner, orientation, attention, mental state, mood, personal hygiene, dress
- Cognitive clues – turning to a companion before answering implies uncertainty
- Speech, language, facial appearance
- Gait, stance, clumsiness, weakness, involuntary movements, sensory symptoms
- Risk factors, lifestyle, tobacco, alcohol, drugs, religion, illness beliefs, fears
- Disability, aids, state benefits, aspects of daily living, driving, employment, sports
- Endocrine or other clues – hypothyroidism, hypopituitarism, bruises
- Relations with GP, hospital staff, attitudes towards treatment, expectations.

## Brief Neurological Examination

Detailed examination is impracticable in a busy practice. We need a robust, safe and rapid approach:

- Impressions (see above), gait, balance, arm swinging
- Head: visual acuity, fundi, pupils, eye and face movements, tongue
- Limbs: posture of arms outstretched, wasting, fasciculation, tone, power, coordination, reflexes, plantars
- Sensation: ask the patient
- Brief general exam, BP lying/standing.

## Detailed Examination

The Queen Square scheme is adapted into Table 4.1.

**Table 4.1** Detailed examination.

---

**History and general assessment**

Complaints, past and family history

Personal (confidential) issues, alcohol drugs, tobacco, travel, occupation

Previous opinions, medical notes

Review of systems

**Examination**

Initial appraisal, mental state, cognition, speech

Stance, gait, balance, hand preference, skull, spine

Cranial Nerves I-XII

**Motor System**

Movements, upper limb posture, wasting, tone, power, reflexes, coordination, diaphragm, neck

**Sensation (sensory chart)**

Posterior columns: vibration (128 Hz, VS), joint position (JPS), light touch (LT), 2-point

Spinothalamic: pain (PP), hot/cold (TM)

**General Physical Examination**

CVS, BP standing/lying, respiratory, abdomen, endocrine, skin, nodes, joints

**Summary, Formulation & Provisional Diagnosis**

---

### Cognition and Mental State

Queen Square Cognitive Screening Tests are excellent; there are many others.

- Orientation and alertness
- Language and Literacy
- Praxis and Memory &c.

Follow with clinical psychometry if need be – see Chapters 5 and 22.

### Skull, Scalp and Spine

Skull & scalp: contour, circumference, old burr holes, pulseless vessels, skull bruits.
For bruits, to abolish noise:

- Say: 'gently close your eyes'.
- Rest stethoscope bell over one closed lid.
- 'Open your other eye, and just stop breathing, briefly'.

Spine: contour, scars, deformity, pain, bruits, hair tufts, dimples, sinuses.

### Cranial Nerves
#### I: Olfaction
Use clove oil, peppermint, eucalyptus &c – or soap, coffee and/or an orange (see Chapter 13).

#### II: Vision, Pupils and Fundi
- Acuity: use a 3 metre Snellen chart. Correct refraction with lenses or pinhole – make one if necessary.

- Fields: finger confrontation is reliable, and/or use 5 mm white/red pinheads. Ask the patient to cover their left eye; fix gaze of their right with your left eye. Fields are not flat: move target along a circumference, *c.* 50 cm away.
- Central defects: Amsler grid, or, use text: '. . ..are there any holes in the print?'
- Colour vision: Ishihara or 100 Hue cards.
  Pupils:
  - dim lights, bright torch
  - approach from temporal side avoids convergence
  - cross-illuminate – second torch lights up a dark iris – many an unreactive pupil constricts
  - relative afferent pupillary defect: swinging light test.
- Fundi: develop your own technique.
  - I seat the patient gazing horizontally at an object, and say: '. . .. its fine if you blink. . ..'
  - For the left fundus, I look through my ophthalmoscope with my left eye and cover my right.

### III, IV and VI Diplopia: 4 Patterns and 4 Formal Rules
Most double vision fits one of four patterns:

### VI: Abducens Palsy
- Complaint: double vision – two images side by side
- Evident convergent squint
- Double vision disappears on looking away from the weak lateral rectus and vice versa; worse towards it – the squinting eye
- No pupil abnormality.

  Remember: a lateral rectus palsy can be caused by a VIth nerve lesion, by muscle or neuromuscular junction disease.

### III: Oculomotor Palsy (complete)
A complete IIIrd causes:

- Ptosis – upper lid drops and covers eye
- Large pupil unreactive to light (contralateral pupil constricts normally)
- An eye (lift upper lid) that's 'Down & Out'.

  A partial IIIrd spares parasympathetic fibres (these fibres run beneath the nerve - separate blood supply). Pupil: normal. Ptosis: incomplete.

### Internuclear Ophthalmoplegia (INO)
INO = damage to brainstem medial longitudinal fasciculus.

- Disconjugate horizontal eye movements – eyes move at different velocities. Look at the patient's forehead: otherwise you fixate on one eye and miss what's happening to the other.
- Incomplete ADDuction of one eye.
- Coarse jerk nystagmus on lateral gaze in the other eye (on ABDuction).

  INO is left-sided when there is failure of left ADDuction (looking right).

### IV: Trochlear Palsy

A rarity, compared with others:

- Double vision on looking down, twisted images, a.k.a. torsional diplopia
- Head tilt: away from side of superior oblique weakness
- No obvious squint.

When diplopia does not fit one of the patterns above, Formal Rules help.

1) False image: usually the less distinct and more peripheral
2) Diplopia: occurs in positions dependent upon contraction of a weak muscle
3) False image: is projected in direction of pull of the weak muscle
4) Image separation: increases in direction of pull of the weak muscle.

Dificulties: these include myasthenia, where diplopia varies; also blurring/false-framing is easily accomplished, sometimes deliberately, by converging too closely. Diplopia is normal at extremes of gaze.

### V: Trigeminal, Sensory and Motor

Most with sensory loss within one or more trigeminal branches complain of symptoms in a defined zone (see Cranial Nerves Figure 13.3). Most of us have had temporary $V_3$ loss, at the dentist.

Motor V lesions are unusual. Look at the centre line of incisor teeth, upper and lower. See if the lower incisors remain central or move laterally as the jaw opens against slight resistance. Then assess the jaw jerk.

### VII: Facial

A complete LMN facial palsy affects all facial muscles on one side. Upper motor neurone (UMN) weakness affects the lower face; this spares blinking and forehead wrinkling. In early UMN facial weakness a hint of slowing of a blink, or grimace is all that may be seen, sometimes with dissociation between voluntary and involuntary movement.

Make suggestions:

- *Frontalis:* 'look upwards' produces furrowing of the brow.
- *Orbicularis oculi:* 'screw up your eyes tightly'
- *Alae nasae:* 'wrinkle your nose'
- *Orbicularis oris:* 'now try to whistle gently'
- *Risorius:* '. . . and now please show me your teeth'
- *Platysma:* 'tension the skin of your neck'.

Involuntary movements (e.g. myokymia, fasciculation and slight hemifacial spasm): illuminate the face well. Finally, as a practical point, gradual emergence of patchy facial weakness is distinctly unusual in Bell's palsy.

### VIII: Auditory

Testing is unnecessary when there is no problem. With some hearing loss, note distance at which a whisper is heard. Rinne & Weber tests are now felt to be of doubtful value.

My approach: occlude gently both external auditory meati with the tips of each index finger. Rustle with each middle finger the skin/hair over the mastoid – a measure of bone conduction. If there is marked difference between each side, sensorineural loss is usually present. Any suspicion of a CPA lesion: MRI and audiometry.

### VIII: Vestibular

Dizziness, vertigo and nystagmus: Chapter 15. Gait & stance, Romberg & Unterberger tests. Common error: over-diagnosis of nystagmus. A few beats at extremes of lateral gaze is normal. Nystagmus must usually be sustained, within binocular gaze to be pathological.

### IX and X: Glossopharyngeal and Vagus

Take both together. Observe uvula & fauces saying 'Aaah'. Look for saliva pooling, food, palate/uvula deviation.

- Voice sounds 'wet' in early bulbar weakness (Chapter 13)
- Listen to a cough
- Watch patient begin to drink, if safe – spluttering, pooling.

An isolated IXth – almost impossible to identify – causes impaired unilateral pharynx sensation.

### XI: Accessory

Trapezii and sternomastoids: scapula winging, weak shoulder shrugging and head turning,

### XII: Hypoglossal

Tongue: wasting and deviation to weak side when protruded. Speed and amplitude diminished in pyramidal lesions and Parkinson's. Fibrillation: diagnose fibrillation only when tongue rests within mouth; twitching occurs in normal people when protruded.

### Gait and Movement Disorders

Assess gait:

- Normal, symmetrical, without limp
- Spastic – narrow-based, stiff, toe-scuffing
- Hemiparetic
- Extrapyramidal – shuffling, festinant (hurrying), with poor arm swinging, slow
- Apraxic – with gait ignition failure, with walking difficulty but preserved ability to move legs rapidly on a bed or seated
- Ataxic
- High stepping, foot drop, myopathic, antalgic, neuropathic
- Otherwise unusual – dystonia, chorea or myoclonus, or apparently theatrical.

Do not miss subtleties – early chorea, a little dystonia. A video on a phone is helpful.

## Motor System
Techniques are important.

### Posture of Outstretched Upper Limbs
- Ask the patient to extend arms symmetrically, palms uppermost and then close the eyes.
- Drift with pronation/descent towards midline is a cardinal sign of an early pyramidal lesion.
- Postural tremor, chorea, pseudochorea and asterixis become apparent. Rest tremor diminishes.
- Apply gentle downward wrist pressure and release: rebound – a cerebellar lesion.
- Fatiguability: inability to maintain the arm outstretched.
- Inspect arms, hands, nails.
- Non-organic problems: often aimlessly waving around.

### Tone
Distinguish between akinetic-rigidity and spasticity.

Extrapyramidal lead pipe rigidity is detectable throughout all passive movements. Take the hand through slow, extension, flexion, rotation movements. This elicits early stiffness in wrist and forearm muscles and cogwheeling. Stiffness becomes more evident when the opposite limb is moved actively a.k.a. synkinesis. By contrast, in spasticity, the early pronator catch or beats of ankle clonus will only become apparent if sought by brisk movements – quickly supinating the forearm or dorsiflexing the ankle: slow movements can miss these signs. A catch of increased tone at an ankle precedes sustained clonus.

### Power, Muscle Bulk, Consistency
MRC 0–5 Power Grades:

- 5: Normal
- 4: 4+, 4−  Active movement against gravity and resistance
- 3: Active movement against gravity
- 2: Active movement, gravity eliminated
- 1: Flicker of contraction
- 0: No visible muscle contraction.

Limitations: inability to record slight weakness & dependence on cooperation. 'I could just overcome hip flexion' is better than $4^+$ and $4^-$. 'Give-way' weakness means poor effort and/or pain. Assess skilled hand & foot movement: 'play piano, wriggle toes'.

Assess fatiguability, if needed. Consider focal or general muscle wasting, fasciculation, muscle bulk/consistency, myotonia.

### Cerebellar Signs
Look for dysmetria (past pointing) and action tremor.

Dysmetria: place the patient's forefinger on the point of your tendon hammer shaft, at the limit of their reach; 'now, please touch the tip of your nose, and back'. Move the shaft to a different position. Do not test finger–nose–finger rapidly – this misses early dysmetria. Follow with other tests – try circular polishing of the dorsum of the opposite hand with a single finger, and alternating forearm pronation/supination.

In the lower limb heel–shin test:

- Raise one leg, touch your opposite ankle with your heel and then move the heel up your shin, to the knee and down again.
- Repeat the sequence. Simply gliding one heel up and down the shin can miss early ataxia.

Foot tapping also elicits incoordination.

Knee jerks with a pendular pattern - slow and swinging - or absent reflexes do occur with cerebellar disease, if seldom.

Dysarthria is usually obvious.

Nystagmus rarely occurs without other cerebellar features.

Remember: a midline cerebellar lesion may cause gait and trunk ataxia without limb ataxia.

### Tendon Reflexes

Ensure the patient is relaxed – with head and trunk supported. Minor asymmetry is common, and reduced knee jerks compared with ankle jerks. Reinforcement: ask the patient to clench their teeth and then relax. Original Jendrassik manoeuvre: hook fingers together and pull.

Do not miss slow relaxing reflexes: hypothyroidism.

### Absent Reflex→Clonus nomenclature

| 0 | Absent with reinforcement | Almost always pathological |
|-----|---------------------------|----------------------------|
| ± | Present with reinforcement | Sometimes normal; may be pathological |
| + | Present | Normal |
| ++ | Brisk | Normal |
| +++ | Very brisk | Pathological if tone increased; can be normal |
| CL | Clonus | >3 beats of ankle clonus = pathological; 2 beats may be normal |

### Spinal levels of tendon reflexes, a.k.a. deep tendon reflexes – DTRs in US

| C5–6 | Supinator |
|------|-----------|
| C5–6 | Biceps |
| C7 | Triceps |
| C8 | Finger jerks |
| L(3)4 | Knee |
| S1 | Ankle |

### Extensor Plantar (Babinski)

Babinski published the 26-line *phénomène des orteils* (toes) in 1896. An extensor is an indication of a brain or cord UMN lesion. A reproducible upgoing toe by any reasonable stroking action on the foot is abnormal. Extensors are exceptional in normal adults.

### Superficial Abdominal Reflexes

Elicit muscle twitches by gentle stroking each quadrant with an orange-stick – not with a needle. Superficial abdominals are lost with pyramidal lesions and hard to elicit or absent in the obese. Preservation of upper superficial abdominal reflexes with absent lower abdominals can occur with a thoracic sensory level in cord compression (T10 = umbilicus).

### Respiration, Diaphragm

Respiration and the diaphragm can be assessed by observing inspiration and expiration and abdominal muscles. Selective diaphragm weakness causes paradoxical upward movement of the umbilicus – well seen with the patient supine during sniffing. Measure vital capacity.

### Lower and Upper Motor Neurone Lesions

See Table 4.2.

**Table 4.2** Lower (LMN) & upper motor neurone (UMN) lesions.

| Feature | LMN | UMN |
| --- | --- | --- |
| Muscle wasting, a.k.a. amyotrophy | Visible | Absent |
| Fasciculation | Visible | Absent |
| Fibrillation | Recordable on EMG, visible in tongue | Absent |
| Tone | Flaccid/normal | Increased/spastic type |
| Weakness pattern | Root, nerve or distal | Pyramidal + dexterity |
| Tendon reflexes | Depressed/usually absent | Exaggerated[a] |
| Clonus | Absent | Present |
| Abdominal reflexes | Present | Absent |
| Plantars | Flexor (normal) | Extensor |

[a] tendon reflexes can be absent/depressed initially with an acute UMN lesion.

## Sensory System

Abnormalities are exceptional when the patient is articulate without sensory complaints. Focus neuro-anatomically:

- Assess posterior columns first – vibration (VS) and joint position sense (JPS).
- Spinothalamic sensation: cold metal and a disposable sharp object.
- Light touch: fingertip or cotton wool. Avoid stroking/tickling.
- Two-point discrimination (0.5 cm finger tips, 2 cm soles): useful & shows you are thorough.
- Chart sensory loss or altered sensation.

## Formulation

Drawing together data is essential. To conclude that a fall with loss of consciousness and residual weakness is 'collapse?cause' or a hemiparesis is 'a CVA' are not formulations any doctor should reach. Tease out the history and build on the signs found, to reach either a diagnosis or at least a direction for investigations. Such attention to detail can be hard in an emergency, but it is in acute neurology that many mistakes occur. For example, a sudden headache can be discounted when the reality is a subarachnoid haemorrhage, whereas thoughtful appraisal usually provides the correct answer. Another common error is the distinction between a seizure and syncope; epilepsy is overdiagnosed. It is sometimes taxing to formulate a diagnosis, but essential to try.

### Difficulties

When a diagnosis is unclear, try to establish relevant and secure details – whether or not features are certain. A fact is a clearly witnessed account of a tonic–clonic seizure. Unequivocal signs are sustained ankle clonus and extensor plantars. Separate these from vague findings such as weakness, or dizziness without vertigo or nystagmus. Recognise, accept and record uncertainty – easier to write than to put into practice.

## Diagnostic Tests

We are surrounded by technology, by defensive practice and the need to provide reassurance by exclusion. Be aware of costs; try to target studies for some real purpose.

### Imaging

This summary is a stepping-stone to widely available resources, such as:

- htpps://radiopaedia.org

Plain X-rays have a limited role – skull, spine and skeleton – and radio-opaque implants and ventricular shunts.

CT (computerised tomography) uses X-rays to generate thin tomographic slices. CT relies upon tissues attenuating X-rays to different degrees. Grey-scale images are adjusted to provide optimal contrast between brain, water (CSF) and bone (Figures 4.1 and 4.2).

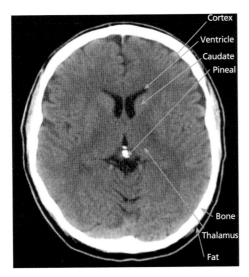

**Figure 4.1** Axial brain CT: brain windows.

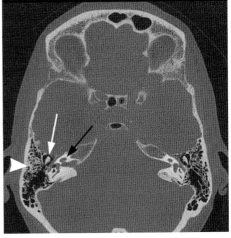

**Figure 4.2** Axial brain CT: bone windows. White arrow: ossicles. Black arrow: cochlea. Arrowhead: mastoid bone trabeculations.

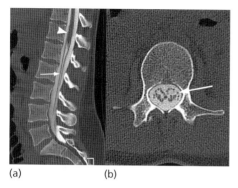

(a)                    (b)

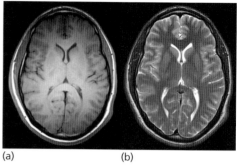

(a)                    (b)

**Figure 4.3** CT Myelogram. (a): Sagittal. (b): Axial. Intrathecal contrast creates high attenuation CSF, outlines vertebral canal contours, cord (white arrowhead) and nerve roots (white arrows).

**Figure 4.4** Axial MR (a) T1w – CSF black. (b) T2w – CSF white, grey matter hyperintense to white matter.

CT myelography images the cord and nerve roots (Figure 4.3).

Magnetic resonance imaging (MRI) uses magnetic fields (1.5 Tesla and 3 Tesla) with radiofrequency pulses to generate signals from protons in water molecules. Two commonly used sequences (Figure 4.4) produce images based on variations in relaxation times of protons, generating T1-weighted (T1w) and T2-weighted (T2w) images.

Many other sequences are used – Fluid Attenuated Inversion Recovery (FLAIR), diffusion-weighted imaging (DWI) and susceptibility-weighted imaging (SWI). Gadolinium is used for contrast. CT and magnetic resonance angiography (MRA, Figure 4.5) are used for vascular imaging.

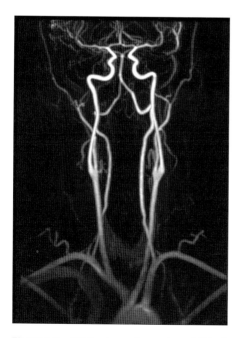

Advanced MRI, functional MRI, and MR spectroscopy are used in specialist units, and also positron emission tomography (PET) and single-photon emission computed tomography (SPECT).

Duplex ultrasound, a.k.a. Doppler, is commonly used to assess extracranial carotid arteries. Transcranial Doppler (TCD) gains information from intracranial vessels and has therapeutic possibilities.,

Digital subtraction catheter angiography (DSA) is the gold standard for vascular anatomy. It is invasive, usually via femoral artery puncture. DSA provides images of arterial, capillary and venous phases (Figure 4.6).

Interventional neuroradiology is used to treat intracranial aneurysms and AVMs and is evolving rapidly. Magneto-encephalography and transcranial magnetic brain stimulation are largely research tools.

**Figure 4.5** MR Angiography: contrast MRA of neck vessels.

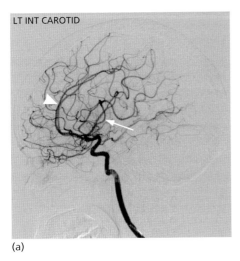
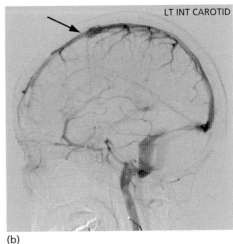

(a)                                      (b)

**Figure 4.6**   DSA: (a) arterial and (b) venous phase. Left internal carotid artery injection. White arrowhead: anterior cerebral artery. White arrow: middle cerebral artery branches. Black arrow: superior sagittal sinus.

## Clinical Neurophysiology

### Electroencephalography
The EEG records via scalp electrodes potentials generated by millions of neurones. Precise sources of these rhythms remain uncertain. Main roles are in epilepsy, in diffuse brain diseases, in ITU and in sleep disorders. Videotelemetry – prolonged EEG recording with simultaneous film – is of value in the assessment of 'attacks' (Chapter 8). Sleep studies: Chapter 20.

### *Alpha, Theta, Delta and Beta Activity in Normal Subjects*
Alpha activity seen over the occipital lobes is 8–14 Hz – some 150 μV amplitude and attenuates on eye opening.

Theta activity of 4–7 Hz is also seen, and becomes prominent during drowsiness.

Delta activity is a slower frequency, less than 4 Hz. Delta waves around 1 Hz appears during the first non-REM sleep period.

Beta activity is a normal largely frontal rhythm faster than 14 Hz.

### *Epilepsy*
Spikes, or spike-and-wave abnormalities (Figure 4.7) are hallmarks of epilepsy. However most with epilepsy have a normal EEG between seizures. Epileptic activity is either generalised or focal.

### *EEG Artefacts*
The most common is high amplitude frontal activity from scalp muscle contraction and eye movements.

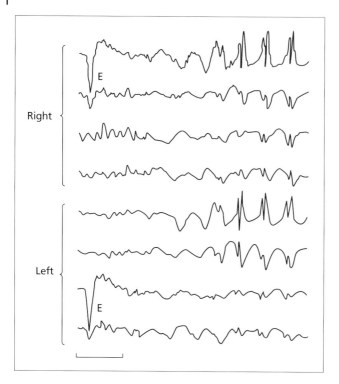

**Figure 4.7**   Normal EEG followed by frontal spike-and-wave. E: eye movement artefact.

Sharp waves describe non-sinusoidal waveforms seen in the normal population – not diagnostic of epilepsy, but may occur in patients with seizures.

Difficulties surround EEG reports. Conclusions can only be reached within a clinical context. Useful questions:

- Is there generalised epileptic activity? Is there localised epileptic activity?
- Is there generalised or localised abnormal slow wave activity, and could slow waves be seen in the normal population?
- Are the sharp waves reported normal?
- In coma, is there any EEG responsiveness to stimulation?

### Diffuse and Focal Brain Disorders

Typical EEG abnormalities appear:

- Periodic lateralised epileptic discharges (PLEDS): viral encephalitis, cerebral abscess, anoxic brain damage.
- Slow waves appear in many encephalopathies.
- Repetitive generalised sharp waves every 0.5–1 seconds: seen in some prion cases.
- High voltage slow wave complexes, every 3–10 seconds: subacute sclerosing pan-encephalitis (SSPE).
- Triphasic slow waves: metabolic disorders, typically hepatic coma.

*Brainstem Death*

The EEG becomes isoelectric (flat) in brainstem death and in deep coma, for example with barbiturates or hypothermia (Chapter 20).

## Clinical Neurophysiology: Nerve and Muscle

See also Chapter 10.

*Electromyography (EMG)*

A concentric needle electrode is inserted into voluntary muscle. Amplified EMG recordings are viewed on an oscilloscope and heard through a speaker. Three main features:

- Normal motor unit recruitment
- Denervation and reinnervation changes
- Myopathic, myotonic, myasthenic features, myokymia, cramps, hemifacial spasm or continuous motor unit activity.

Much depends upon observations of the neurophysiologist.

*Normal Motor Unit Recruitment*

Normal muscle at rest is silent electrically. When a single anterior horn neurone fires, all muscle fibres connected to it contract. The contraction of each muscle fibre within the motor unit is not synchronous. Interference pattern describes the appearance and sound of motor units running together during contraction.

*Chronic Partial Denervation*

If one anterior horn cell (A) fails, for example in motor neurone disease (MND), adjacent anterior horn cells B and C produce sprouting axons that re-innervate muscle fibres originally supplied by A. In chronic partial denervation, the EMG reflects this: reduced numbers of polyphasic, long duration, high voltage muscle action potentials (MAPs).

*Fibrillation, Fasciculation and Positive Sharp Waves*

When a muscle is denervated, spontaneous contraction of individual fibres begins to occur after 7–14 days. These contractions produce tiny fibrillation potentials of amplitude <10–200 μV. Fibrillation in a limb is invisible, but visible in the tongue, typically in MND. Positive sharp waves are bi-phasic potentials with a longer duration (<10 ms) than fibrillations and usually with amplitudes of 10–200 μV, also seen in denervation.

Fasciculation describes the visible twitching of a muscle seen in various situations. In normal people, benign fasciculation is common in calf and other muscles. In denervated muscle, fasciculation potentials are produced by spontaneous discharges of motor units, and visible – often widespread in MND.

*Myopathic EMG*

This is characterised by:

- Individual units of low amplitude, of short duration and polyphasic
- Rapid motor unit recruitment to a full interference pattern at lower than normal voluntary effort, and
- A crackly audible pattern.

### Myotonic EMG Changes

Myotonic muscle (*dystrophia myotonica*; Chapter 10) responds to stimulation with high frequency action potentials. The discharge frequency diminishes as the seconds pass to create a whine, likened to a dive-bomber of propeller-driven vintage. A softer sound can be heard through a stethoscope over a contracting myotonic muscle. Complex repetitive discharges, a.k.a. pseudo-myotonic, commence and end abruptly; they occur in chronic neuropathies and myopathies.

### Hemifacial Spasm, Cramps, Myokymia and Stiff Person Syndrome

- Hemifacial spasm (Chapter 13) is probably an example of ephaptic transmission, that is transmission between adjacent VIIth nerve fibres. EMG: bursts of normal motor unit discharges, without denervation.
- Normal muscle cramps produce high frequency discharges. In myophosphorylase deficiency (McArdle's disease; Chapter 10), cramps occur but these discharges are not found.
- Myokymia (Chapter 13) refers to two facial phenomena:
  - Quivering movements around the eye, common and invariably innocent.
  - Worm-like wriggling, persistent and typically around the chin – occurs in brainstem gliomas and MS.
- In stiff person syndrome (Chapter 7), continuous motor unit activity is found simultaneously in opposing muscle groups, as one might expect from the stiffness.

### Peripheral Nerve Conduction Studies

Five measurements are of value in neuropathies and peripheral nerve entrapment:

- Motor conduction velocity (MCV) – normal values 41–49 m/s or greater
- Sensory conduction velocity – normal 40–50 m/s
- Distal motor latency (DML) – less than 4.4 m/s in median nerve, less than 3.3 m/s in ulnar
- Sensory (nerve) action potentials (SAPs or SNAPs) – 2–15 mV, depending on nerve
- Compound muscle action potentials (MAPs or CMAPs).

Nerve conduction studies use supramaximal stimulation, that measures conduction in fastest fibres – a blunt instrument compared with the finesse of EMG interpretation. Technique: see Figure 4.8.

### Polyneuropathy

In axonal neuropathies, MCV is initially preserved but there is reduction in CMAP amplitude. SAPs are lower than normal. In demyelinating neuropathies, nerve MCV is markedly slowed. SAPs are lost or diminished (Chapter 10).

### Entrapment Neuropathies

Hallmarks: increased distal motor latency such as in carpal tunnel syndrome, slowing of conduction across the site of entrapment with diminution of relevant sensory action potentials. Denervation when entrapment is severe.

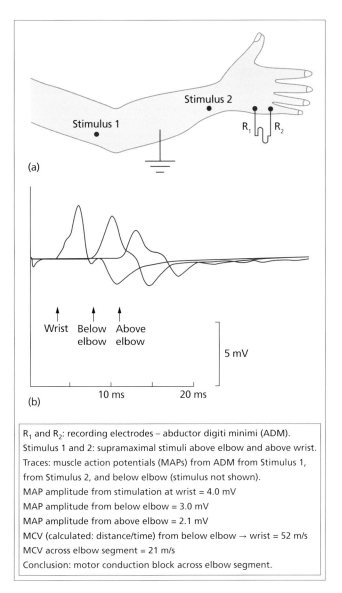

**Figure 4.8** Ulnar nerve conduction: nerve compression at elbow. *Source:* Hopkins (1993).

### F waves

These are low-amplitude muscle responses to a peripheral stimulus produced by antidromic discharges of anterior horn cells. Prolonged latencies or disappearance occur in root lesions and polyneuropathies.

### Hoffman (H) Reflexes

These are neurophysiological equivalents of a stretch reflex. Usually the tibial nerve is stimulated at the knee and contraction of gastrocnemius and soleus recorded: delayed when peripheral conduction is slowed, such as in polyneuropathies.

## Neuromuscular Transmission
### *Repetitive Stimulation: Myasthenia and Myasthenic–Myopathic Syndromes*
A muscle surface electrode records this. In myasthenia, responses decrease in amplitude. Also, a phenomenon known as jitter can also be recorded by single fibre studies.

In Lambert–Eaton syndrome the converse is seen – facilitation (increase) of motor responses with high frequency stimulation.

## Cerebral-Evoked Potentials
Evoked potentials record the amplitude and time for a visual, auditory or other sensory stimulus to reach the cortex. See Chapters 11 and 15.

## Specialised Investigations

Various tests that may be unfamiliar to a newcomer to neurology are listed below:

| | |
|---|---|
| Serum copper & caeruloplasmin | Wilson's disease & rare cord disease |
| CAG repeat assay | Huntington's (Ch. 8) |
| Genetic tests | Neuropathies and ataxias (Chs 10, 17) |
| Antiganglioside antibodies | Acquired neuropathies (Ch. 10) |
| Antineuronal antibodies | Paraneoplastic syndromes (Chs 17, 21) |
| Anti-endomysial & anti-gliadin antibodies | Coeliac disease (Ch. 17) |
| Anti-GAD antibodies | Stiff person syndrome (Ch. 8) |
| Anti-acetylcholine receptor, anti-MuSK antibodies *et al* | Myasthenic syndromes (Ch. 10) |
| Striated muscle antibodies, genetic tests | Myopathies, dystrophies (Ch. 10) |
| Aquaporin 4 antibodies | Devic's (Ch. 11) |
| Voltage-gated K channel antibodies *et al* | Autoimmune limbic encephalitis (Ch. 9) |
| Porphyrins, amino-acids | Porphyrias, amino-acid disorders |
| Leucodystrophies, various | V. long chain fatty acids, enzyme & genetic tests (Ch. 19) |

## Cerebrospinal Fluid Examination

CSF is the clear, colourless, almost acellular fluid (Table 4.3) around the brain, cord, nerve roots and within the ventricles, withdrawn at lumbar puncture (LP). Cervical puncture is now rarely performed. Ventricular CSF is sometimes examined.

### Indications for LP and CSF Examination
Principal indications are:

- Suspected meningitis and encephalitis – in some cases
- Suspected subarachnoid haemorrhage – blood products
- Pressure measurement (e.g. idiopathic intracranial hypertension)
- Therapeutic CSF removal (e.g. idiopathic intracranial hypertension)

**Table 4.3** Normal CSF.

| Observation | | Comment |
|---|---|---|
| Appearance | Crystal clear, colourless | Clear when held to light, a.k.a. 'gin clear' |
| Pressure | 60–150 mm CSF | Patient must be relaxed, recumbent with needle patent for CSF to oscillate in manometer |
| Cell count | <5/mm$^3$. | *No polys*: mononuclears only |
| Protein | 0.2–0.4 g/L | Slightly raised protein <0.7 g/L rarely pathological |
| Glucose | ⅔ to ½ of blood glucose | CSF glucose <½ blood glucose suspicious |
| Culture | Sterile | Do not accept contaminants |
| IgG | <15% of total CSF protein | Usually only on request |
| Oligoclonal bands | Absent | Parallel blood sample |

- Assays in MS, neurosyphilis, sarcoidosis, Behçet's, chronic infection, malignant meningitis, polyneuropathy & some dementias.
- Intrathecal contrast injection and drugs.

In suspected CNS infection, meticulous attention should focus on examination for cells, cell types and microbiological tests.

### Informed Consent, LP Risks, CSF Removal

The procedure should be explained and its potentially painful nature. Written consent should be obtained.

The principal risks relate first to the removal of CSF. CSF often continues to leak around the punctured lumbar dura. This leads to low pressure (low volume) headaches (Chapter 12) and exceptionally to intracranial subdural haematoma.

Secondly, there are local complications at the LP site:

- Infection and meningitis
- Trauma –pain, nerve root damage
- Bleeding, spinal epidural haematoma
- Arachnoiditis (Chapter 16).

LP should follow the established procedure. LP should not be performed in the presence of raised intracranial pressure without prior brain imaging and a clear risk appraisal. Inappropriate intrathecal injection of drugs can have fatal consequences.

### LP: Contraindications

- Suspicion of a mass lesion within the brain or spinal cord. Caudal herniation of the unci and cerebellar tonsils (coning) may occur if an intracranial mass is present and the pressure below is reduced by removal of CSF. Spinal cord compression may worsen, or even develop, if an unsuspected cord tumour is present. Such complications can develop within minutes of LP. Unconscious patients and those with papilloedema must have brain imaging (MRI if feasible), before LP.

- Any cause of suspected raised intracranial pressure, without careful consideration.
- Local infection near the LP site.
- Congenital lumbosacral region abnormalities (e.g. meningo-myelocoele).
- Platelet count $< 40 \times 10^9$/L; other clotting abnormalities; anticoagulant drugs.

Contraindications are relative: there are circumstances when LP is carried out despite them, for example with papilloedema when idiopathic intracranial hypertension is suspected.

CSF pressure and naked-eye appearance should be recorded: clear, cloudy, colourless, yellow (xanthochromic), red – and if red, whether or not the colour begins to clear after the first or subsequent sample. Patients should lie flat for 24 hours after LP to avoid subsequent headaches, and drink plenty, both manoeuvres of uncertain value. Analgesics may be needed for post-LP headaches and occasionally treatments for prolonged low pressure headaches (e.g. epidural autologous blood patches; Chapter 12). Post LP headaches often last several days but may continue for weeks or more.

## Biopsy: Brain, Nerve and Muscle

Biopsy of brain, with or without meningeal biopsy is carried for diagnosis of brain tumours, for other mass lesions and other indications, such as chronic infection and vasculitis. Stereotactic procedures are employed increasingly (Chapter 21). Risks are infection, haemorrhage, epilepsy and/or damage to surrounding brain. Morbidity: below 2%.

Peripheral nerve biopsy (sural or radial) is sometimes performed in chronic neuropathies and vasculitis. Risks are few: infection is rare but painful paraesthesiae sometimes follow. A numb patch on the foot is to be expected following sural nerve biopsy.

Muscle biopsy (deltoid or quadriceps) is a standard procedure in many muscle diseases.

## Neuropsychological Testing

Cognitive Screening Tests have been mentioned. Detailed testing is sometimes of great value, and outside the remit of a general neurologist. Reports tend to vary in emphasis, some dwelling on psychiatric diagnoses while others focus upon cognitive function.

Intellectual function overall: the Wechsler Adult Intelligence Scale Revised (WAIS-R) is divided into subtests. The Verbal IQ with the National Adult Reading Test (NART) provides a measure of the premorbid optimal level of function – reading vocabulary is relatively resistant to neurodegenerative processes that degrade cognition. Performance IQ gives a measure of present overall cognitive, especially, non-verbal ability.

Specific tests address memory functions, language, literacy, calculation, perceptual function, frontal/executive function, attention validity/credibility and effort. The formulation draws together the results: problems with concentration and effort must be given appropriate weighting, especially when pain, depression and anxiety are present.

# The Vocabulary of Neurology

This is an overview of patterns we see in practice.

## Focal Cortical Disorders

The cortical mantle is highly differentiated. A working knowledge of the cortex is essential, despite the availability of imaging. Beware theories that appear highly specific – the neural network concept is often a more accurate model than attempting to pinpoint a focal lesion – many functions depend upon interactions between cortex and subcortical structures. Here, I summarise some definitions of language disorders and introduce temporal lobe, frontal and parietal problems. There is overlap with Chapter 5 where memory and perception are addressed and common cortical disorders such as aphasia and dementia.

### Language and Speech Disorders

Language means that combination of sounds or writing used for interactive communication. A phoneme is its shortest unit.

- Dysphasia describes any disorder of language
- Dysgraphia: disorders of written language
- Dyslexia: disorders of reading ability – often used for the common developmental problem rather than an acquired problem caused by a stroke, or other focal lesion
- Dysarthria is disordered articulation – production and/or coordination of speech. Anarthria is complete inability to articulate.
- Dysphonia is disordered voice production, caused by passage of expired air over poorly vibrating or paralysed vocal cords. Aphonia is complete inability, or apparent inability to produce sounds.

### Temporal Lobes

Many small (<2 cm) unilateral temporal lesions are silent. Epilepsy is common (Chapter 8). Upper quadrantic hemianopia is seen when the forward-looping fibres (Meyer's loop) are damaged. A lesion in the posterior dominant anterior temporal lobe can cause a posterior (Wernicke) aphasia (Chapter 5), or much less commonly, and usually when bilateral, word deafness, that is inability to understand speech, caused by damage to auditory areas in or near Heschl's gyrus.

Non-dominant anterior temporal lobe lesions are sometimes associated with inability to recognise faces (prosopagnosia). Unilateral mesial temporal lobe lesions can also produce subtle changes in memory, more marked for verbal material in the dominant, and faces and topographical features in the non-dominant hemisphere.

Bilateral temporal lobe lesions, such as post-herpes simplex encephalitis can cause profound memory loss for recent events. Bilateral damage in primates can cause hypersexuality, hyperphagia, and aggression (Klüver–Bucy syndrome). Sometimes, elements of this occur in Man, such as temper dyscontrol, but the usual outcome is amnesia and aimlessness.

**Frontal Lobes**

Many lesions remain silent. Frontal regions have connections with the basal ganglia and limbic systems, networks that mediate emotional, social and motivational behaviours. Lesions involving the dorsal frontal convexities can cause impassivity and apathy – more medial lesions may even cause mutism, while orbito-frontal lesions are more likely to produce disinhibition. However, localisation is distinctly imprecise.

Lesions involving dominant inferior frontal gyrus cause anterior (Broca's) aphasia.

Substantial damage such as traumatic frontal brain injury, direct or *contra-coup* can cause disabling problems:

- Abandonment of social inhibitions – from inopportune comments to more profound, such as urination, exposure or masturbation
- Inappropriate jollity (*witzelsucht*) – tales overlong, unwanted, with loss of empathy
- Apathy (abulia), lack of initiative, poor planning (dysexecutive problems)
- Irritability, anger or the converse – placidity in the face of irritation
- Distractability, or the converse – obsessions
- Continuing one action when another is appropriate, a.k.a. motor perseveration
- Utilisation behaviour: the patient sees a stethoscope and begins to use it.

Release of primitive programmes from early infancy, such as grasp, rooting or sucking reflexes can emerge. Bilateral frontal lesions, such as small vessel disease can lead to gait apraxia and failure to initiate walking (gait ignition failure), with urinary incontinence.

Alleged brain damage with behavioural change has become a common plea in claims following minor head injury. The patient and relatives are asked leading questions about features such as impulsivity, temper, fiscal ability, multi-tasking, planning, depression and anxiety – all common problems in any event. There is no evidence that these are caused by brain injury following a minor blow to the head, with normal imaging. Frontal lobe seizures are described in Chapter 8.

**Occipital Lobes**

Field defects are mentioned in Chapter 14. Neglect or even denial of virtually complete visual loss (cortical blindness or Anton's syndrome) are sometimes seen following bilateral infarction. An explanation for 'blind sight' (perception of objects when the occipital cortex is destroyed) is preservation of anterior visual pathways via the lateral geniculate bodies that are below the level of awareness. Epilepsy, with episodes of flashing lights or, rarely, more formed features, can occur with occipital lobe lesions.

**Parietal Lobes**

These integrate visual and somatosensory information, such as awareness of body parts and their relation to objects. A complex nomenclature has evolved. Attempts to associate precise areas to particular functions are bedevilled by variation between individuals, and because the cortex is not divided into discrete compartments. The following are seen with lesions of either parietal lobe:

- Attention defects in the contralateral visual field and neglect of the opposite side
- Lower quadrantic homonymous field defects

- Astereognosis – inability to recognise common objects placed in the palm despite normal sensation
- Agraphaesthesia – inability to recognise numbers drawn on the palm
- Pseudo-athetosis (waving about) and/or drift of an outstretched contralateral hand
- Contralateral cortical sensory loss – impaired two point discrimination despite intact peripheral sensation.

Sensory epilepsy is sometimes a feature.

### Dominant Parietal

Inability to execute a skilled movement despite no discernable weakness may be seen – apraxia. The patient may not respond to suggestions 'imitate combing your hair' or 'pretend to turn a key': a.k.a. 'ideational' apraxia. Alternatively, the patient may have difficulty imitating a meaningless gesture made by the examiner: 'ideomotor' apraxia. Typically, they are bewildered, moving the hand in a non-purposive way or attempting to grasp the examiner's hand.

Lesions may produce impairment of literacy skills: alexia, agraphia and acalculia. The rare constellation of these with finger agnosia (inability to name individual fingers and right–left disorientation) is known as Gerstmann's syndrome. Auditory short-term verbal memory can be impaired. Neglect of contralateral limbs is typically less prominent with a dominant than non-dominant parietal lesion.

### Non-dominant Parietal

Patterns include:

- Neglect of opposite limbs. Neglect can extend to denial that limbs belong to the patient.
- Inability to draw shapes such as a house or a clock face. The left side of a picture drawn (such as numbers 1–5 on a clock face) tend to be omitted with a right parietal lesion, a.k.a. constructional apraxia.
- Visual apperceptive agnosia – inability to perceive objects under poor viewing conditions or from an unusual angle.

## Motor Abnormalities: Brain and Spinal Cord

Hemiparesis, hemiplegia, paraparesis, cerebellar syndromes and disorders of movement are summarised here.

### Hemiparesis

This is the weakness on one side usually from a pyramidal tract lesion. Hemiplegia means total paralysis. See Examination (above). Hemiparesis without other UMN signs is highly unusual in organic weakness.

### Cerebellar Syndromes

Features of cerebellar disease are well defined. With a lateral cerebellar lobe lesion, there is rebound and dysmetria in the ipsilateral limbs, dysarthria and nystagmus. With a vermis lesion, there is ataxia of stance, trunk & gait, sometimes with negative Romberg.

There are two practical points:

First, if an expanding cerebellar mass lesion is suspected or found on imaging, there must be speedy liaison with a neurosurgeon. While all brain mass lesions are potentially serious, many tumours above the tentorium can be dealt with in an expectant manner. With a cerebellar mass progression can take place over hours or less. Secondly, to misdiagnose as non-organic the ataxia of stance and gait of a midline lesion does happen. See cerebellar syndromes: (Chapter 17).

## Movement Disorders

These can be divided into akinetic-rigid syndromes, where poverty of movement predominates, and dyskinesias in which excessive movement is the principal feature. Akinetic-rigid syndromes include idiopathic Parkinson's, Parkinson-plus, drug-induced & post-encephalitic parkinsonism, manganism (v.rare), childhood akinetic-rigid syndromes and Wilson's disease.

Dyskinesias include tremors, chorea, hemiballismus, myoclonus, tics, dystonias, paroxysmal and drug-induced dyskinesias. The distinction between the two groups is artificial. For example, Parkinson's can be primarily tremulous; Wilson's disease can have features of akinesia with an unusual tremor.

No amount of writing surpasses seeing a movement disorder, either in the flesh or on video. See: Chapter 7.

Diagnostic difficulties occur. First, when akinetic-rigidity becomes apparent, early idiopathic Parkinson's disease tends to be over-diagnosed. The reality, evident some years later, is another akinetic-rigid syndrome. Parkinson's is almost always asymmetrical, and also should be diagnosed with caution if rest tremor is not apparent. Progressive supranuclear palsy (PSP) or multiple system atrophy (MSA) tend to be symmetrical from the onset. Consider Wilson's disease in akinetic-rigidity, or dyskinesia below 40.

Benign essential tremor (BET), though common, can cause difficulty. Usually, tremor occurs when the limbs adopt a particular posture. However, forms of BET mimic benign tremulous Parkinson's disease, and even cerebellar action tremor.

Early chorea is easy to miss – mistaken for fidgeting. Minor dystonia can also escape recognition. Non-organic movement disorders are difficult; many labelled initially as functional have organic disease.

## Paraparesis

Spastic paraparesis, meaning lower limb weakness of cord or, rarely, cortical origin, is a pivotal diagnosis. Prior to MRI, clinical examination had a major role in differentiating between cord compression and other causes of paraparesis.

The clinical picture begins with subtle features:

- Scuffing the toes of shoes, often worse on one side
- Stiffening of gait (spastic gait) with retention of a narrow base
- Noticeable beats of ankle clonus (e.g. on a step or kerbstone)
- Changes in lower limb sensation.

Spinal pain is common in cord compression. With a thoracic meningioma, pain at tumour level develops with an emerging spastic paraparesis and a sensory level, rising from below. The patient complains of numbness or altered sensation commencing in the feet, that marches upwards, over days, weeks or longer. Brown-Séquard features (pyramidal signs on one side, spinothalamic on the other) may appear.

These features apply equally to tetraparesis (*syn.* quadriparesis).

The five principal features of a pyramidal lesion may not all be present. Pain may not be present in cord compression. Marked asymmetry can sometimes cause difficulty.

Two questions arise when signs of spastic paraparesis are found:

- Is the paraparesis caused by cord compression?
- Is the paraparesis the result of a condition in which it is part of the picture? Examples are:
  - MS
  - MND
  - Subacute combined degeneration of the cord
  - Syringomyelia
  - Cortical lesions such as a parasagittal meningioma, hydrocephalus and other brain lesions can occasionally cause paraparesis.

Paraparesis is also caused by many rarities, such as vascular anomalies of the cord, adrenoleucodystrophy and copper deficiency (see Chapter 16). There can be difficulties with the initial diagnosis: within primary care, especially when restricted to a brief telephone call, emergence of difficulty in difficulty in walking is not taken seriously, and early features of a paraparesis can pass unrecognised.

### Brainstem Syndromes

Anatomy is outlined in Chapter 2. Figure 4.9 is a helpful diagram, repeated here in a clinical context: think of the level within the brainstem and of the dorso-ventral plane. The usual hallmark is coexistence of damage to motor and/or sensory fibres and to cranial nerve nuclei. Syndromes involving oculomotor nerves III, IV and VI indicate upper or mid brainstem disease. Mid and lower brainstem disease affects nuclei VII–XII.

Bulbar and pseudobulbar palsy describe common brainstem syndromes (Chapter 13). Both cause dysarthria, dysphagia, drooling and respiratory problems. Bulbar palsy means disease of the lower cranial nerves (IX, X, XII), their nuclei and muscles. Pseudobulbar palsy is shorthand for UMN lesions of lower

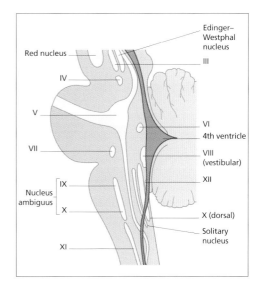

**Figure 4.9**  Brainstem: lateral schematic view. *Source:* Hopkins (1993).

cranial nerve nuclei. MS, brainstem stroke and MND cause pseudobulbar palsy, the latter usually both pseudobulbar and bulbar. Advanced Parkinson's causes poverty of movement of these muscles.

## Anterior Horn Cell Disease

Relatively few diseases afflict the anterior horn. All are serious. The commonest is MND; spinal muscular atrophies, Kennedy's disease, poliomyelitis and other viruses, notably West Nile are also causes. LMN signs of wasting and weakness develop. Amyotrophy is also a word used to describe wasting; it means myo (muscle) atrophy. Typically in all these diseases, initially at least, weakness can be highly selective. For instance, MND can present with weakness of one or two finger extensors. Neurophysiology is often diagnostic.

## Sensory Abnormalities: Patterns at Different Levels

Sensation is difficult to evaluate. Eponyms abound – positive Tinel (carpal tunnel), *tic douloureux*, causalgia, *anaesthesia dolorosa*, lightning pains, Lhermitte, Brown-Séquard, dissociated sensory loss, suspended sensory loss, sacral sparing, thalamic pain and astereognosis.

An approach that some find valuable is that if a sensory symptom is the principal complaint, such as the pain of trigeminal neuralgia (Chapter 13) or nocturnal tingling of the hands in median nerve entrapment at the wrist (Chapter 10), the quality of symptoms tend to be diagnostic. In other situations, the history and neurological signs suggest the diagnosis. The sensory signs that point to the level in a spastic paraparesis with cord compression are an example.

Figure 4.10 summarises principal patterns of sensory loss.

## Peripheral Nerve Lesions

A lesion of an individual nerve produces symptoms and signs within its distribution. Demarcation is clear-cut. Areas of sensory loss are discussed in Chapter 10. The quality of sensory disturbance varies between numbness, tingling and painful pins and needles. Painful tingling in the distribution of a damaged nerve when it is percussed, is known as a positive Tinel's sign, for example in some carpal tunnel cases.

Neuralgia (Chapter 23) describes severe pain in the distribution of a nerve or root. In trigeminal neuralgia (*tic douloureux*; Chapter 13), the paroxysmal nature of pain, and its distribution are diagnostic.

Causalgia (Complex Regional Pain Syndrome, Chapter 23) describes chronic pain after nerve section or crush injury, sometimes following amputation. *Anaesthesia dolorosa* is pain in an anaesthetic area.

## Polyneuropathy

Symmetrical, four limb, distal tingling, numbness or deadness are typical of polyneuropathy (Chapter 10).

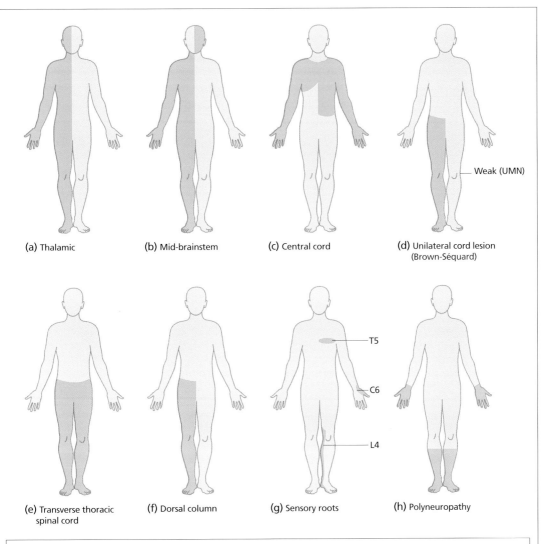

(a) Thalamic      (b) Mid-brainstem      (c) Central cord      (d) Unilateral cord lesion (Brown-Séquard)

(e) Transverse thoracic spinal cord      (f) Dorsal column      (g) Sensory roots      (h) Polyneuropathy

(a) Thalamic lesion: sensory loss throughout opposite side (rare).

(b) Brainstem lesion (rare): contralateral sensory loss below face and ipsilateral loss on face.

(c) Central cord lesion (e.g. syrinx): 'suspended' areas of loss, often asymmetrical and 'dissociated' (i.e. pain and temperature loss but light touch remaining intact).

(d) 'Hemisection' of cord or unilateral cord lesion = Brown-Séquard syndrome: contralateral spinothalamic (pain and temperature) loss with ipsilateral weakness and dorsal column loss below lesion.

(e) Transverse cord lesion: loss of all modalities below lesion.

(f) Isolated dorsal column lesion (e.g. demyelination): loss of proprioception, vibration and light touch.

(g) Individual sensory root lesions (e.g. C6, cervical root compression; T5, shingles; L4, lumbar root compression).

(h) Polyneuropathy: distal sensory loss.

**Figure 4.10** Principal patterns of sensory loss.

### Sensory Root and Root Entry Zone

Spinal and Vth nerve dermatomes are shown in Figure 4.11. There is sometimes overlap between adjacent dermatomes. Root pain is typically perceived both within the dermatome and within the myotome but tends to be less demarcated than pain with a single nerve lesion. For example, with an S1 root lesion from a lumbosacral disc, the sensory disturbance is down the back of the leg, without clear dermatome demarcation. Stretching the root by straight leg raising typically makes matters worse.

When a root entry zone is affected, within the cord, such as in *tabes dorsalis*, intense stabbing pains involve one or more spots, typically on the ankle, calf, thigh or abdomen – the lightning pains of *tabes*, seldom seen today.

Neuralgia, persistent burning root pain can follow shingles (post-herpetic neuralgia, Chapter 23).

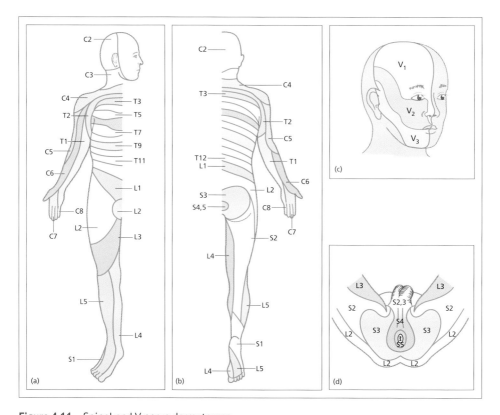

**Figure 4.11**  Spinal and V nerve dermatomes.

### Cord Lesions: Sensory Changes

#### Posterior Columns
Patients describe:

- Band-like sensations, around trunk or limbs
- Limb clumsiness, deadness

- Numbness and burning
- Electric shock-like sensations.

Joint position sense, vibration, light touch and two-point discrimination become diminished below the lesion. Stamping gait and pseudochorea of the outstretched hands are products of failing position sense.

Lhermitte's sign is a sudden electrical sensation down the back, into the limbs produced by bending the head forward. Lhermitte's suggests posterior column damage or occasionally caudal medulla. Lhermitte's is seen in:

- MS, typically in exacerbations
- Cervical myelopathy, radiation myelopathy, trauma
- Subacute combined degeneration of the cord
- Occasionally: Behçet's, Chiari malformations.

**Spinothalamic Tracts**

A lesion within these tracts produces changes in pain and temperature sensation below its level. With progressive compression from outside the cord, such as by an enlarging thoracic meningioma (extramedullary cord compression), the sensory level will tend to commence in the feet and rise to the level of the tumour – because of lamination of spinothalamic fibres in the cord. The patient may notice they cannot gauge water temperature with a foot. Extramedullary cord compression tends to affect both principal cord sensory pathways – both posterior column and spinothalamic.

When a lesion is within the cord (intramedullary) such as a syrinx (Chapter 16) sensory loss can initially be confined entirely to the spinothalamic pathways. The sensory loss is described as dissociated. Suspended sensory loss describes another aspect also seen with a syrinx: the dissociated sensory loss does not extend to the lower limbs – it is thus hanging, on the thorax or abdomen.

Sacral sparing is the phrase used to capture preserved sacral and perineal sensation when a central cord lesion expands centrifugally, damaging first centrally placed fibres and reaching last the spinothalamic sacral fibres on the periphery of the cord.

As a cavity develops within one side of the cord, dissociated sensory loss on one side occurs with pyramidal signs such as a spastic lower limb on the other. This carries the eponym Brown-Séquard, from a treatise in 1849 on traumatic hemisection of cord. Brown-Séquard findings mean spinothalamic signs on one side with pyramidal and dorsal column signs on the other. They point to a cord lesion, on the same side as the pyramidal and dorsal column loss. The patient may report: 'I cannot feel the bathwater with my left foot, but it is my right that drags'.

**Brainstem Lesions and Sensation**

Various patterns are seen: trigeminal sensory loss (Chapters 2 and 13), dissociated (spinothalamic) sensory loss in the limbs, and/or lower limb numbness. The site of a lesion is usually determined more from signs from cranial nerve nuclear damage than by the sensory loss.

### Thalamic Lesions

Destructive lesions of the complex thalamic nuclei are relatively unusual causes of sensory symptoms. When the ventral posterior lateral (VPL) and ventral posterior medial (VPM) thalamic nuclei (Chapters 2 and 5) are damaged, such as following a thrombo-embolic stroke, contralateral hemi-anaesthesia follows immediately. Sometimes, however, during the weeks or months following the stroke, highly unpleasant disabling persistent pain (post-stroke central pain, a.k.a. thalamic pain, Chapter 23) develops in partially anaesthetic limbs. Pain is usually permanent.

## Mononeuropathy, Polyneuropathy

See Chapters 10, 13, and 16.

Common mononeuropathies are easy to recognise once seen, such as ulnar, median, radial, common peroneal (lateral popliteal), lateral cutaneous nerve of the thigh and sural nerve lesions. Cranial nerves are discussed in Chapter 13.

Multiple mononeuropathy means two or more peripheral nerve lesions. Principal causes are leprosy, diabetes, hereditary neuropathy with liability to pressure palsies (HNPP), and vasculitis such as polyarteritis.

Polyneuropathy a.k.a. peripheral neuropathy describes conditions in which nerves die back, usually symmetrically to cause peripheral (hands and feet) sensory loss, muscle weakness and wasting with loss of tendon reflexes.

### Neurogenic Muscle Wasting

The crux is to distinguish between:

- Generalised thinning, normal in old age and seen in cachexia – power is normal
- Widespread wasting seen in MND, polyneuropathy
- Focal wasting with denervation.

Seek out sites of predilection:

- Small hand muscles (T1)
- Guttering of forearm flexors
- Wasted anterior tibial compartment – lateral to the leading edge of the tibia
- Wasted extensor digitorum brevis muscles – small oyster-like muscles below each lateral malleolus.

Muscles with normal bulk, consistency and power are usually normal electrophysiologically and histologically.

### Root Lesions

Characteristics are:

- Root pain
- Wasting and muscle weakness

- Sensory loss, and
- Loss/depression of deep tendon reflex(es).

A root lesion is often called radiculopathy when this is part of an inflammatory, vascular or neoplastic process with derivatives such as polyradiculomyelopathy. I prefer the shorter English word root. A cervical or lumbar root lesion usually implies compression, often from a disc. Movements, root values, muscles and nerves are summarised in Table 4.4.

**Table 4.4** Movement, root value, muscle & nerve.

| Movement | Root | Muscle | Nerve |
|---|---|---|---|
| Shoulder abduction | C5, (C6) | Deltoid (also supraspinatus) | Axillary |
| Elbow flexion (supinated) | (C5), C6 | Biceps | Musculocutaneous |
| Elbow flexion (mid-prone) | C5, (C6) | Brachioradialis | Radial |
| Wrist extension | (C6), C7, (C8) | Triceps | Radial |
| Tip of thumb & index finger flexion | C7, C8 | Flexor pollicis and digitorum profundus I, II | Median |
| Tip of ring & Vth finger flexion | C8 | Flexor digitorum profundus IV, V | Ulnar |
| Thumb abduction | T1 | Abductor pollicis brevis | Median |
| Finger abduction | T1 | Dorsal interossei | Ulnar |
| Finger flexion | (C7), C8, (T1) | Long and short flexors | Median and ulnar |
| Hip flexion | L1, L2, (L3) | Iliopsoas | Nerve to iliopsoas |
| Hip adduction | L2, L3, L4 | Adductor magnus | Obturator |
| Knee extension | L3, L4 | Quadriceps femoris | Femoral |
| Ankle dorsiflexion | L4, L5 | Tibialis anterior | Deep peroneal |
| Big toe extension | L5, (S1) | Extensor hallucis longus | Deep peroneal |
| Ankle eversion | L5, S1 | Peroneal muscles | Superficial peroneal |
| Ankle inversion | L4, L5 | Tibialis posterior | Tibial |
| Ankle plantar flexion | S1, S2 | Gastrocnemius, soleus | Posterior tibial |
| Knee flexion | S1, (S2) | Hamstrings | Sciatic |
| Hip extension | S1, (S2) | Gluteus maximus | Inferior gluteal |

Root pain caused by distortion or stretching of meninges surrounding a root is perceived both in the myotome and the dermatome. This is relevant in C7 root compression: pain can be felt deep to the scapula (C7 muscles) while the sensory disturbance runs to the middle finger (C7 dermatome). The triceps jerk is lost. See Chapters 10 and 16.

### Cauda Equina Syndrome

The *cauda equina* (horse's tail) is the leash of roots emanating from the lower end of the cord. *Cauda equina* compression (e.g. central L4/L5 disc) affects all lumbo-sacral roots streaming caudally. There is loss of bladder and bowel control, buttock and thigh (saddle) numbness with weakness of ankle dorsiflexion (L4), toes (L4, L5), eversion and plantar flexion (S1). S1 reflexes are lost (ankle jerks). A central disc can progress rapidly over hours, or less, sometimes with little back pain – a neurosurgical emergency.

A lesion of the *conus medullaris*, the lowermost cord, such as an MS plaque can cause difficulty. Weakness, sensory loss and loss of sphincter control also occur, and with an acute conus lesion tendon reflexes can also be lost, as with the *cauda equina*. Extensor plantars and sensory loss typical of a cord lesion, such as a sensory level or Brown-Séquard signs should enable distinction clinically, before imaging.

### Myopathy

Muscle disease tends to produce symmetrical abnormalities (Chapter 10).

Inflammatory disease, such as polymyositis, causes induration, pain and weakness. Dystrophies and most metabolic muscle diseases present typically with weakness alone; pseudohypertrophy (excessively bulky muscles) may develop. Slow relaxation is a feature of myotonic conditions. Fatiguability is characteristic of myasthenia gravis, and the reverse, an increase in power on exercise is sometimes seen in LEMS.

### Subacute Paralysis

This describes increasing limb weakness, up to an arbitrary 3 weeks. Cord compression, poliomyelitis, Guillain–Barré, other neuropathies, MS, myasthenia, LEMS, botulism are potential causes (Chapters 9, 10, and 11). Respiratory impairment is easy to miss with limb weakness. Initial paralytic symptoms are regarded as non-organic in about one-quarter when patients first seek help.

## Abnormal Illness Behaviour and Somatic Symptom Disorder

Symptoms that are unexplained or only partially explained by organic disease are common. Deliberate exaggeration and even fabrication were thought to be more frequent than current views suggest, perhaps now erring towards political correctness. The reality is that many have symptoms that are worrying or uncomfortable but do not reflect any serious disease – for example, unexplained fatigue, give-way weakness and non-organic sensory loss, or 'attacks'. The problem is serious: about one-third of apparent status epilepticus and a fifth of recurrent attacks referred to epilepsy clinics are non-organic (see also Chapter 22).

One approach is to accept that the majority do have the symptoms of which they complain. This comment excludes those involved in legal claims, where non-organic features are especially prominent and of a more doubtful nature. The second suggestion is to exclude organic disease with all reasonable certainty. A third is to understand the psychiatric diagnoses, such as depression that might explain such symptoms. Abnormal illness behaviour or somatoform disorder (now known as Somatic Symptom Disorder in DSM-5) are other potential explanations. However, in many cases of apparent illness behaviour, no formal psychiatric diagnosis is apparent.

Factitious disorder – to gain medical attention – and malingering – for material gain – are also possible, if rare explanations.

## Acknowledgements

I am most grateful to Matthew Adams, Robin Howard, Martin Rossor, Simon Shorvon & Jason Warren for their help with our chapter in *Neurology A Queen Square Textbook* Second Edition, upon which this text is based.

The late Dr Anthony Hopkins (1937–1997) my consultant colleague at St Bartholomew's Hospital in the 1980s and 1990s provided me with inspiration – and also talked much common sense.

## References

Clarke C. Neurological diseases. In *Clinical Medicine*, 6th edn. Kumar PJ, Clark M, eds. Elsevier, 2005.
Hopkins AP. *Clinical Neurology: A Modern Approach*. Oxford Medical Publications, 1993.

## Further Reading

Clarke C, Adams M, Howard R, Rossor M, Shorvon S, Warren J. The language of neurology, symptoms, signs and basic investigations. In *Neurology A Queen Square Textbook*, 2nd edn. Clarke C, Howard R, Rossor M, Shorvon S, eds. John Wiley & Sons, 2016. There are useful references.

Also, please visit https://www.drcharlesclarke.com for free updated notes, potential links and references as these become available. You will be asked to log in, in a secure fashion, with your name and institution.

# 5

# Cognition, Cortical Function and Dementias

This chapter is an introduction to cognition, the cortex and its disorders followed by dementia investigations and the syndromes themselves.

## Cognitive Functions and Clinical Practice

Cognition, like other aspects of brain function has topographical organisation, but unlike the sensory and motor systems, one needs to know less about precise anatomy, that varies between individuals.

In other words, whilst a neurologist needs to know the course of the pyramidal tracts, or a peripheral nerve – what I call 'the wiring' – anatomical knowledge of precise aspects of cortical function is of less clinical value. Similarly, obsession with exact localisation of brain lesions, beloved before the era of imaging, has dwindled.

However, specific profiles are helpful, exemplified by the different forms of dysphasia/aphasia in left hemisphere strokes, the spatial neglect that follows non-dominant hemisphere insults and the profound amnesia of Wernicke–Korsakoff syndrome.

I outline some of the terminology – the language to describe various deficits – in essence my clinical overview. I appreciate that there are different approaches.

## Attention and Neglect

Attention is the overall ability to direct and gate awareness, to select and focus upon incoming data. First, one needs to be awake, and aware.

- Awareness is maintained by the ascending reticular activating system.
- Frontal and networks such as vision enable us to focus on particular types of stimuli.
- When awareness is depressed, for organic or psychological reasons, cortical function tends to be impaired.
- Neglect syndromes, that is deficits of selective attention occur with disease in the non-dominant parietal lobe. There is neglect, typically of left space in a right-handed person.

*Neurology: A Clinical Handbook*, First Edition. Charles Clarke.
© 2022 John Wiley & Sons Ltd. Published 2022 by John Wiley & Sons Ltd.

## Memory – Its Subdivisions

Explicit memory means something that can be consciously accessed – one recalls an event by thinking about it. Implicit memory is accessed automatically, for example skills when driving a car – we do not think about them, we simply execute them.

Explicit memory has two components:

- Short-term memory = information that is encoded for immediate retrieval
- Long-term memory is divided into memory for events from past experience, known as episodic memory, and semantic memory, meaning conceptual knowledge.

Episodic memory is divided into:

- retrograde memory – retrieval of events past– prior to an injury or an illness
- anterograde memory – encoding of new events, for subsequent retrieval, and
- memory for different features, such as for words, faces or topography.

Semantic memory covers a vast area – of facts, the meaning of words, and numbers and mathematics. It is distinguished from episodic memory by the absence of a memory of when or how the knowledge was acquired.

## Anatomy

The medial temporal lobes (hippocampal formation, parahippocampal gyrus and entorhinal cortex) are critical for episodic memory. The diencephalic system, meaning the thalamus and its limbic connections including the fornix and mamillary bodies, and the basal forebrain also have important roles. For example, Wernicke–Korsakoff cases typically have petechial haemorrhages and degeneration in the mammillary bodies and medial dorsal thalamic nuclei. Posterior cortical areas including the posterior cingulate, retro-splenial and temporo-parietal association cortex are intimately connected, via the diencephalic system, with the medial temporal lobes.

Short-term memory has separate systems for temporary storage of verbal, visuospatial and auditory information.

Verbal short-term memory is supported by the fronto-parietal network, largely in the left hemisphere. Visuospatial short-term memory depends on the right cerebral hemisphere, and auditory memory on the temporal regions.

Information within our memory store may need to undergo cognitive manipulation, rather than just being stored and retrieved. In other words, one has to think about it, or in more neuropsychological terms one uses executive processes, to weigh up what we are doing, for example making sense of an ambiguous message or an unfamiliar route.

This variable interaction, between the executive system and short-term memory stores, constitutes working memory. For example, digit span forwards (131,132,133. . .) relies less on executive processes than backwards, as we then need to interrogate earlier memory of the forward sequence.

One can also think of these storage mechanisms as slave systems, under some control of the fronto-subcortical executive. One corollary is that the executive does not usually allow us to remember unimportant facts.

Neurochemically, ascending cholinergic pathways subserve memory. In many dementias these pathways, which normally exert influences on the medial temporal lobe and neocortex, become disrupted.

## Amnesias

Deficits of verbal, visual and topographical memory become evident early in many dementias. Patients become unable to recall conversations, messages and names, and experience difficulty with route finding – sometimes in locations that were once familiar.

Amnesias are common following a traumatic brain injury (TBI). Post-traumatic amnesia describes the duration after a head injury before continuous memory returns. This duration may be used to grade severity of TBI, though this is of limited value.

Severe deficits of anterograde and retrograde memory with preserved immediate recall were originally described in thiamine deficiency with chronic alcoholism (Wernicke–Korsakoff syndrome, Chapter 19). Patients are marooned in the present with no capacity to lay down new memories, though they may retain some implicit memory. Bilateral temporal lobe resection for epilepsy and herpes simplex encephalitis (Chapter 9) are other causes.

Transient global amnesia (Chapter 6) describes sudden memory loss lasting for a matter of hours, with recovery.

## Paramnesias

Paramnesias are false or distorted recall – seen in acute confusional states or in dementia. When prompted to fill a gap in their everyday record, the patient describes events that did not occur, or accounts of events that could not have occurred (confabulation). Confabulation is seen after frontal lobe and fronto-limbic damage.

Reduplicative paramnesias are beliefs that a place or person has been transposed. A house is believed to be a replica of the real one (topographical paramnesia), or a person has been replaced by an impostor with identical appearance (Capgras delusion, Chapter 22).

## Perception and Its Disorders

Processing involves visual analysis, a structural representation of an object, and ability to perceive its meaning. Visuospatial disorders are common features of many dementias.

The peri-striate cortex (*syn.* visual association cortex), illustrated in Chapter 14 – consists of ventral 'What is that object?' and dorsal 'Where is that object?' regions (or visual processing 'streams').

Progressive visual dysfunction occurs in many dementias and specifically in the rare posterior cortical atrophy. Dysfunction may manifest as a problem with acuity, depth perception (stereopsis), and discrimination of form. Achromatopsia – deficient colour perception – and/or akinetopsia – impairment of motion detection – can follow a posterior circulation stroke.

Misperceptions can also occur: patterns on fabric change, body parts, especially faces can appear distorted (metamorphopsia), persistent or transposed (palinopsia) or multiple (polyopia). Impaired face perception (prosopagnosia) can follow occipito-parietal damage.

Cortical blindness follows bilateral occipital cortex damage, typically vascular. Denial of blindness (visual anosognosia, a.k.a. Anton's syndrome) occurs with lateral occipito-parietal damage.

Apperceptive visual agnosia means inability to perceive the geometry that enables object identity, resulting in a failure to recognise common items or familiar people. Difficulty distinguishing coins, banknotes and playing cards are examples.

Disruption of the dorsal visual processing stream results in visual disorientation: a patient may have difficulty locating a knife and fork, threading a needle, reading text or keeping within traffic lanes while driving. Some cases fail to perform visually guided movements (optic ataxia) and/or to direct the eyes (ocular apraxia) – components of Balint's syndrome (Chapter 14). Ultimately, such cases are regarded as functionally blind.

Other perceptive disorders and their anatomical correlates include:

- Cortical deafness – a rare sequel of bilateral damage of auditory pathways.
- Auditory agnosia – for music and/or environmental noises (either temporal lobe).
- Dysgeusia (taste) – distortion or loss of taste (insular cortex).
- Olfactory identification difficulties – (often early features of Alzheimer's and Parkinson's disease).
- Impaired tactile perception of shape (astereognosis), for example of numbers traced on the skin (tactile agnosia) – deficits that may emerge after parietal lobe damage.

## Hallucinations – False Perceptions

Hallucinations are perceptual experiences without an external sensory stimulus – in other words, people see objects that are not there, hear voices, or believe there is a smell. Pseudo-hallucination is used to indicate that someone has insight into the fact that the object in question is not real.

Visual hallucinations are frequent in delirium. The patient sees people or animals that tend to appear in dim light, transiently or emerge from behind objects.

Hallucinations may be outside the visual fields – a.k.a. extra-campine hallucinations (simply from Latin – outside the field). The Third Man delusion describes the presence of another person, well-recognised in extreme isolation, for example single-handed at sea.

Other hallucinations include:

- olfactory hallucinations, for example a sudden odd smell – temporal lobe epilepsy
- auditory hallucinations, such as direct orders from God are typical of schizophrenia – and unusual in neurological diseases.
- musical hallucinations can occur in acquired deafness.

Hallucinations arise from various mechanisms, often hard to define:

- Abnormal excitation or disinhibition of sensory cortex by irritative processes, such as seizures, migraine or drugs.

- Loss of sensory input, that causes abnormal release of sensory cortex. For example peripheral visual loss, with deafferentation of visual cortex can produce visual hallucinations, in the absence of a cognitive problem (Charles Bonnet syndrome Chapter 14).

Hallucinations may also occur after midbrain damage, a.k.a. peduncular hallucinations – dream-like or cartoon-like images, a result of reticular activating system dysfunction.

Visual cortex dysfunction tends to produce elementary hallucinations, such as fortification spectra – like battlements, sometimes shimmering – in migraine. More complex hallucinations, with distortions of self-perception, such the Alice in Wonderland syndrome, can also occur in migraine, but more typically follow psychoactive drug use or temporal lobe disease.

Visual hallucinations also follow dysfunction of neurotransmitter pathways such as in dementia with Lewy bodies, with acetylcholine deficiency.

## Voluntary Action Failure: Apraxias

Failure in cognitive control/guidance of voluntary actions produces apraxia – a disturbance of movement that cannot be explained by motor or sensory deficits.

Apraxia classification is hard to remember because of its terminology. Ideomotor apraxia refers to an inability to produce unfamiliar, novel or meaningless actions, whilst ideational apraxia affects previously learned actions.

Ideomotor apraxia is a prominent feature of Alzheimer's – difficulty imitating hand positions or assembling a simple puzzle.

Ideational apraxia is exemplified by being unable to use common utensils, or attempts to use them inappropriately, such as by trying to write with scissors. When asked to wave goodbye or salute (symbolic gestures) or imitate using a screwdriver, an awkward or partial approximation is produced, and there is failure to recognise gestures, such as blowing a kiss.

Constructional apraxia is an impaired ability to copy drawings or designs. This occurs with parietal lesions and in degenerative diseases.

Dressing apraxia describes becoming muddled when dressing – a form of visuospatial disorientation, seen after a right hemisphere lesion, and in dementias.

Gait apraxia is difficulty initiating walking – a disordered or shuffling gait. When seated patients can show that they understand the movement of walking, or even running, by moving their legs appropriately. The problem occurs with frontal lobe lesions, hydrocephalus and dementias. Some gait apraxia is common in old age and contributes to falls.

Purists consider constructional, dressing and gait disorders not to be true apraxias, but the terms describe common problems.

Three other apraxias:

- Orofacial (or orobuccal) apraxia is exemplified by loss of ability to whistle and difficulty initiating chewing or swallowing. When asked to cough or yawn the response may be incomplete or exaggerated, but can remain normal when performed spontaneously.
- Apraxia of speech is recognised by difficulty forming words and their syllabic building blocks, while retaining knowledge of all spoken and written language.

- Asymmetrical limb apraxia a.k.a. limb-kinetic apraxia causes rigidity with cortical sensory signs. Actions are coarse or uncoordinated and movements incomplete. Patients cannot make movements using both hands, such as clapping – the more affected hand mirroring the other (alien limb phenomenon). Forced grasping for objects or purposeless actions such as repeatedly removing and replacing spectacles, may occur. This occurs characteristically in cortico-basal degeneration (Chapter 7).

The neuroanatomy of apraxia is vague. Sites of importance are:

- dominant temporal lobe: conceptual knowledge of gestures
- frontal and sub-frontal regions: control of gait and gestures
- dominant parietal lobe: organisation of actions.

## Speech and Language

Many find the classification of speech disorders difficult. Language competency depends on a discrete set of abilities:

- sensory decoding of the spoken message
- appreciation of meaning
- the capacity for repetition
- production of correctly articulated and correct speech.

The words dysphasia and aphasia often used interchangeably – speech and language impairments, most frequently follow focal lesions of the dominant (left) cerebral cortex. As imaging has progressed, precise localisation of specific functions has been found to vary between individuals. Study of aphasias in dementias also casts doubt on the value of pinpointing the focal lesion. For a historical perspective, Ludwig Lichtheim (Breslau, nineteenth century) and others postulated:

- a cortical centre for word concepts
- a posterior centre for interpreting word sounds and
- an anterior centre for speech output.

Before classifying aphasias further, it is useful to appreciate the differences between 'anterior' and 'posterior' aphasia – by listening to and seeing patients (see video references).

- The more common anterior aphasia, a.k.a. Broca's aphasia (Paul Broca, Paris nineteenth century) is an expressive, or motor aphasia, seen frequently following a left hemisphere stroke, with inferior frontal gyrus damage. This is speech production failure: output is any combination of sparse, effortful and agrammatic (disjointed and telegraphic) speech. Comprehension is relatively preserved. Patients who recover say that they knew what they wanted to say but could not produce the words.
- Posterior aphasia, a.k.a. Wernicke (Carl Wernicke, Germany nineteenth century): receptive, posterior or sensory aphasia may also follow a left hemisphere stroke – in the posterior temporal region. This is speech output regulation failure. Speech is fluent, often

excessively. At its worst there is a profuse outpouring of unintelligible jargon (word-like sounds without meaning). Patients who recover say that they found speech, both their own and of others like a foreign language, which they could not stop themselves from speaking. Wernicke's is sometimes mistaken for psychiatric illness.

There are also specific types of receptive aphasia:

- Word deafness: difficulty understanding and repeating spoken words despite normal comprehension of written material.
- Transcortical sensory aphasia: impaired comprehension of single spoken words with a preserved ability to repeat them.
- Conduction aphasia: selective impairment of speech repetition.

Specific expressive aphasias include:

- Nominal aphasia, a.k.a. anomic aphasia, impaired word retrieval – pauses in conversation to retrieve a word, and inability to name objects – seen in many conditions.
- Dysprosody, that is the pattern of stress and timing – the melody of speech.

Damage to the basal ganglia, thalamus and subcortical pathways can also produce aphasias. Breakdown in speech production occurs in many dementias, such as motor neurone disease with dementia. This can progress to cortical anarthria – no speech at all.

## Reading, Writing and Numeracy

Premorbid attainments are heavily influenced by education and by limitations such as developmental dyslexia or dyscalculia.

### Reading

Alexia (difficulty reading) and agraphia (difficulty writing) were originally described following strokes in the posterior cerebral hemispheres.

Acquired dyslexia can be classified into:

- Peripheral dyslexia: disturbed visual analysis of written words produces peripheral dyslexia, sometimes with preserved writing ability. Visuo-perceptual and visuospatial impairments are common. Patients tend to read letter by letter.
- Central dyslexia: these fall into two categories:
  - Phonological dyslexia results from an inability to translate combinations of letters into sounds. Such patients have difficulty reading 'non-words' (such as 'plaz').
  - Deep dyslexia: a patient may look at a word, such as black and producing a related word such as dark.
  - Surface dyslexia is a tendency to regularise pronunciation of vowel combinations. The word 'soot' is seen to rhyme with 'root' rather than 'foot'. Such dyslexia occurs typically with English, and not in languages with regular spelling systems, such as Italian and Spanish.

## Writing

Agraphia *syn.* dysgraphia, impairments of writing and spelling are divided (in theory) into:

- Central dysgraphias: here the core defect lies in knowledge of spelling.
- Peripheral dysgraphias: here the problem is with motor programming and execution of writing.

Mixed forms are common. Dysgraphia is generally a feature of left parietal lobe disease. Peripheral dysgraphia is seen in dementias and in left temporal lobe atrophy.

## Numeracy

Dyscalculia depends on either a core defect of computation, or difficulty processing numbers – hard to distinguish. There is difficulty handling change, and day-to-day accounts. There may be specific difficulties – calculating scores in games, reading and writing numbers. Like dysgraphia, dyscalculia is typically a feature of dominant parietal lobe disease.

Gerstmann's syndrome – a rarity – is dysgraphia and dyscalculia with finger agnosia and right–left disorientation resulting from an angular gyrus lesion in the dominant hemisphere.

# Knowledge and the Cognitive Executive

Knowledge storage and retrieval depends not only on semantic memory – both temporal lobes – but also on executive function, that allow us to choose and reflect on information, and often regarded as one of the core aspects of intellect.

The cognitive executive describes this ability to control behaviour, to coordinate operations, in order to adapt and direct them towards relevant goals. Like the executive system, these functions depend chiefly on the frontal cortex and subcortical connections. Failure of this complex system of control attracts various labels, including 'executive dysfunction' and the '(frontal) dysexecutive syndrome'.

Examples of problems arising from a diminished capacity to modulate cognitive inputs according to context are:

- Difficulty in assessing feedback from or consequences of behaviour, resulting in personality changes of which patients are usually unaware. They may develop poor social judgement, lack of empathy, impulsivity or reduced expressivity. Impulsivity, inappropriate behaviour – sometimes of a sexual nature. Insensitive remarks are common and profoundly damaging to interpersonal relationships. Patients fail to reflect not only on their own beliefs, desires, intentions and perspectives, but also those of others (the 'Theory of Mind' deficit).
- Reduced capacity for abstract thought, and an inflexible approach to daily tasks. Obsessions, rituals, clock-watching and hoarding develop. Analogies pass unrecognised and proverbs interpreted literally.
- Reduced ability to search for answers to simple questions and verbal fluency tests, such as generating words beginning with a given letter, or belonging to a category.

- An emergence of novel interests, such as religious, philosophical or artistic pursuits, on a background of little previous interest.
- Failure to generate activity, apathy (abulia), including for personal hygiene, leading to reliance on others.
- Slowness of thought (bradyphrenia), passivity, and perseveration: patients spend all day watching TV or absorbed in jigsaws, and disengage reluctantly.
- Utilisation behaviour, such as donning glasses or peeling an orange when placed before them; hyper-orality, and mimicry of others' speech (echolalia) or actions (echopraxia) are related phenomena.

Executive difficulties are exposed by tasks that demand planning, abstract thought, and consideration of alternatives. There may be inconsistency between performance on different tests and between testing sessions.

The precise frontal neuroanatomy remains vague.

- Disinhibition, sociopathic behaviour and altered drives correlate with mainly right anterior temporal and inferior frontal lobe (ventro-medial, orbito-frontal) damage.
- Abulia occurs with dorsolateral frontal and anterior cingulate damage.

### Emotion

Disturbances of emotion and expression are integral to medicine, and have a neurochemical and thus organic substrate, even if this is hard to define. There remains a tendency to label problems as 'psychological', as if they do not have a physical cause, implying they were less real than organically based disabilities.

Disturbance of mood, in particular depression, is common. Since neurologists tend to seek neuro-anatomical explanations, such affective changes are caused at least in part, by damage to limbic circuits (Chapter 22) and their cortical projections. For example, the right amygdala and orbito-frontal cortex are implicated in normal emotion processing.

## Dementias

With ageing populations, degenerative neurological diseases and especially dementia have become common in many societies.

Definitions of dementia vary but a key feature is that the disorder of cerebral function must involve more than one cortical domain and produce loss of independence in normal daily activities. In practical terms any substantial cortical problem should be investigated. This section addresses basic investigations, followed by the descriptive neurology of the main forms of dementia.

### Investigation of dementia

In most established cases of dementia the diagnosis will be evident. The role of investigation is therefore largely confirmatory, though it may uncover rare, unexpected and, occasionally treatable causes.

Basic principles include:

- Exclusion of delirium
- Exclusion of a genetic or reversible metabolic cause
- Routine tests – bloods (thyroid, calcium), CXR, ECG
- Basic cognition (MMSE, Addenbrooke's, Queen Square Cognitive Tests)
- Brain imaging (MR/CT)
- Neuropsychometry
- EEG, CSF, specialised tests, consideration of brain biopsy

I deal here with the typical investigations carried out in a district general hospital, and mention first three common pitfalls, from clinical experience:

- Routine bloods – it is easy to miss, for example, hypothyroidism unless this is requested and results scrutinised.
- Unless quantitative psychometric testing is carried there will be no baseline for the future. One sees cases occasionally diagnosed as dementia simply because they appear to be demented.
- Brain imaging: review this personally. Regional and global cerebral atrophy may not have been fully assessed.

**Brain Imaging**

MR brain imaging is the test of choice, although CT may be the only practical proposition. FDG-PET can reveal regional dysfunction in a radiologically normal brain. Radiolabelled specific ligands may become useful but are not yet in routine use. For study of the many imaging changes in dementias, websites are of value, such as:

htpps://radiopaedia.org

**Electroencephalography**

EEG is usually unhelpful – typically normal initially in Alzheimer's, though as disease progresses alpha rhythm degenerates. EEG tends to remain normal in FTD. In CJD periodic complexes may develop.

**CSF Examination**

Alzheimer's is associated with a reduction in CSF Aβ 1–42 and an increase in tau and/or phospho-tau, but CSF protein biomarkers specific for other dementia pathologies have not entered routine practice. Elevated protein 14-3-3 is associated with rapid neuronal destruction in classic CJD, but it is not diagnostic.

**Additional Investigations**

In exceptional cases, brain biopsy may be carried out – when there is unresolved suspicion of a treatable process, such as vasculitis.

Biopsy of other organs has an occasional role. Skin biopsy may detect Lafora, Kufs or other rare rarities, and cerebral AD arteriopathy with subcortical infarcts and leuco-encephalopathy (CADASIL). Nerve biopsy may help in rare dementias such as amyloidosis.

Muscle biopsy including histochemistry and respiratory enzyme analysis – mitochondrial disease. Bone marrow examination can identify sea-blue histiocytes in Niemann–Pick disease type C and may help in paraneoplastic syndromes. Small bowel biopsy may reveal Whipple's disease.

## Alzheimer's Disease

Alzheimer's is the most common cause of cognitive decline, responsible for more than 60% of all dementias.

The prevalence of Alzheimer's is age-dependent – more than doubling every 5 years over 60. At 65–69 around 1% suffer from Alzheimer's, rising to about 20% at 85 and over. There are over 750 000 people with this dementia in the UK.

Alzheimer's is also the most common cause of young (under 65) onset dementia. Alzheimer's before the age of 50 is rare and raises the possibility of a genetic cause.

### Neuropathology

Diagnostic features are extracellular amyloid plaques and intracellular neurofibrillary tangles, with heaviest deposition of plaques in the cortical association areas. Amyloid may also be seen in cerebral blood vessels – a.k.a. amyloid angiopathy.

The building block of each plaque is beta-amyloid (Aβ), a peptide of 40–42 amino-acids, formed from cleavage (by γ-secretase) of amyloid precursor protein (APP). APP is encoded by the *APP* gene, while γ-secretase activity depends on presenilins 1 and 2 (encoded by *PSEN1* and *PSEN2*, respectively).

Neurofibrillary tangles are breakdown products of neuronal microtubules. Tau, the protein that stabilises microtubule assembly, becomes hyperphosphorylated in Alzheimer's and aggregates into a tangle of paired helical filaments within neurones. Tangles appear in the entorhinal cortex, progress to involve the hippocampus and limbic structures and then become widely distributed (Figure 5.1).

### Genetics

The majority of cases of Alzheimer's are sporadic – of cause unknown and unpredictable. However, in less than 1% of cases there is a family history, with an early age of onset. Mutations in three genes (*PSEN1*, *APP*, and *PSEN2*) cause Alzheimer's.

A first degree relative of a patient with sporadic Alzheimer's carries a slightly increased risk. This is largely due to the risk-modifying effect of carrying the ε4 (rather than the ε2 or ε3) allele of the apolipoprotein E gene (*ApoE*), though other genes have been discovered.

These have contributed to Alzheimer's pathogenesis, particularly the amyloid cascade – outside the scope of this chapter.

Current guidelines do not recommend testing for *ApoE* or other mutations in a patient with possible Alzheimer's, or in their relatives.

## Clinical Features

The most common complaint, often from a spouse or friend, is of problems with episodic memory. Patients become repetitive, forgetting that they asked a question or said something.

Amyloid β

Tau

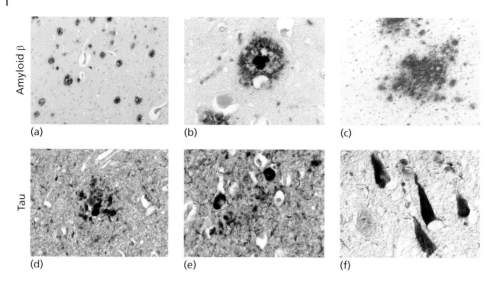

(a)    (b)    (c)

(d)    (e)    (f)

**Figure 5.1** Alzheimer's disease autopsy: abundant amyloid plaques in neocortex (a). Neuritic plaques with a dense core and peripheral halo (b). Diffuse plaques - large protein deposits (c). Neurites - with abnormal tau (d). Multiple intraneuronal inclusions, neurofibrillary tangles - either small globose, perikaryal (e), or band/flame shaped (f).

Messages are forgotten, items misplaced and route-finding becomes challenging. Forgetfulness may be suggested by loss of recollection for context, such as a family visit being recalled but not how long ago or who was there. Such lapses may occur during normal ageing and/or with anxiety, but what singles out Alzheimer's are their severity, frequency and progression.

Atypical presentations also occur, including predominant or even isolated visuospatial deficits (posterior cortical atrophy, PCA), dyspraxia or aphasia (primary progressive aphasia, PPA). Frontal (dysexecutive) Alzheimer's is rare.

Alzheimer's patients become less confident, apathetic and less spontaneous. Depression commonly coexists with Alzheimer's but can also mimic it – and vice versa. Cognitive problems are frequently attributed to depression.

Whilst these symptoms reflect impairment of episodic memory, deficits in other cortical domains also emerge as the pathology progresses beyond the temporal lobes. Cortical deficits caused by Alzheimer's tend to become generalised, with an emphasis on posteriorly represented (visual, spatial, numerical and praxic) functions, though subtle early impairments of language and executive function may be present.

Problems with driving may be noticed, and accidents follow due to visuospatial difficulties, misjudgments or slowed reactions.

The early stages of Alzheimer's are not typically associated with marked behavioural and personality change. A well-preserved social façade is common. However, as Alzheimer's progresses, behavioural problems develop – agitation, delusions and occasionally aggression.

Myoclonus may occur later in the disease, especially in the fingers, and a generalised increase in tone (*Gegenhalten*). Motor function is typically preserved, to the extent that whilst an Alzheimer's patient cannot look after themselves, they can wander far away.

Marked sleep–wake cycle reversal sometimes develops. Seizures occur in less than 5%, late, as do incontinence and dysphagia.

Survival is typically 4–8 years from diagnosis – but extends to about 15 years in a minority. Pneumonia is a common cause of death.

## Imaging

MR brain imaging may be normal at first, but often shows marked and disproportionate medial temporal lobe atrophy initially stages. Generalised atrophy follows and ventricular enlargement (Figure 5.2).

## Therapy

A stark reminder from a major dementia research unit emphasises that 'there is no evidence that current treatments alter the underlying disease progression'. Drug therapy is summarised here. The overall management of dementia is dealt with later.

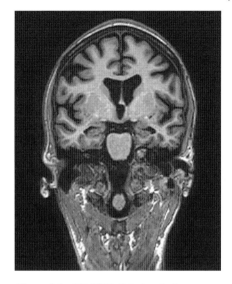

**Figure 5.2**   MR T1W: Alzheimer's disease – widespread cerebral atrophy. *Source*: Professor Peter Garrard.

### *Cholinesterase Inhibitors in Alzheimer's*

The rationale is that by inhibiting breakdown of acetyl choline there is enhancement of cortical acetyl choline levels.

Three drugs are licensed:

- donepezil (Aricept)
- galantamine (Reminyl)
- rivastigmine (Exelon)

A modest temporary benefit follows in mild Alzheimer's. NICE recommends that these drugs should be used in mild-to-moderate disease, but should be stopped when benefit is no longer evident. Peripheral cholinergic side effects, are common but usually transient. Cholinesterase inhibitors may have detrimental effects on mood, sleep and behaviour in later stages.

Memantine (Ebixa and others) is an MNDA receptor agonist that blocks effects of elevated levels of glutamate by preventing calcium influx into neurones. Its cognitive enhancing effect is modest. It is sometimes used when cholinesterase inhibitors are thought to have lost their effects.

## Frontotemporal Dementia

In the nineteenth century a progressive aphasia with focal temporal atrophy (Figure 5.3) was described by Arnold Pick (Prague). The term Pick's disease survives, but frontotemporal dementia (FTD) is now more commonly used. Though classifications vary, there are two main FTD phenotypes:

- Behavioural Variant (bvFTP)
- Primary Progressive Aphasia (PPA) – divided into semantic dementia (SD), progressive non-fluent aphasia (PNFA) and logopenic aphasia (LPA).

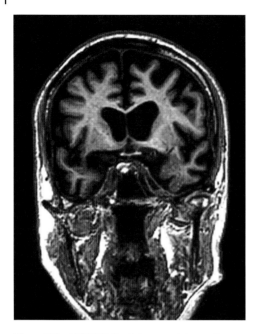

**Figure 5.3** MR T1W: frontotemporal dementia – asymmetry is typical. *Source*: Professor Peter Garrard.

All are less familiar to a general neurologist than Alzheimer's.

The bvFTD presents with personality and behavioural change, that may cause disinhibition, obsessionality and loss of interest or empathy. Patients appear to have forgotten the rules of social engagement. Anger, impulsivity, and disorderly behaviour ensue, in the presence of preserved memory – distinct from Alzheimer's. Imaging may be normal initially but usually reflects focal, often asymmetric, frontal and temporal atrophy. Distinction between FTD and psychiatric illness can be difficult.

SD presents with word finding difficulty and loss of understanding of the meanings of words. Speech is initially fluent and grammatically correct but notably empty of content. Surface dyslexia is often demonstrable, and behavioural changes similar to bvFTD may be present. Progressive asymmetrical (usually left) anterior–inferior temporal lobe atrophy is almost universal.

PNFA presents with hesitant, effortful, agrammatic or telegraphic speech. Comprehension and insight are typically preserved. Orofacial apraxia is sometimes seen.

Variants and combinations of these syndromes occur, as well as syndromes that overlap with MND and PD.

### Genetics and Prognosis

A family history of dementia is found in about one third of FTD patients. Mutations in the tau (*MAPT*) and progranulin (*GRN*) genes, and hexanucleotide repeat expansions at C9orf72 are the commonest. All FTD syndromes are progressive, though at variable rates, with a life-expectancy of 3–15 years following diagnosis.

### Parkinson's Disease Dementia (PDD) and Dementia with Lewy Bodies (DLB)

These conditions form a clinical continuum, defined by Lewy bodies in the cortex, limbic region and subcortical nuclei.

Some 30% of PD patients eventually develop dementia (PDD), while essential features of DLB are early cognitive decline, often with hallucinations and the later emergence of parkinsonism.

Management presents particular difficulties. Levodopa may make cognitive problems and hallucinations worse, though the response to cholinesterase inhibitors is often more marked than in Alzheimer's. Neuroleptic drugs should be avoided in both because they can cause severe extrapyramidal reactions. New generation agents such as quetiapine or clozapine can be useful.

**Dementia with Other Movement Disorders (Chapter 7)**

Cognitive decline is a feature of what used to be referred to as Parkinson's-plus syndromes. These are characterised by neuronal inclusion bodies of tau protein isoforms with four microtubule binding domains ('four-repeat tauopathies'):

- Progressive supra-nuclear palsy (PSP) is frequently accompanied by slowness of thought, perseverative speech patterns, executive deficits and utilisation behaviours.
- Cortical-basal degeneration (CBD) can cause orofacial and limb apraxia and progressive aphasia.

Huntington's disease has cognitive impairment as a core feature.

Spinocerebellar ataxias can be accompanied by cognitive decline (Chapter 17).

**Vascular Dementia (VaD) – Vascular Cognitive Impairment (VCI)**

Cerebrovascular disease (Chapter 6) causes dementia both in its own right and in association with Alzheimer's. Dementia develops within 1 year in about one third of stroke survivors. Despite both frequency and importance, there is little consensus about VaD. Vascular cognitive impairment (VCI) is used to deal with this vagueness.

Pathology: a varied spectrum – atheroma in large and small arteries, lacunar and larger infarcts, lipohyalinosis of small arteries and arterioles, cavitation of white matter (leuco-araiosis), scattered cortical microinfarcts, foci of old haemorrhage and amyloid angiopathy are seen.

Clinical features: diverse – executive and attentional problems, behavioural changes, particularly abulia and cognitive slowing with or without memory and other focal cortical deficits.

Traditionally, emphasis was placed on stepwise accumulation of deficits and recurrent cortical strokes, a.k.a. multi-infarct dementia, a construct that is unusual in clinical practice.

One VCI imaging presentation, also known as Binswanger's disease, is a patient who presents with indolent cognitive decline but who lacks a history of clinical vascular episodes – and rather obviously this may mimic Alzheimer's. Memory impairment is frequent, with slowness of thought and dysexecutive features. There are however added features – brisk facial and limb reflexes. Gait is wide based, apraxic or a *marche à petits pas* (short stepping). Parkinsonism, urinary incontinence and pseudobulbar palsy develop. Hypertension is common.

**Imaging**

Interpretation of MR brain imaging in VCI is confounded by the occurrence of ischaemic changes in the symptomless population that become more prominent as years go by. In VCI, typically extensive periventricular white matter changes are seen which spare subcortical U-fibres and the corpus callosum.

Other vascular causes of brain damage:

- Anti-phospholipid syndrome: a potential rare cause of ischaemic damage. There is possibly a direct effect of the antibody on neural tissue.
- Sickle-cell disease: multiple focal infarcts can occur and possibly there is an effect of chronic hypoxia.
- Cerebral autosomal dominant arteriopathy with subcortical infarcts and leuco-encephalopathy (CADASIL) – *Notch3* gene (Figure 5.4).

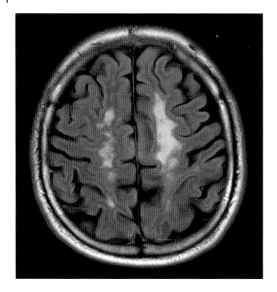

**Figure 5.4** CADASIL. Typical vascular changes (MR T1W). *Source*: Professor Peter Garrard.

### Differential Diagnosis of Probable VCI

The potential for clinical confusion between VCI, Alzheimer's and the four-repeat tauopathies should be evident, but there is also an extensive differential diagnosis for the associated imaging changes, including MS – which can present with pure cognitive decline, PML, HIV, lymphoma, post-irradiation degeneration, hereditary leucodystrophies, repeated trauma, CO poisoning and hypoxia. Most will be recognisable from the clinical context.

## Prion Diseases

Prion diseases (a.k.a. transmissible spongiform encephalopathies) infect both man and animals.

Human diseases are:

Creutzfeld–Jakob disease(CJD), variant CJD (vCJD), Gerstmann–Sträussler–Schinker disease (GSS), familial fatal insomnia (FFI) and Kuru.

All prion diseases are fatal. Prions are transmissible agents. There is accumulation in the brain of an abnormal isoform of the cell surface glycoprotein prion protein (PrP). The isoform, $PrP^{Sc}$, is derived from its normal cellular precursor, $PrP^{C}$. The abnormal isoform is the principal, possibly sole transmissible constituent.

Whilst rare, these conditions are considered here because of their biological interest.

### Aetiology and Classification

Human prion diseases have three distinct aetiologies. They occur sporadically, can be acquired by eating or iatrogenic exposure to prions or via autosomal dominant inheritance – a result of mutations in the prion protein gene (*PRNP*).

The main human prion disease is sporadic CJD. It may arise from somatic mutation of *PRNP* or spontaneous conversion of PrP$^C$ to PrP$^{Sc}$ as a rare random event. There is no evidence of an environmental source.

Prion diseases show phenotypic variability, explained by the existence of distinct prion strains. Four main types are seen in CJD:

- PrP$^{Sc}$ types 1–3 in sporadic and iatrogenic CJD.
- PrP$^{Sc}$ type 4 in all vCJD cases. A similar type 4 PrP$^{Sc}$ is seen in bovine spongiform encephalopathy.

A common *PRNP* polymorphism at codon 129, where either methionine or valine can be encoded (M129V), is a key determinant of susceptibility to acquired and sporadic prion diseases.

### Sporadic Creutzfeldt–Jakob Disease

Sporadic CJD is a rapidly progressive dementia typically with myoclonus. The onset is usually between 45 and 75 years. Progression follows, over weeks, to akinetic mutism and death. Most die within 6 months. Prodromal features include fatigue, insomnia, depression, weight loss, headaches, general malaise and ill-defined pains. Presenting features include pyramidal and extrapyramidal signs, cerebellar ataxia, and cortical blindness (the 'Heidenhain variant' when prominent). About 10% present with ataxia.

Routine blood tests and routine CSF examination are normal. The CSF protein 14-3-3 is usually elevated. However, this is also elevated after cerebral infarction, haemorrhage, encephalitis and in some patients with Alzheimer's.

MRI shows high signal in the striatum and/or cerebral cortex in FLAIR or DW images Cerebral and cerebellar atrophy develops.

EEG can show pseudo-periodic sharp wave activity.

Brain biopsy may be considered occasionally, with strict prion control precautions.

Neuropathology: spongiform change, neuronal loss and astrocytosis with positive PrP immunohistochemistry. Most sporadic CJD cases are homozygous for the common M129V polymorphism.

### Iatrogenic Creutzfeldt–Jakob Disease

Transmission of sporadic CJD has occurred by accidental inoculation with human prions during medical procedures, contaminated instruments, dura mater, corneal grafting and via human growth hormone.

There is a progressive cerebellar syndrome and behavioural disturbance, or a CJD-like dementia. The incubation period can be short (2–4 years for dura mater grafts) or longer (typically 15 years or more) with peripheral infection. Diagnosis is confirmed by PrP immunocytochemistry or Western blot of brain tissue for PrP$^{Sc}$ types 1–3.

### Variant CJD

vCJD was first described in 1996. Its occurrence in young adults and distinctive neuropathology differentiated it from sporadic CJD. A link with BSE was confirmed by typing prions. Under 200 cases have occurred in the UK, the last in 2016.

Early features are non-specific, and cases were frequently referred to a psychiatrist. Depression, anxiety and social withdrawal were typical, with delusions. Other features included emotional lability, aggression, insomnia and auditory and visual hallucinations. A prominent early feature in some was persistent dysaesthesiae or pain in the limbs or face. In most cases a progressive cerebellar syndrome developed. Cognitive impairment followed with progression to akinetic mutism. Myoclonus was seen in most, and chorea. Cortical blindness developed in a minority. Age at onset was from 12 to 74 (mean 28) years. Death followed in 1–2 years.

EEG frequently showed generalised slow wave activity, but without the pseudo-periodic pattern seen in sporadic CJD.

MRI FLAIR showed bilateral increased signal in the posterior thalamus, a.k.a. the pulvinar sign in some, not specific for vCJD.

Tonsillar biopsy became the usual diagnostic procedure. *PRNP* analysis was essential. Most cases of vCJD had the MM genotype at *PRNP* codon 129.

Neuropathology: widespread spongiform change, gliosis and neuronal loss, most severe in the basal ganglia and thalamus. Abundant PrP amyloid plaques in cerebral and cerebellar cortex. Western blot analysis (brain): PrP$^{Sc}$ type 4.

### Secondary (Iatrogenic) vCJD

Since 2004, 4 transfusion-associated cases of vCJD occurred amongst 23 people who received blood from a donor who subsequently developed vCJD. Features were those of vCJD.

### Kuru

Kuru is of historical interest – an effect of cannibalism. This prion encephalopathy reached epidemic proportions in the Eastern Highlands of Papua New Guinea. When first described in the 1950s kuru was a major cause of death amongst women and small children, who engaged in consumption of a dead relative as a mark of respect. Kuru has disappeared since cessation of this solemn ritual cannibalism. There was progressive cerebellar ataxia, with dementia seldom a prominent feature, leading to death in 3 months to 3 years.

### Inherited Prion Diseases

These are exceptionally rare adult onset AD prion diseases associated with *PRNP* coding mutations.

Gerstmann–Sträussler–Schinker disease (GSS) is an AD chronic cerebellar ataxia with pyramidal features and dementia. Onset is usually in the 3rd–4th decades. There are multicentric PrP-amyloid plaques.

Inherited prion disease kindreds show phenotypic variability, encompassing both CJD-like and GSS-like cases and mimics of other neurodegenerative conditions. Inherited prion diseases are a cause of young onset dementia. *PRNP* should be analysed in all suspected cases of CJD, and considered in all young onset dementia and ataxias.

Clinical features in inherited prion diseases are dementia, cerebellar ataxia, pyramidal and extrapyramidal signs, chorea, myoclonus, seizures and muscle wasting.

The most frequent isoforms are PrP E200K, and PrP P102L – both of which can mimic Alzheimer's.

Fatal familial insomnia, another rarity, is associated with the D178N mutation, and causes untreatable insomnia, dysautonomia and motor signs. There is selective atrophy of the anterior-ventral and mediodorsal thalamic nuclei.

### Prevention

Prion diseases can be transmitted by inoculation, but they are not contagious. Case-to-case spread has occurred only by cannibalism or iatrogenic inoculation. Prions resist conventional sterilisation: surgical instruments can act as a vector.

vCJD prion infection has been transmitted, even if very seldom, by blood transfusion. UK policy continues to enforce leuco-depletion of all whole blood and sourcing plasma products from outside the UK – a controversial issue.

## Dementia in Young Adults

Dementia is exceptional before 50 and demands intensive investigation. In some there will be a background of cognitive impairment in childhood. Wilson's disease, porphyrias, mitochondrial disease and late-onset of many storage diseases that usually present in childhood, are all potential causes.

## Controversial Entities

### Alcohol

Alcohol is associated with dementia but it is hard to know to what extent cognitive decline is caused by its toxicity rather than by factors such as malnutrition (thiamine deficiency – Wernicke–Korsakoff syndrome), drug abuse, or hepatic encephalopathy. However, chronic heavy alcohol abuse alone can itself produce dementia. Improvement occurs with prolonged abstinence.

### Traumatic Brain Injury

Head trauma is certainly linked to dementia following repeated injury over many years, for example in boxers, and occasionally footballers and rugby players who develop cognitive deterioration and parkinsonism. These sportsmen have had frequent and either clinically minor and/or disregarded head injuries. This condition a.k.a. *dementia pugilistica* is influenced by the severity of these repeated insults – and probably also by ApoE status. Dementia is more common with the ε4 allele. Pathological appearances overlap with the tauopathy of Alzheimer's, but also have distinct features.

Single insult TBI has been identified as a risk factor for the later development of Alzheimer's in some epidemiological studies, though the causal relationship is debated. The likely explanation is that with a very common disease such as Alzheimer's, one might expect that those who have pre-existing damage, from any cause and thus less cognitive reserve, would develop features of Alzheimer's earlier than the normal population, if they were going to develop Alzheimer's in any event. This is keeping with the observation that dementia can follow other causes of single insult brain damage, such as following encephalitis, carbon monoxide poisoning, hypoxia or damage caused by neurosurgery, but the dementing process is not caused by these insults. Claims that minor head injuries or even serious traumatic brain injuries lead to Alzheimer's neuropathology are unsubstantiated.

**Autoimmune Hashimoto and Coeliac Disease**

The issue is the possible role of autoimmunity as a cause of cognitive decline. This remains contentious and considered unlikely by many. These conditions can certainly lead to cognitive decline because of systemic disturbances such as hypothyroidism or the effects of malabsorption.

*Normal Pressure Hydrocephalus*

In the 1960s the triad of gait apraxia, urinary incontinence and cognitive decline associated with ventricular enlargement was heralded as a form dementia reversible by shunting. The validity of this concept has been questioned and alternative pathologies such as Alzheimer's, and/or VCI are suggested as explanations. It has even been suggested that some with Alzheimer's improve transiently following a shunt. Opinion on the very existence of NPH remains divided.

**Other Causes of Dementia**

Numerous conditions can lead to cognitive decline and hence be listed as causes of dementia. It is important to consider and exclude delirium – confusion in the elderly can follow an otherwise unnoticed urinary infection. Many conditions are mentioned within specific chapters but are assembled below:

| | |
|---|---|
| Degenerative | Alzheimer's, FTD, PDD, DLB, CBD, MND dementia |
| Metabolic | Uraemia, dialysis, hypoglycaemia, hepatic failure, cardiac failure, respiratory failure, obstructive sleep apnoea |
| Intoxication and nutrition | Alcohol, CO, heroin, heavy metals, organic solvents, organophosphates, lithium, methotrexate, alpha-interferon, thiamine, $B_{12}$, nicotinic acid, multiple vitamin deficiencies |
| Endocrine | Thyroid, adrenal, parathyroid, pituitary failure |
| Infection, inflammation, | HIV, TB, fungal meningitis, neurocysticercosis, JC virus, SSPE, encephalitis lethargica, Whipple's, Lyme (?), prion diseases, MS, Behçet's, channelopathies, coeliac, Hashimoto's, neurosarcoid, limbic encephalitis |
| Epilepsy | Non-convulsive status, repeated focal seizures, Rasmussen's |
| Neoplasms &c | Frontal and other tumours, CNS lymphoma, carcinomatous meningitis, metastases, paraneoplastic syndromes, post-radiotherapy, hydrocephalus |
| Vascular | Post-stroke, multiple strokes, lacunes, hyperviscosity, sickle-cell, AVMs, Susac's, cerebral vasculitis |
| Traumatic brain injury | Subdural haematoma, repeated head injury, late effects of TBI (?) |
| Genetic (metabolic, vascular, degenerative) | Wilson's, porphyria, storage disorders, urea cycle disorders, leucodystrophies, CADASIL, amyloidosis, Fabry's, familial Alzheimer's, FTD, Huntington's, familial prion diseases. |

## Management of Dementia

Care provided by the NHS for dementia is in stark contrast to many other degenerative diseases and cancer, where support at home can be excellent. The effects of dementia, and in particular the later, behavioural changes, produce significant psychological and financial burdens on families and carers – around half of whom are women aged over 75. In the later stages total dependency is usual and 24-hour care is needed. Profound loss of memory leads to inability to recognise surroundings or objects, family and friends. Almost all comprehensible speech is lost. Input from the social care and charitable sectors only partially alleviates these problems, and there is significant regional variation in both quality and availability of such inputs. Some practical considerations are summarised below.

### Safety, Legal Aspects and Financial Planning
Patients usually function best in familiar surroundings. A home evaluation and modifications should be organised.

Powers of Attorney, the wishes of the patient and their Will should be raised at an early stage. Financial planning is essential. Advance directives can also be considered. It may be helpful to alert local police and shopkeepers, if the community setting is appropriate. Bank cards may need to be revoked.

Fitness to drive: UK law directs that if a licence holder becomes aware that they have a disability they must inform the DVLA. Alzheimer's patients sometimes curtail their driving when they realise their passengers feel unsafe. However, both lack of insight and poor judgement with FTD can become a major issue. If the patient does not approach the DVLA, and the physician remains concerned, then the DVLA can be informed directly. I suggest that in this unusual situation, the doctor should give a written view to family.

Gait instability, falls and wandering. Wandering is a frequent problem and tracking devices are a popular and useful intervention. Behavioural measures such as increasing interaction, encouraging exercise, improving the structure of the day may help. Sometimes, locking doors becomes the only solution.

### Carers
Carers are a vulnerable and often elderly population. To cope with dementia becomes a burden for everyone:

- Depression, low self-esteem and poor sense of well-being are common. Carers have more chronic conditions and GP attendances than their peers.
- Social isolation is frequent. Carers have less time for their hobbies and social life. They may have difficulty coping with embarrassing social consequences.
- Costs of care and lost earnings can weigh heavily on a spouse.

Local support groups and national associations are helpful. Carers are sometimes reluctant to seek help. Their needs change during the course of the illness but can continue after the death of the patient.

### Behavioural Management
Major behavioural changes are seen early in FTD, but frequently develop in Alzheimer's. Anxiety, and worrying about trivia exacerbate these problems.

A daily routine and gentle but firm discipline helps – at times of washing, dressing and eating when irritation is typical.

Sleep cycles become disturbed; patients can be up all night and sleep all day – exhausting for everyone. A routine should be established with a fixed bedtime, and no stimulants after mid-morning. Hallucinations tend to occur in dimly lit surroundings.

As dementia progresses, a multidisciplinary programme becomes essential, typically achieved only in residential care.

Strategies include scheduled toileting to reduce urinary incontinence, and music during meals and bathing to reduce disruptive behaviour. Exercise, massage and pet therapy are all used to reduce abnormal behaviours.

Urinary and faecal incontinence need to be dealt with.

Dysphagia and/or orobuccal apraxia (e.g. in PNFA): a nasogastric tube, or PEG may need to be considered.

Weight loss and immobility contribute to vulnerability to pressure sores and infection. Issues of withholding life-prolonging treatment, including CPR, need to be discussed.

Whilst there are currently no disease-modifying treatments for FTD. Drugs such as quetiapine or clozapine are useful, cautiously at low doses.

### Co-morbidity

Dementia cases have a low threshold for developing delirium and take longer to recover than those who are cognitively normal. Urinary or respiratory infection is the typical cause.

Depression is common and treatable. SSRIs are usually the best drugs.

Seizures either partial or generalised can occur in dementia. Anti-epileptic drugs such as valproate or carbamazepine usually supress attacks in small doses.

The usual cause of death is pneumonia.

### Autopsy and Brain Donation

Diagnostic accuracy in dementia without histology – the usual situation – is at best 75%. Neuropathological examination can usually provide an accurate diagnosis and resolve any genetic issues. Tissue donation is helpful for research.

## Acknowledgements

Professor Peter Garrard, Professor of Neurology at St George's, University of London, gave me invaluable help by editing and commenting personally on this chapter. He also provided images of high quality.

Professor Martin Rossor was the Lead Author of Dementia & Cognitive Impairment in the Second edition of *Neurology A Queen Square Textbook*. His colleagues John Collinge, Nick Fox, Simon Mead, Catherine Mummery, Jonathan Rohrer, Jonathan Schott & Jason Warren contributed. This chapter draws in part on their original text and I am most grateful.

## Further Reading

Rossor M, John Collinge, Nick Fox, Simon Mead, Catherine Mummery, Jonathan Rohrer, Jonathan Schott and Jason Warren. Dementia and cognitive impairment. In *Neurology A Queen Square Textbook*, 2nd edn. Clarke C, Howard R, Rossor M, and Shorvon S, eds. John Wiley & Sons, 2016. There are numerous references.

Also, please visit https://www.drcharlesclarke.com for free updated notes, potential links and references as these become available. You will be asked to log in, in a secure fashion, with your name and institution.

## Websites

https://www.nhs.uk/conditions/dementia/help-and-support/

## Broca's aphasia

https://www.youtube.com/watch?v=JWC-cVQmEmY

## Wernicke's aphasia

https://www.youtube.com/watch?v=3oef68YabD0

# 6

# Stroke and Cerebrovascular Disease

Stroke means a clinical event – for example, sudden and enduring weakness on one side, that is an acute or progressive focal deficit almost invariably from brain vascular disease. Three-quarters follow thrombo-embolic cerebral arterial infarction. A fifth of these events follow intracranial haemorrhage, either intracerebral or subarachnoid. A few follow arterial dissection, vasculitis or are associated with cerebral venous thrombosis. MS can exceptionally present as a stroke; so can a tumour or a subdural haematoma.

Stroke requires immediate assessment because intervention has revolutionised outcomes following infarction. It is thus vital to distinguish infarction from haemorrhage. Common causes and emergency management are dealt with first. Subarachnoid haemorrhage and venous thrombosis require different approaches.

In United Kingdom stroke causes around 10% of deaths, around 38 000 annually; about 100 000 people have a stroke. Stroke is important throughout life – a fifth occur before 60 – and *in utero,* stroke is a cause of cerebral palsy.

A transient ischaemic attack (TIA) is rapid loss of focal function lasting less than 24 hours with complete recovery. A TIA requires urgent assessment because it may herald a stroke.

The essential vascular anatomy is outlined in Figures 6.1–6.3.


## Pathophysiology: Ischaemic Stroke

Inter-related mechanisms are:

- thrombosis, embolism, hypoperfusion and infarction
- at the centre of an infarct, damage is most severe. At the periphery, collaterals may or may not preserve the zone surrounding the centre, a.k.a. the ischaemic *penumbra* – a word meaning a type of shadow, but here a zone where perfusion can be critical
- metabolic changes and raised intracranial pressure.

*Neurology: A Clinical Handbook*, First Edition. Charles Clarke.
© 2022 John Wiley & Sons Ltd. Published 2022 by John Wiley & Sons Ltd.

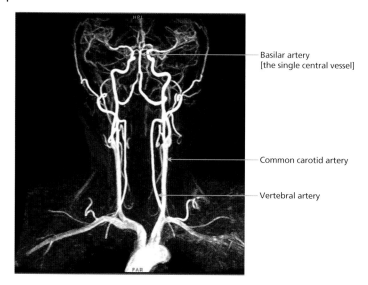

**Figure 6.1**   MRA: Origins of common carotid and vertebral arteries. *Source*: Courtesy of Professor Raymond Cheung.

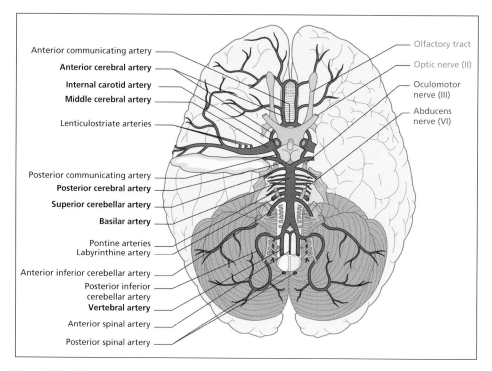

**Figure 6.2**   Principal cerebral arteries. *Source*: Courtesy of Professor Thomas Champney.

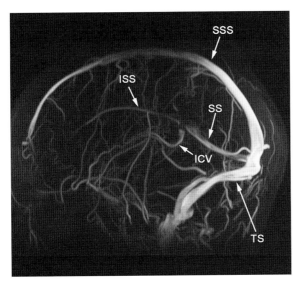

**Figure 6.3**   Venous sinuses: MR venogram. SSS: superior sagittal sinus, ISS: inferior sagittal sinus, SS: straight sinus, TS: transverse sinus, ICV: internal cerebral vein.

### Thrombosis, Embolism, Collaterals and the Ischaemic *penumbra*

Outcome of an arterial occlusion depends upon several variables. Imagine a symptomless 95% internal carotid artery stenosis. A thrombus forms to occlude this vessel:

- if collaterals are adequate – and the clot does not embolise – there may be no symptoms.
- if there are no collaterals infarction of the entire carotid territory can follow. When there are some collaterals, vulnerable areas infarct – typically those most distant, with poorest perfusion.
- an embolus is an alternative: a platelet thrombus forms on an ulcerated plaque within the stenosis
  - this embolus might lodge at the anterior cerebral artery (ACA) origin, but because of the contralateral collateral circulation, this may have no clinical effect, or
  - it might lodge at the origin of the middle cerebral artery (MCA). Collaterals maintain some cortical areas, temporarily. MCA lenticulostriate deep perforators are blocked: deep territories infarct, to cause a hemiparesis. Pneumonia and hypotension follow. Collaterals in the *penumbra* no longer cope, and a hemiplegia follows.

### Metabolic Changes and Raised Intracranial Pressure

When neurones become ischaemic, excitatory toxic neurotransmitter activity increases. The process soon becomes irreversible. Oedema causes further decrease in blood flow, compromising both *penumbra* and surrounding brain. Massive MCA infarction, or cerebellar infarction can ensue, with coning.

## Risk factors: Age, Hypertension, Tobacco, Lipids, Alcohol

Stroke incidence doubles with each decade past 55 years. Hypertension is most important. Tobacco remains another leading problem: smoking predisposes to carotid stenosis, particularly. Diabetes mellitus increases stroke risk about three-fold. High total cholesterol and LDL correlate with atherosclerosis. Alcohol has a curious, a.k.a. J-shaped relationship: heavy drinking carries a high risk of all stroke, ischaemic and haemorrhagic. Moderate consumption reduces, if slightly the risk, above abstemption. Carotid stenosis greater than 75% carries an annual stroke incidence of less than 2% – unexpectedly low – but about 10% for myocardial infarction.

### Cardiac Disease

Atrial fibrillation (AF) is important. AF is common in the over 60s. There is a 5% annual stroke risk. Age and hypertension increase this. Valve disease: vegetations on native or prosthetic valves are also causes. After an MI, systemic emboli occur in about 3%.

Paradoxical embolus – venous thrombosis entering the arterial circulation – is well-recognised. A triad suggests this:

- a DVT has been confirmed or there is a good reason for it, such as thrombophilia
- the stroke happens when a paradoxical embolus is likely, for example during a Valsalva
- the stroke is typically cardio-embolic.

The most common shunt is a patent foramen ovale (PFO) – present in around 50% of strokes below 40.

### Ischaemic Stroke and the Blood

Many clotting abnormalities can predispose to stroke and TIAs. In practical terms if there is neither polycythaemia nor an evident clotting problem, a blood-related cause is unusual. The following are possibilities: sickle cell disease, thrombocythaemia, antiphospholipid antibody syndrome, thrombotic thrombocytopenic purpura, paroxysmal nocturnal haemoglobinuria, leukaemia, myeloma, activated protein C (APC) resistance, factor V Leiden mutation, protein C deficency, protein S deficency, antithrombin III deficiency, prothrombin G20210A mutation, malignancy, vasculitis, homocystinuria, malaria, OCP, DIC, nephrotic syndrome.

APC resistance is the commonest clotting abnormality – a venous risk factor – and not a cause of arterial stroke. Antiphospholipid antibody syndrome is dealt with in Chapter 26.

## Stroke and TIA

It is common knowledge that 'he's had a stroke' usually implies sudden unilateral weakness, typically with aphasia if weakness is right sided. Focal features include aphasia alone, a visual field defect, ataxia, facial weakness, diplopia, cognitive change, or a balance problem. The cause may not be evident without imaging. Also, whilst stroke implies a sudden event, weakness can be gradual (progressive, subacute) over hours, days or weeks. Descriptions of stroke syndromes imply that they should be recognisable clinically – they may not be: do not make pronouncements before thorough investigation.

## Transient Ischaemic Attack (TIA)

TIA lasts less than 24 hours with complete recovery – often caused by thrombo-embolism.

- Hemipshere TIA: contralateral weakness and/or dysphasia are typical. Sensory loss alone seldom occurs.
- Amaurosis fugax: monocular blindness, usually a curtain/shutter lasting several minutes is typical of carotid stenosis and retinal thromboembolism. A retinal cholesterol arterial embolus (a Hollenhorst plaque, Chapter 14) may be visible, exceptionally.
- Vertebrobasilar TIAs cause diplopia, facial or tongue numbness, dysarthria, vertigo and visual loss. Isolated vertigo (Chapter 15) is rare.

### Thrombo-embolic TIA Patterns, Carotid Stenosis and Alternative Diagnoses

TIA symptoms are usually negative, abrupt and persist typically from several to 30 minutes. A TIA can point to carotid stenosis, but can occur with other risk factors, for example with polycythaemia or endocarditis.

When there is carotid stenosis, high-frequency attacks – several a week – point to severe stenosis. TIAs sometimes cause limb jerking, suggesting a focal seizure, followed by weakness. Anterior circulation thromboembolic TIA are frequently followed by stroke – 20% within a month and 50% within a year. A TIA can also follow a lacunar infarct, or a microhaemorhage.

Cases often referred to a TIA clinic have other aetiologies. TIA-like episodes (TIALES) occur in migraine, in cervical artery dissection, giant cell arteritis and in focal epilepsy, or have no apparent cause. A tumour, subdural haematoma, and MS can cause a TIALE, so can hypoglycaemia, syncope and malaria. A TIALE occasionally occurs in a climber above 5000 m, possibly from brain edema.

Transient global amnesia (TGA) describes a dramatic amnesia often misdiagnosed as a TIA. The patient, who is usually over 50 suddenly appears bewildered and asks repetitive questions such as 'Where am I. . .what's going on?' Personal identity remains intact, but there is inability to recall recent events and confusion. Recovery is usual within hours and there is no subsequent stroke risk. In the majority there is no recurrence. Various precipitating events have been suggested such as emotional stress, and immersion in cold water. Occasionally an underlying cause is found – a tumour, or hypertension – and rarely TGA is a possible prelude to dementia.

### Lacunes

Lacunes are small (1–15mm) single or multiple infarcts (Figure 6.4 and Figure 6.5). Risk factors are hypertension, diabetes and high cholesterol. Some are symptomless, but others announced by a TIA or stroke. Lacunar strokes include pure hemiparesis, hemisensory loss, ataxia and clumsy hand-dysarthria. Repeated infarcts cause peri-ventricular

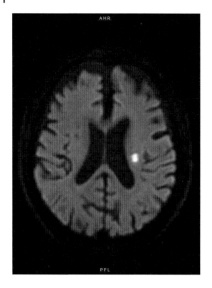

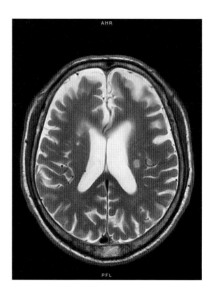

**Figure 6.4**  MR DWI: single lacunar infarct. *Source*: Courtesy of Professor Raymond Cheung.

**Figure 6.5**  MR T2W: multiple white matter lesions. *Source*: Courtesy of Professor Raymond Cheung.

change, a.k.a. leukoaraiosis, with gait apraxia (gait ignition failure, *marche à petit pas*), imbalance and dementia.

## Typical Stroke Patterns

### Internal Carotid Artery (ICA) Disease

ICA disease causes symptoms either by embolism, by thrombus on an ulcerated plaque, haemodynamic failure or complete occlusion. A neck bruit is sign of ICA stenosis. If flow is diminished this can disappear. Horner's syndrome may develop when the artery is acutely thrombosed, or with dissection. Embolism from a carotid is most likely to produce a partial or complete MCA syndrome. Atheroma elsewhere is commonly present.

### Total and Branch Middle Cerebral Artery (MCA) Occlusion

The MCA may be blocked by embolism or thrombosis *in situ*. If there are inadequate collaterals the entire territory infarcts (Figure 6.6, below), a.k.a. front-to-back infarction: conjugate eye deviation (frontal), aphasia, hemiplegia, hemisensory loss and hemianopia. Cerebral oedema at 48–72 hours, coning and death can follow.

Upper MCA branch occlusion causes hemiparesis, hemisensory loss, ocular deviation and aphasia. Lower branch occlusion affects the temporal lobe – receptive aphasia. Small occluded distal cortical branches tend to cause focal weakness. With deep MCA infarction – striatum and internal capsule – collateral circulation may protect the cortex (Figure 6.7).

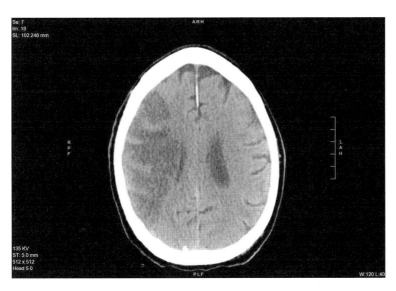

**Figure 6.6**   Cerebral edema following right MCA occlusion (CT). *Source*: Courtesy of Professor Raymond Cheung.

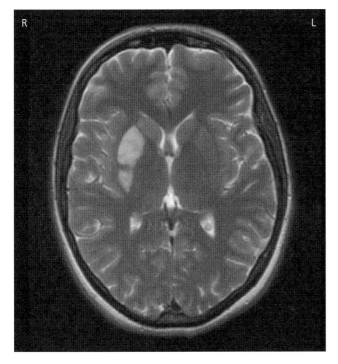

**Figure 6.7**   MR T2W: deep MCA (striato-capsular) infarction.

### Anterior Cerebral (ACA) and Posterior Cerebral Artery (PCA) Occlusion

With ACA occlusion contralateral hemiplegia is typical. PCA occlusion (Figure 6.8) is typically embolic; hemianopia is common. PCAs also supply the thalami and temporal lobes – confusion/aphasia can ensue. If both PCA territories are infarcted – an embolus at the top of the basilar – cortical blindness and confusion follow.

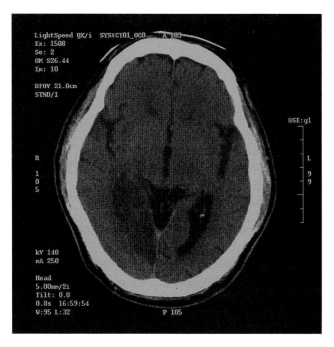

**Figure 6.8** Unenhanced CT: acute PCA oclusion. *Source*: Courtesy of Professor Raymond Cheung.

### Vertebral Artery

The lateral medullary syndrome, a.k.a. Wallenberg's follows posterior inferior cerebellar artery (PICA) thrombosis (Figure 6.9). Features: Horner's, dissociated (temperature and pain) sensory loss on the ipsilateral face and opposite side of the body, nystagmus, ipsilateral limb ataxia and ipsilateral palatal and vocal cord paralysis, or extensive brainstem and cerebellar damage. A common site for vertebral atheroma is at its subclavian origin.

### Basilar Artery

Thrombosis *in situ* can occur in the basilar or follow vertebral artery dissection and/or thrombosis. Various patterns, usually with quadriparesis follow:

- Within the medulla
  - bulbar (LMN) or pseudobulbar palsy (UMN) – brisk facial reflexes, spastic tongue, spontaneous laughter/crying.

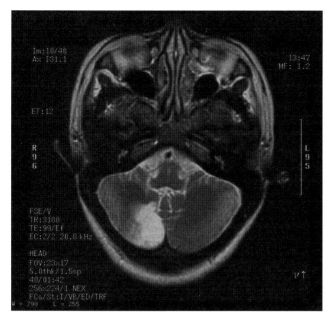

**Figure 6.9**   MR T1W: PICA infarction. *Source*: Courtesy of Professor Raymond Cheung.

- Above the medulla:
  - pontine infarction – VIth palsy, gaze paresis, internuclear ophthalmoplegia, pinpoint pupils.
  - midbrain infarction – loss of vertical eye movement, pupil abnormalities, coma or locked-in syndrome.
  - Posterior cerebral artery infarction leads to hemianopia or cortical blindness.

### Border Zone Ischaemia

In zones between major arteries, the brain is vulnerable to perfusion failure, such as following cardiac arrest:

- Parieto-occipital cortex, between MCA and PCA territories: infarction causes visual field defects, incoordination of hand/eye movement.
- Deep border zones within the *centrum semi-ovale* and between ACA and MCA – hemiparesis/hemiplegia.
- In the hippocampi – an amnestic syndrome.

### Vascular Dementia

Alzheimer's and vascular dementia (Chapter 5) may co-exist – generally, this diagnosis is made in an dementia case with multiple white matter lesions. However sometimes recurrent small strokes cause cognitive impairment, gait apraxia/initiation failure and postural instability.

## Intracerebral Haemorrhage (ICH)

Brain haemorrhage causes about 10% of strokes. ICH typically follows intracerebral arterial rupture. Haematoma expands along white matter tracts, and/or into the ventricles, with mass effect dependent upon clot volume. ICH is typically sudden and devastating, but a small haemorrhage can cause a TIA. Tiny bleeds pass unnoticed. Following major ICH, about half die.

Hypertension leads to disease of small perforating arteries. Control of hypertension has reduced ICH dramatically. Related issues are aneurysms and SAH – about 20% of ICH. A vascular malformation, tumour and amyloid angiopathy can cause an ICH, cocaine, and amphetamines can cause haemorrhage. A recent infarct can become haemorrhagic. Anyone on an anticoagulant with new neurology must be assumed to have bled. A microbleed that would have been silent in a non-anticoagulated patient enlarges to become apparent. Other coagulopathies, thrombocytopaenia, or liver/renal failure may also cause bleeding.

### Deep Haemorrhage

Haematomas form in the putamen (Figure 6.10), caudate or thalamus.

- Putamen: sudden contralateral hemiparesis, conjugate gaze deviation towards the side of the bleed. Aphasia or other cortical dysfunction follows. Herniation ensues if mass effect becomes critical, or the bleed ruptures into the ventricles.
- Caudate and intraventricular haemorrhage and can mimic subarachnoid bleeding – headache and meningism with few focal signs.
- Thalamic haemorrhage produces sensory change in the contralateral limbs and/or aphasia. Forced downward gaze with small pupils can follow midbrain compression.

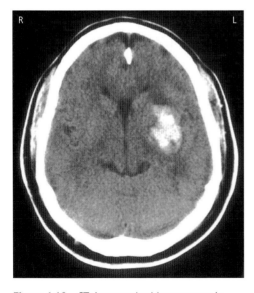

**Figure 6.10**  CT: intracerebral haematoma in putamen.

### Lobar Haemorrhage

In the frontal lobe, eye deviation and contralateral hemiparesis is common. In the posterior frontal and fronto-parietal region, hemisensory loss is found, with aphasia in the dominant hemisphere. Parietal lobe haemorrhage causes hemisensory loss and neglect/inattention. Bleeding into the dominant temporal lobe can cause a Wernicke's aphasia.

Haemorrhagic transformation of infarction and a haemorrhagic tumour can also occur. Cerebral amyloid angiopathy (CAA) is deposition of amyloid-β in small cortical arteries. CAA can cause a lobar ICH in the elderly, or progressive cognitive decline, and occasionally a TIA.

### Pontine and Cerebellar (Infratentorial) Haemorrhage

Pontine haemorrhage causes coma with pinpoint pupils, loss of horizontal eye movements and quadriparesis. Hyper-pyrexia and irregular respiration can ensue. A large haematoma is often fatal.

Cerebellar haemorrhage (Figure 6.11) – about 10% of ICH – causes an acute head-ache, vomiting and unilateral ataxia. Gaze palsies may occur and/or skew deviation. Brainstem compression and hydrocephalus follow. Decompressive craniectomy can be life-saving.

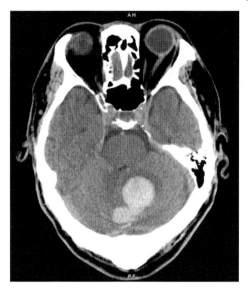

**Figure 6.11**   CT: cerebellar haemorrhage.
*Source*: Courtesy of Professor Raymond Cheung.

## Stroke & TIA management

### NICE Guidance: Stroke & TIA – Diagnosis and Initial Management

Everyone in general practice, any form of emergency medicine and neurology should be aware of NICE Guidance and its implications. The NICE headings are outlined below.

### Rapid Recognition of Symptoms and Diagnosis

This focuses on tools such as the Face, Arm, Speech Test (FAST), and Recognition of Stroke in the Emergency Room (ROSIER), and exclusion of hypoglycaemia. Any suspected stroke requires immediate admission, ideally to a stroke unit. With a confirmed thromboembolic TIA, aspirin is recommended unless contraindicated. Suspected TIA cases should be seen by a specialist service within 24 hours.

### Imaging for Suspected TIA or Non-disabling Stroke

CT and MR should be carried out ASAP. Carotid imaging/ultrasound and surgery should be available urgently:

- Carotid stenosis greater than 50% should be considered for surgery, but not stenosis of a lesser degree.

### Specialist Care

All cases should be admitted to an acute stroke unit. Immediate non-enhanced CT brain imaging should be carried out, and vascular imaging if thrombectomy might be indicated.

### Alteplase (Thrombolysis) and Thrombectomy *et al*

- Alteplase is recommended for acute ischaemic stroke in adults if treatment is started within 4.5 hours of symptoms, and intracranial haemorrhage has been excluded.
- Thrombectomy is considered when there is a confirmed occlusion within the anterior circulation.

- Recommendations relate to aspirin, a proton pump inhibitor, statins, prosthetic valves and anticoagulation with AF. Arterial dissection: consider either anticoagulants or anti-platelet agents.
- Cerebral venous sinus thrombosis should usually be treated with anticoagulation.
- In haemorrhagic stroke, anyone on an anticoagulant should have clotting returned to normal ASAP.

**Maintenance/Restoration of Homeostasis, Nutrition and Hydration**
Avoidance of hypoxaemia, control of blood sugar and blood pressure. Adequate nutrition and hydration are essential and regular swallowing assessment.

**Emergency Neurosurgery, Early Mobilisation, Positioning**
This deals with items such as surgical decompression, cerebellar haemorrhage and important nursing aspects.

## Stroke and TIA Investigations

The usual investigations are below:
- Full blood count – anaemia, polycythaemia, thrombocythaemia and thrombocytopaenia, ESR and CRP.
- Urea and electrolytes: guide acute management; end-organ damage from hypertension.
- Glucose – diabetes is common; hypoglycaemia can cause focal signs.
- Lipid analysis.
- Syphilis and HIV serology.
- Serum proteins and immunoglobulins – myeloma or other gammopathy.
- Multiple blood cultures and repeated urine exams – if endocarditis possible. Thick film, if malaria possible.
- Thyroid function tests.
- CXR, ECG, transthoracic/transoesophageal echocardiography.
- Special investigations include:
  - thrombophilia assessment – rarely useful in arterial stroke
  - antiphospholipid antibodies can be associated with many vasculopathies
  - venous thrombophilia may be relevant as a rarity
  - autoantibodies – markers of systemic vasculitis
  - screening for mitochondrial and NOTCH III (CADASIL) mutations, leucocyte galactosidase A (Fabry's), and homocysteine in exceptional circumstances.

### Progressive Stroke

About one-third of ischaemic stroke cases progress in the first 24 hours, and more following ICH as the bleed enlarges. In ischaemic stroke, causes include extension from thrombus propagation, recurrent embolism, failure of collaterals and/or enlargement of the *penumbra* and local effects of cytotoxic oedema. Other factors include:

- Metabolic disturbances, for example low or high blood sugar, hyponatraemia
- Hypotension, or hypertension, arrhythmias, myocardial infarction, cardiac failure
- Infection, dehydration, hypoxia
- Cerebral oedema and/or hydrocephalus, haemorrhagic transformation of infarction
- New infarction/embolism or haemorrhage in a new location.

## Common Complications of Stroke

- Dysphagia, or simply an unsafe swallow. All should be nil-by-mouth until safe. Nasogastric feeding may be necessary.
- DVT in hemiparetic limbs is common, silent respiratory & urinary infection.
- Pressure sores – turning, positioning & mattresses. Early mobilisation: essential.
- Shoulder pain, largely preventable by positioning and early physiotherapy.
- Swelling of the hand or foot of a hemiparetic limb: elevation and passive movements help.
- Spasticity: early mobilisation &and local botulinum toxin.
- Depression.
- Post-stroke pain (Chapter 23) - – a deep burning pain throughout the weak side. Dystonia is a rare late complication of basal ganglia stroke.

## Secondary Prevention

Targets for highly effective measures following TIA and stroke include:

- lifestyle – abstain from tobacco, take exercise, reduce weight
- BP control, lowering cholesterol, diabetes treatment
- prevention of cardiac embolism – anticoagulation for AF, carotid endarterectomy or stenting
- inhibition of platelet aggregation - – antiplatelet agents.

## Intracranial Aneurysms

Rupture of an intracranial aneurysm causes 85% of non-traumatic SAH. 5% are caused by an AVM, cerebral vasculitis, a tumour, dural arteriovenous fistula, dural sinus or venous thrombosis, carotid or vertebral artery dissection, or coagulopathy. Non-aneurysmal peri-mesencephalic haemorrhage – an unexplained phenomenon – accounts for about 10%. SAH is least frequent in the Middle East and commonest in Japan, Australia and Scandinavia. F:M ratio around 1.8:1.0.

Aneurysms are typically saccular: there is protrusion of intima through a defect in the arterial muscular layer. A circle of Willis aneurysm, a.k.a. berry aneurysm, is the usual cause. Mycotic aneurysms develop in endocarditis.

Large aneursyms greater than 25 mm tend to rupture more frequently than those smaller than 7 mm. Over 5 years around 50% of known large aneurysms rupture, but fewer than 5% of small aneurysms.

Most cases of aneurysmal SAH are sporadic, but familial aneurysms account for 10%. There are associations with AD polycystic kidneys, Marfan's, pseudoxanthoma elasticum, Ehlers–Danlos, $\alpha_1$-antitrypsin deficiency and cocaine. These account for less than 5%. Hypertension and tobacco are important. Smoking with high BP increases SAH risk 10-fold.

## Clinical Features: Thunderclap Headache

Headache (Chapter 12) is present in almost all. Headache is typically sudden, of unique severity, with vomiting. Thunderclap headache is not specific for SAH – only about 1 in 10 thunderclap cases turn out to have had a bleed. Exceptionally, bacterial meningitis can present with SAH.

Headaches predating SAH by days or weeks, a.k.a. sentinel headaches occur occasionally. Loss of consciousness, confusion or prolonged coma occurs in about 30%. Death can follow SAH, in minutes to hours.

Meningeal irritation is found in most. SAH still tends to be misdiagnosed – as migraine or a benign acute headache. Neck stiffness can be missed in an acute headache unless it is sought. A few SAH cases remain ambulant – in these, low back pain/sciatica from irritation by blood products can develop within a week.

Signs vary, from coma with or without papilloedema and/or retinal haemorrhage, to a severe headache with a stiff neck and focal signs. Hemiparesis, IIIrd or VIth nerve palsies are caused either by the aneurysm itself, intraparenchymal extension of blood or later by vasospasm. Focal signs may be absent. Rupture of a basilar artery aneurysm (Figure 6.12) can lead to immediate coma and death within hours.

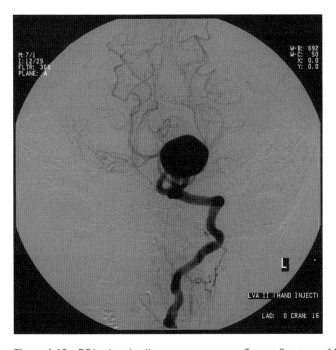

**Figure 6.12** DSA: giant basilar artery aneurysm. *Source*: Courtesy of Professor Raymond Cheung.

Clinical features can help localise an aneurysm:

- A painful complete IIIrd nerve palsy suggests a PCOM artery aneurysm (Figure 6.13)
- An anterior communicating artery (ACOM) aneurysm can present with frontal symptoms - bilateral lower-limb weakness, extensor plantars, incontinence and abulia.
- An anterior choroidal or MCA aneurysm can cause hemiparesis and aphasia.

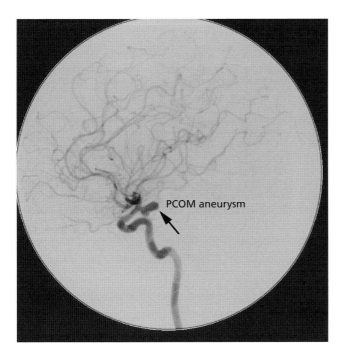

**Figure 6.13**   Catheter angiogram: bi-lobed PCOM artery aneurysm.

Ocular haemorrhages are seen in 25%:

- Retinal haemorrhages around the fovea
- Subhyaloid (preretinal) haemorrhages
- Vitreous haemorhage (Terson's syndrome) is usually bilateral.

Spinal SAH, a relative rarity, causes sudden back pain, with or without root pain and/or paraparesis, but with features of intracranial SAH.

### Investigation and Management

CT brain imaging, promptly, is essential with any possible SAH. Intracranial blood is seen in over 90% in the first 48 hours – typically around basal cisterns, Sylvian fissures and/or cortical sulci (Figure 6.14)

If the CT is normal, lumbar puncture should be considered, assuming no contraindications. Xanthochromia – yellow to the eye, confirmed by spectrophotometry – is present in most between 12 hours and 2 weeks.

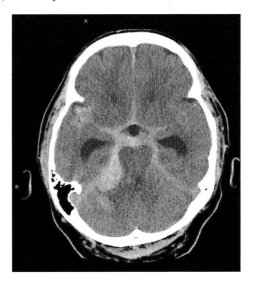

**Figure 6.14**   CT: SAH – blood around brainstem.
*Source*: Courtesy of Professor Raymond Cheung.

All SAH cases should be referred promptly to a neurovascular unit. Digital subtraction angiography (DSA) is one principal investigation, but 3-D CT angiography and MR angiography are also used. An aneurysm can be obscured by vasospasm, hypoperfusion and poor technique. Repeat imaging detects an aneurysm in some. About 5% of SAH cases have no known source of haemorrhage despite thorough imaging – typically young males with blood in peri-mesencephalic cisterns. Full supportive care is essential. Avoid aspirin. Start oral nimodipine: this reduces risks of cerebral infarction.

### SAH Complications, Treatment & Outcome

Following SAH that may be either catastrophic or appear relatively benign, complications are frequent:

- Rebleeding, arterial vasospasm, hydrocephalus
- Seizures, cardiac arrhythmias
- Pulmonary oedema, hyponatraemia – either cerebral salt-wasting, or SIADH.

Intravascular coiling is now used extensively. Age, co-morbidities, location and aneurysm size require specialist assessment. Mortality: 50% in the first month. Around one third remain dependent and many have cognitive problems. However, some eventually return to employment.

## Cerebral Venous and Venous Sinus Thrombosis

These thromboses are seldom recognised clinically – they tend to be imaging diagnoses. Thromboses develop within cortical veins, within dural sinuses and/or deep veins. This can follow sepsis. In about one quarter no cause becomes apparent. Potential causes are below:

- Pregnancy, OCP, HRT, heparin-induced thrombocytopenia & thrombosis (HITT), polycythaemia, paroxysmal nocturnal haemoglobinuria, sickle cell, factor V Leiden, Protein C and S deficiency, antithrombin III, prothrombin gene mutation, DIC, antiphospholipid syndrome.
- Post-Covid-19 immunisation: cerebral venous and venous sinus thrombosis, sometimes fatal, mainly in young females below 50 years has been reported. Further information will be forthcoming.
- Behçet's, SLE, sarcoid, GPA, inflammatory bowel disease, thrombangiitis obliterans
- Septicaemia, endocarditis, TB, malaria, aspergillosis, facial cellulitis, mastoiditis, paranasal sinusitis, ophthalmic infection, intracranial abscess, meningitis.
- Carcinoma, carcinoid, lymphoma, myeloma, nephrotic syndrome, traumatic brain injury, low CSF pressure, meningioma, congenital heart disease, cardiac failure, dural AVM, severe dehydration.

Features vary:

- A cortical venous thrombosis presents typically with headache, seizures and focal signs.
- Sagittal sinus thrombosis (SST) and/or lateral sinus thrombosis are usually seen in the context of severe illness/sepsis. SST can present in isolation with headache, papilloedema with grossly normal CT imaging – features initially identical to idiopathic intracranial

hypertension, before spread of thrombus to cortical veins and/or venous sinuses produces focal signs and/or stupor.

- Venous sinus thrombosis can cause isolated headache, sometimes thunderclap, as the only initial feature. Cortical venous thrombosis seldom causes an isolated stroke.
- Cavernous sinus thrombosis (Chapter 14) typically follows local sepsis. Early features are ocular pain, headache, fever, proptosis, conjunctival engorgement and ophthalmoplegia. Mortality is high.

### Imaging, Treatment and Outcome

With cortical venous thrombosis, focal haemorrhagic infarction with surrounding oedema is typical. Thrombus in the major venous sinuses may be visible on both CT and MR. Angiography may be needed. Confirmed cases should be anticoagulated, though the evidence-base is uncertain. Sepsis needs immediate treatment. Many cases are gravely ill. Outcome: variable – some make good recoveries.

## Arteriovenous Malformations

An AVM is a tangle of arteries, veins and A-V fistulae (Figure 6.15) that arises in embryonic life.

Many AVMs are discovered coincidentally, but typically an AVM presents with intracranial haemorrhage – intracerebral, subarachnoid or intraventricular. AVMs can also cause seizures, in about 25%. An AVM can also cause non-haemorrhagic focal symptoms, such as progressive hemiparesis, or a visual field defect. Even dementia has been described. A brainstem AVM can resemble MS. Migrainous headaches can occur. A cranial bruit is present in about 25% – common with a dural AVM.

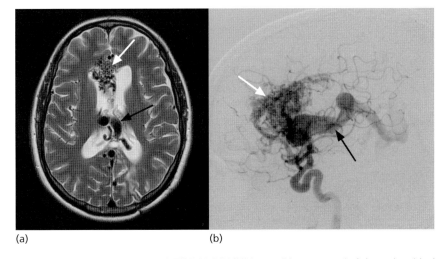

(a)                                        (b)

**Figure 6.15** Frontal AVM (a) MR T2W (b) DSA. Nidus – white arrows; draining vein – black arrow.

All cases should be evaluated by a neurovascular team. The aim is to eradicate/reduce the risk of future haemorrhage. Techniques include resection, endovascular glue embolisation and stereotactic radiosurgery. Untreated AVMs carry a small annual risk of rupture of the order of 2% – some are best left alone. Cord AVMs are mentioned in Chapter 16.

## Cavernous Malformations

Cavernous malformations a.k.a. cavernous angiomas, cavernous haemangiomas, or cavernomas occur in around 1 in 200 people. Cavernomas are typically raspberry-like, 2–20 mm in diameter – a tangle of intertwined vascular channels. Cavernomas are usually silent but they can cause seizures, or bleed. Silent haemorrhage seen on imaging is common. Occasionally a progressive hemiparesis occurs, caused by recurrent small bleeds. When a cavernoma has been found – by chance or following a seizure – there is a low risk of bleeding, less than 2% annually. Cavernomas are seen best on MRI (Figure 6.16) and tend to be occult on CT. Stereotactic radiosurgery is considered following multiple haemorrhagic episodes or poorly controlled seizures. Most are left alone.

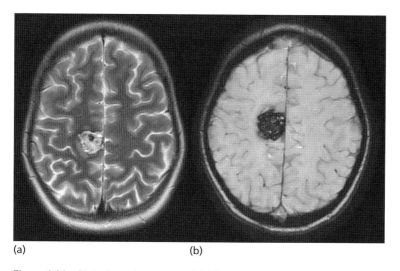

(a)                              (b)

**Figure 6.16**  Right frontal cavernoma (a) MR T2 (b) MR SWI.

## Non-atherosclerotic Vascular Disease and Other Causes of Stroke

Most with ischaemic arterial stroke and ICH have atherosclerosis. However, important non-atherosclerotic vasculopathies include extracranial arterial dissection and vasculitides.

### Carotid and Vertebral Artery Dissection

Dissection of the vertebral or carotid arteries should be considered as a cause of stroke in patients below 50. Mechanism: through an intimal tear, of uncertain cause, there is penetration of arterial blood and extension in the vessel wall to form an intramural haematoma. This narrows the lumen. Blood within the vessel wall may itself lead to arterial occlusion but frequently the dissection exposes a thrombogenic surface on which intraluminal clot develops, that can then embolise.

The majority of these strokes occur in young people. Neck extension, during hair washing or painting a ceiling are sometimes preceding complaints, but are probably only provoking events rather than causes. Dissection is also sometimes attributed to neck manipulation – but it may be neck pain from the dissection that took the patient initially to a therapist.

Dissection following major head and neck trauma is surprisingly unusual, suggesting that these young stroke cases have some collagen defect that induces vulnerability, perhaps fragments of Marfanism. Fibromuscular dysplasia, seen in middle-aged females can sometimes lead to dissection. Dissection in the majority is in the extracranial carotid and vertebral arteries. Dissection is unusual in older patients, perhaps because atherosclerosis renders their arterial walls more robust.

These cases typically present with a stroke. There may also be an apparent precipitating event with headache – or a migraine-like event. Sometimes weeks elapse before the embolus causes a stroke. Although many stroke syndromes can follow dissection, a Horner's syndrome is one hallmark of a carotid dissection. Occasionally too, carotid dissection causes a unilateral XIIth nerve lesion – tongue deviation. Following vertebro-basilar dissection, a lateral medullary syndrome can follow embolic occlusion of the PICA.

MRI and/or CT angiography provide sensitive means to confirm dissection, but may require specialist neuroradiological interpretation.

NICE guidelienes recommend either antiplatelet agents or anticoagulation following a typical carotid or vertebral dissection. Most neurologists anticoagulate these cases for some months.

## Vasculitis and Other Rarities

It is exceedingly rare for vasculitis to present simply as stroke, but various medical conditions can lead to cerebrovascular disease. Systemic vasculitis is summarised in Chapter 26.

### Infective Vasculitis

Infective vasculitis occurs in bacterial, fungal, TB or viral infection. There are nearly always preceding features of a meningo-encephalitis.

In syphilis an obliterative endarteritis of small cerebral vessels can follow primary infection, with a variable latency. Headache and encephalopathy occur before stroke. Lyme borreliosis can have similar features, but is often difficult to define.

Viral infection is responsible for some cerebral vasculitis previously considered idiopathic. Hepatitis B and C and herpes zoster are examples. Zoster is the most well-known: $V_1$ shingles is followed by a stroke several weeks later. The infarct is usually in carotid territory and ipsilateral to the rash; there may also be encephalitis. In children, stroke can, if rarely follow chickenpox.

COVID-19 has been reported with large vessel stroke in cases under 50 presumably following endothelial damage.

Parasites can cause endarteritis. Neurocysticercosis can cause a stroke: cysts lodge in the subarachnoid space leading to meningeal inflammation. In cerebral malaria, haemorrhagic stroke occurs, particularly in children. A TIA with a high swinging fever is almost diagnostic of malaria in countries where it is common.

With HIV there are many mechanisms to explain the increased stroke incidence – primary infection, encephalopathy, premature atheroma and drugs.

### Thrombotic Thrombocytopenic Purpura

This is characterised by microangiopathic haemolytic anaemia, thrombocytopenia and systemic microinfarction from thrombi. Renal failure, fever and TIAs, and/or diffuse encephalopathy occur. Large cerebral vessel infarction can also occur and so do ICH, and posterior leuco-encephalopathy. Treatment: plasma exchange and/or anticoagulation.

### Behçet's Disease, Susac's and Sneddon's Syndrome

Behçet's: neurological manifestations are meningitis, encephalitis, stroke-like events and dural sinus thrombosis. The brainstem can be involved.

Susac's is a rare microangiopathy in young women – of the brain, retina and cochlea. There is obliteration of retinal arteries with focal scotomata and stepwise visual loss. Tinnitus and sudden hearing loss occur. Other features are dementia, pyramidal and cerebellar signs.

Sneddon's is a rarity – chronic skin lesions, livedo reticularis and stroke. Skin biopsy shows inflammatory changes in small and medium arteries.

### Mitochondrial Disease and Fabry's

MELAS (mitochondrial myopathy, encephalopathy, lactic acidosis and stroke-like episodes) can sometimes present with a stroke in a young person. Imaging may show multifocal abnormalities typically in the parieto-occipital and temporal lobes. Other features of a mitochondrial cytopathy are present (Chapter 10).

Fabry's disease is an X-linked lyposomal disorder – deficiency of α galactosidase A. Features include painful neuropathy, stroke and renal failure. A young ischaemic stroke may very rarely be the presenting feature.

### CADASIL and CARASIL

CADASIL is the acronym for Cerebral Autosomal Dominant Arteriopathy with Subcortical infarcts and Leucoencephalopathy. This is characterised by extensive white matter abnormalities and lacunar infarction. Patients may present migraine, dementia and/or progressive gait difficulty. MRI often shows characteristic involvement of the temporal white matter. Diagnosis: skin biopsy and genetic testing – mutation of the NOTCH III gene (Chapter 5). CARASIL (autosomal recessive form of CADASIL) is very rare and has similar features.

## Hypertensive Encephalopathy and Eclampsia

When the systemic BP exceeds the upper limit for cerebral autoregulation, oedema develops in the hyperperfused brain. Patients present with headache, fits, focal TIA-like events, stroke and stupor. BP is usually very high, such as 250/150 mmHg. Imaging shows a posterior leuco-encephalopathy, focal infarcts or haemorrhage. Eclampsia has similar features.

### Migraine and Stroke

There is a small but definite increase in stroke in patients with migraine. This needs to be interpreted with caution as vascular disease predisposes to migraine. For example, carotid dissection may cause a typical migraine attack. There are possible links between migraine and antiphospholipid syndrome, sickle cell disease and PFO, all of which can lead to stroke. Other migraine associations include mitochondrial disease and CADASIL.

There remain occasional cases who develop cerebral infarction at the peak of a typical migraine attack. No other reason is found. These rare strokes tend to follow features of the patient's aura: infarction usually involves the occipital cortex.

In most stroke cases with a history of migraine, the stroke is unrelated. However, stroke risk is increased in hypertensive female migraineurs who smoke and take an oral contraceptive pill.

### Moyamoya Angiopathy

Moyamoya ('puff of smoke') angiopathy refers to an angiographic appearance in which carotid occlusion is associated with a fine and friable network of basal collateral vessels. Moyamoya is a distinct condition, prevalent in Japan and occasionally elsewhere. A progressive intracranial arteriopathy develops, with stenosis and occlusion of the basal vessels, usually the termination of both internal carotid arteries and MCAs. In children, Moyamoya can present with TIAs, ischaemic stroke, chorea, severe migraine and/or seizures. The term Moyamoya also describes similar radiological appearances with another cause, such as radiotherapy or sickle cell disease.

### Reversible Cerebral Vasoconstriction and Posterior Reversible Encephalopathy Syndromes (RCVS & PRES)

There is transient but reversible constriction of intracranial arteries, typically with resolution within three months. Presentation is frequently with thunderclap headache and seizures. RCVS can be spontaneous, associated with a serious illness such as haemolytic uraemic syndrome, with eclampsia, or secondary to vasoactive substances. Posterior reversible encephalopathy syndrome (PRES) is similar – there is debate about whether or not PRES and RCVS differ. CT/MR imaging can be normal. Angiography shows segmental narrowing and dilatation – a string of beads pattern. Management: supportive, BP and seizure control. Complications: repeated seizures, SAH, ICH and ischaemic infarction. Prognosis: good in uncomplicated cases.

## Acknowledgements

I am most grateful to Nicholas Losseff, Matthew Adams, Martin Brown, Joan Grieve & Robert Simister for their contribution to *Neurology A Queen Square Textbook* Second Edition upon which this chapter was based.

I am most grateful to Professor Raymond TF Cheung, Director, Acute Stroke Service, University of Hong Kong, Hong Kong SAR, was also most helpful, both for his review of the chapter and in the provision of images.

## Further Reading

Losseff N, Adams M, Brown M, Grieve J, Simister R. Stroke & cerebrovascular diseases. In *Neurology A Queen Square Textbook*, 2nd edn. Clarke C, Howard R, Rossor M, Shorvon S, eds. John Wiley & Sons, 2016. There are numerous references.

NICE Guidelines. Stroke & transient ischaemic attack in over 16 s: diagnosis & initial management. www.nice.org.uk/guidance/ng128

## Personal References

Humphrey PRD, Clarke CRA, Greenwood RG. Cerebral venous thrombosis. In *Cerebral Vascular Disease*. In Butterworths International Medical Reviews, 1983.

Johnson SRD, Hammond A, Griffiths L, Greenwood R, Clarke CRA. Subarachnoid haemorrhage - can we do better? *J R Soc Med* 1989; 82: 721–772.

Murphy MF, Clarke CRA. Superior sagittal sinus thrombosis & essential thrombocythaemia. *Brit Med J* 1983; 287: 1344.

Also, please visit https://www.drcharlesclarke.com for free updated notes, potential links and references as these become available. You will be asked to log in, in a secure fashion, with your name and institution.

## Websites

https://www.nhs.uk/conditions/stroke/
https://www.stroke.org.uk/

# 7

# Movement Disorders

These disorders were once a neglected field, but they have been revolutionised by our understanding of neuroanatomy and neurochemistry, levodopa, genetics and neurosurgical treatments with radiostimulation. However, two issues separate movement disorders from traditional neurology:

- they are intensely visual – chorea once seen is never forgotten
- the desire to localise the causative lesion is often frustated/impossible.

Attempts are made to classify these conditions into dyskinesias, meaning added abnormal movements, and akinetic-rigid syndromes, such as parkinsonism where poverty of movement predominates. However elements of dyskinesias and poverty of movement can be present in a single condition, such as Huntington's. Chorea predominates in some, while poverty of movement appears in others. I deal first with parkinsonian syndromes and Parkinson's disease – disorders that present frequently to a general neurologist. Videos can be sourced via https://www.drcharlesclarke.com and elsewhere from the internet.

## Parkinsonian Syndromes and Parkinsonism

### Parkinsonism: Motor Features

Parkinsonism means features seen in Parkinson's disease (PD) and related disorders.

Characteristics are:

- slowness (bradykinesia), poverty and small amplitude movements (hypokinesia, akinesia)
- difficulty initiating movements, difficulty with simultaneous actions
- fatiguing and decrement of repetitive movements; rest tremor.

Most with parkinsonism have rigidity. Unlike spasticity, stiffness is equal in flexors and extensors, like bending a lead pipe. Tremor can add a ratchety, cogwheel feel to the stiffness, a.k.a. cogging.

Tremor is usual, typically a 4–6 Hz rest tremor, described in the hand as pill-rolling – between thumb and index finger. Tremor usually lessens with movement, to reappear in a

*Neurology: A Clinical Handbook*, First Edition. Charles Clarke.
© 2022 John Wiley & Sons Ltd. Published 2022 by John Wiley & Sons Ltd.

new position, a.k.a. re-emergent tremor. Some have a postural tremor. Rest tremor, particularly with a jaw tremor, is usually a pointer either to PD or drug-induced parkinsonism. Rest tremor, and jaw tremor are uncommon in other parkinsonian syndromes. Postural abnormalities, such as a stoop also develop.

Pathological classification of parkinsonism recognises:

- alpha-synucleinopathies – Lewy body diseases such as Parkinson's disease and multisytem atrophy (MSA)
- tauopathies – including progressive supranuclear palsy (PSP) and corticobasal degeneration (CBD)
- others – such as parkin mutations.

## Parkinson's Disease

The stoop, festinant – hurrying – gait and shaking will be familiar. PD was once felt to be a single entity: a progressive levodopa-responsive form of parkinsonism associated with neuronal loss and intracytoplasmic, eosinophilic, alpha-synuclein inclusions, a.k.a. Lewy bodies. Sites include pigmented brainstem nuclei – substantia nigra and locus caeruleus. This Lewy body pathology is widespread: serotonergic raphe nuclei, mesolimbic, mesocortical and tubero-infundibular pathways, nucleus basalis of Meynert, the cortex, hypothalamus, dorsal Xth nerve nucleus, olfactory tract and sympathetic ganglia are all invoved. However, it is now apparent that there are some forms of PD without Lewy bodies.

Prevalence of PD worlwide is 180/100000. Average age at onset is around 60, rising thereafter. Fewer than 5% begin before 40. Life expectancy is reduced. Causation in most remains unknown.

Most PD is apparently sporadic, but genetic forms are increasingly recognised: the *PARK* genes list now extends to over 25. For example *LRKK2* (PARK8), Park 3 and Park 5, are typical of sporadic PD. Park 1, Park 2, Park 6 and Park 7 are associated with young onset PD, typically below the age of 40.

Meta-analyses of sporadic PD show that the strongest association is with variation within the alpha-synuclein gene. One hypothesis is that exogenous alpha-synuclein fibrils enter neurones, and then promote recruitment of endogenous alpha-synuclein and Lewy body formation. Thence, Lewy body pathology is transmitted from one neurone to another.

### PD: Premotor Features

PD is a motor disorder, but there are premotor features. About 75% of nigro-striatal dopaminergic reserve must be lost before motor features emerge. Sequential fluoro-dopa PET scans have explored this premotor phase. Constipation, dysphagia, olfactory impairment, postural hypotension and REM sleep behaviour disorder (RBD, Chapter 20) can precede the motor disorder, particularly in males. RBD causes a person to act out frightening dreams. About 25% of men with RBD develop Parkinson's within a decade.

## PD: Typical Motor Presentation

Most PD cases come to light with motor features, typically asymmetrical. In some this starts in one arm, with impaired dexterity, and rest tremor. Others drag one leg or shuffle. The partner notices slowing, poverty of facial expression or impaired arm swing. Change in voice and/or micrographia develop. Pain in one limb, a frozen shoulder and back discomfort occur.

Examination reveals hypokinesia, usually with rigidity, and tremor; the earliest can be finger tremor. Sometimes, a rest tremor appears only on walking, when reduced arm swing, stoop and gait abnormality are also seen.

Features that suggest of another parkinsonian disease are symmetry of signs in the limbs, eye movement disorders and ataxia, apraxia and pyramidal signs. Early freezing of gait, although seen in PD should raise these other possibilities.

PD can be graded (Hoehn and Yahr scale). Unilateral PD is Stage 1, and progresses to Stage 2 (bilateral) within 10 years, or less, fully developed disease is Stage 4, and a bedbound immobile state Stage 5.

## PD: Non-motor Features

Many non-motor features develop:

- Depression affects many (Chapter 22). Cognitive impairment can occur early. After 20 years, most have dementia.
- Urinary urgency and nocturia are common (Chapter 25). Sialorrhoea develops.
- Pain is common, such as an aching arm.

## Investigations

Diagnosis is primarily clinical. Young onset cases under 40 years should be screened for Wilson's disease. Routine brain MRI is normal in PD. Dopamine transporter (DaT) imaging can confirm nigrostriatal disease when there is doubt.

## PD Treatment: Levodopa + DDIs: Madopar and Sinemet

Most neurologists wait until symptoms affect daily life before starting levodopa. Levodopa with peripheral dopa decarboxylase inhibitors (DDIs) carbidopa or benserazide (co-careldopa, Sinemet; co-beneldopa, Madopar) are the most effective drugs. Levodopa is transferred via proximal small bowel and across the blood–brain barrier, by an active transport system. Once in the brain, no longer protected from the peripheral DDI that cannot follow it, levodopa is metabolised in surviving presynaptic dopaminergic terminals to dopamine and released to stimulate dopamine receptors.

Two levodopa phenomena follow:

- Patients notice early morning akinesia – a wearing off – and around the same time overshoot – meaning dyskinesia when the dose is working. Generally, these problems develop in 10% of PD cases each year. Younger patients develop problems more severely.

- Gradually, a threshold level develops, so that levodopa works in an all-or-none fashion. The patient fluctuates, from ON and mobile, to OFF with parkinsonian features, sometimes over minutes.

Various tremulous levodopa dyskinesias develop. Attempts to control them with fractionation of doses or controlled release preparations are partially successful.

**Other Side Effects of Levodopa**
Levodopa can cause vomiting, by stimulating receptors in the *area postrema* in the fourth ventricle, and aggravate postural hypotension.

**Monoamine Oxidase B Inhibitors**
Selegiline and rasagiline are irreversible inhibitors of monoamine oxidase B (MAO-B), the iso-enzyme responsible for catabolising dopamine to homovanillic acid. Unlike MAO-A inhibitors, MAO-B inhibitors can be given safely with levodopa. Used alone in early disease, selegiline has been shown to delay the need for levodopa by about 9 months. These drugs have few side effects when given alone, but can potentiate any of the side effects of levodopa. Safinamide is a newer drug.

**Catechol-*O*-Methyl Transferase Inhibitors**
Entacapone and tolcapone (COMT inhibitors) block conversion of levodopa to 3-*O*-methyldopa, its principal metabolite. Both extend the elimination of levodopa, and its duration of action. A combined tablet contains levodopa, carbidopa and entacapone (Stalevo).

**Dopamine Agonists**
Dopamine agonists stimulate receptors directly. These include the ergoline drugs – bromocriptine, pergolide and cabergoline, and the non-ergoline ropinirole and pramipexole. A transdermal non-ergoline agonist (rotigotine) is also used. Apomorphine is also available – the only agonist given subcutaneously. While these agonists are sometimes given before levodopa, in an attempt to delay development of fluctuations and dyskinesias, they have a weaker anti-PD effect. Apomorphine is generally reserved for levodopa-induced complications. Dopamine agonists are often used as add-on drugs – the levodopa dose can be reduced. Some clinicians recommend dopamine agonists *de novo*. One advantage is that these drugs rarely cause fluctuations or dyskinesias but almost inevitably levodopa needs to be added later.

*Adverse Effects: Dopamine Agonists*
Dopamine agonists stimulate both peripheral and central dopamine receptors. Peripheral side effects include nausea and, rarely, aggravation of cardiac disease or peptic ulceration. All can cause ankle swelling. The ergot derivatives can cause an angry erythematous rash – erythromelalgia (Chapter 23). Ergot agonists can rarely cause lung fibrosis and effusions, retroperitoneal fibrosis and heart valve fibrosis.

Central effects include postural hypotension, excessive daytime somnolence and neuropsychiatric problems. Agonists can cause vivid dreams, and hallucinations. Impulse control disorders occur occasionally with levodopa but are commoner with agonists: hypersexuality, compulsive gambling, shopping or eating (see Chapter 22). Agonists can also cause jealousy (Othello syndrome). Punding – repeated stereotyped pointless complex behaviours, such as sorting – can occur but tends to be seen more with lengthy levodopa use.

### Anticholinergics and Amandatine

Anticholinergics such as benzhexol were the drugs used first in PD. They help sialorrhoea and reduce detrusor hyper-reflexia but they can also precipitate urinary retention.

Amantadine was used originally against influenza. It has an amphetamine-like effect. and was once used in early PD, but the effect would wane after 6 weeks. Amantadine has an anti-dyskinetic effect in some patients on levodopa, without worsening parkinsonism. It also helps freezing, in a minority. Amantadine can cause ankle oedema, livedo reticularis and hallucinations.

### Surgery for PD

For some with motor fluctuations, dyskinesias or troublesome tremor despite the available drugs, functional neurosurgery can be dramatically helpful. Thalamotomy and pallidotomy were used for many years but have been largely replaced by deep brain stimulation (DBS) with an implanted pacemaker in the thalamus, subthalamic nucleus or globus pallidus. The trend is towards earlier surgery in PD.

## Parkinson's, Dementia and Lewy Body Pathology

All PD patients have a high risk of dementia – established PD progresses over the years to PD with dementia (PDD). However, the coexistence of features of PD and dementia within 1 year is termed dementia with Lewy bodies (DLB), the commonest cause of dementia after Alzheimer's (Chapter 5). Mean survival of either DLB or PDD is less than 5 years. Histology shows Lewy bodies – often with senile plaques and neurofibrillary tangles – in both cerebral cortex and brainstem. It is impossible to distinguish PDD and DLB pathologically.

Progressive disabling cognitive impairment is a diagnostic requirement for both PDD and DLB. In DLB the following are common:

- Fluctuating cognition with pronounced variations in attention and alertness
- Recurrent visual hallucinations.

Other features of DLB are REM behaviour disoder (RBD) and neuroleptic sensitivity. There is impaired dopamine transporter uptake in the striatum on DaT scanning. Management is difficult (Chapter 22). Quetiapine is usually well tolerated. Clozapine is also used. The cholinesterase inhibitors rivastigmine and donepezil have modest effects.

## Multiple System Atrophy (MSA)

MSA causes a combination of either parkinsonism (MSA-P), cerebellar dysfunction (MSA-C), and/or autonomic failure – orthostatic hypotension, erectile dysfunction and urinary incontinence and/or incomplete bladder emptying (Chapter 25) – and, pyramidal signs.

This alpha-synucleinopathy was once known as Shy–Drager syndrome, striato-nigral degeneration, and/or a form of sporadic olivo-ponto-cerebellar atrophy (sOPCA).

Other features include RBD, snoring, stridor, emotional incontinence, finger myoclonic jerks, impaired sweating, heat intolerance, Raynaud's, cold dusky hands, antecollis, postural instability, and dysphagia. Characteristic dysarthrias – a high-pitched, quivery, strained and hypophonic in MSA-P and slurring in MSA-C. Dementia is an MSA exclusion criterion, because patients with dementia, parkinsonism and autonomic failure are more likely to have Lewy body pathology + dementia.

MSA pathology: widespread neuronal loss with ubiquitin and alpha-synuclein positive intracytoplasmic inclusions, a.k.a. glial cytoplasmic inclusions.

Prevalence is about 4/100 000, mean age at onset 57 and survival about 7 years. Autonomic failure can antedate other neurology. Pure autonomic failure (PAF) describes the situation when autonomic failure alone persists for more than 5 years (see Chapter 24). Such patients have some Lewy bodies in autonomic ganglia and *substantia nigra*. Treatment is rarely helpful.

## Progressive Supranuclear Palsy (PSP)

Sometimes known as Steele–Richardson–Olszewski syndrome, PSP is a sporadic tauopathy. PSP causes axial, symmetrical limb akinesia and rigidity. Falls, typically backwards and without warning occur. Dysarthria – growling, groaning, dysphagia and frontal cognitive deficits develop. Supranuclear gaze paresis is necessary for the diagnosis. The Doll's head manoeuvre remains intact initially. Frontalis overactivity, levator inhibition and blepharospasm also develop.

Pathology involves neuronal loss and gliosis, with straight neurofibrillary tangles and tufted astrocytes particularly in *substantia nigra*, dentate, pallidum, subthalamic nucleus and cerebral cortex. The term tauopathy describes the increase in the 4 repeat isoform of tau.

Prevalence is about 5/100 000, mean age at onset around 60 years and survival about 7 years. Some with PSP have the clinical picture above. One third have more PD-like features (PSP-P), with some levodopa response and resting tremor. Falls and gaze palsy develop later. A few PSP cases present with pure akinesia and gait freezing, with little other evidence of parkinsonism or gaze palsy.

## Corticobasal Degeneration

CBD is also a tauopathy. It shares with PSP over-representation of the H1/H1 tau haplotype, and excess of the 4 repeat tau isoform, suggesting some shared genetic susceptibility.

Many with CBD have difficulty using one limb that progressively becomes useless because of the combination of akinesia, rigidity, fixed dystonia, myoclonus, jerky tremor, cortical sensory loss and, above all, apraxia. Sometimes there is an alien limb phenomenon – the limb wanders off with a mind of its own. Progression is to all four limbs and a supranuclear gaze paresis develops. There is difficulty initiating voluntary saccades, known as oculomotor apraxia (Chapter 14), but when the eyes move they do so with normal velocity. Pathology includes swollen, a.k.a. ballooned cortical neurones predominantly in frontal and parietal areas, neurofibrillary tangles and astrocytic plaques. Mean age at onset: 63 with 8 years survival.

## Investigations: MSA, PSP, CBD

Brain imaging in disorders of movement is rarely helpful. A review of imaging on the internet can help with the rarities:

- MSA and hot cross bun sign: MSA cases develop putaminal atrophy, a hyperintense slit-like lateral rim to the putamen, or posterior putaminal hypointensity. Pontine atrophy with hyperintensity of the middle cerebellar peduncles a.k.a. hot-cross bun appearance of the pons in cross-section, and/or cerebellar atrophy may be seen.
- PSP and hummingbird sign: PSP cases may have this feature a.k.a. hummingbird sign – an increased pons to midbrain ratio on sagittal cuts and atrophy of the superior cerebellar peduncles on axial cuts.
- CBD: there can be asymmetrical or unilateral frontal and parietal atrophy.

FDG-PET scans provide evidence of nigral pathology, but cannot distinguish between these conditions. A normal scan can provide evidence in favour of psychogenic or a drug-induced movement disorder, essential or dystonic tremor. Autonomic tests indicate autonomic failure (Chapter 25), but not whether this is caused by Lewy body pathology, by MSA or by treatment.

### Ethnic and/or Region-Specific Parkinsonism
- X-linked dystonia-parkinsonism, a.k.a. Lubag, with striatal mosaicism, essentially limited to Filipinos is caused by a mutation in the *TAF1* gene. Cases respond to levodopa and DBS may help.
- A parkinsonism–dementia–ALS complex in Guam, characterised by neurofibrillary tangles rather than Lewy bodies may be environmental – it is disappearing.
- An atypical parkinsonism/PSP-like condition occurs in the Caribbean Guadeloupe archipeligo – cause unknown.

### Other Causes of Parkinsonism
Vascular parkinsonism: deep white matter vascular changes can present with parkinsonism, particularly shuffling, and/or apraxic gait. In many there is probably co-occurrence of PD with vascular disease.

Genetic causes include the Huntington's disease Westphal phenotype, Wilson's disease, SACs 1-3, in which tremor and levodopa-responsiveness occur, and in the rare frontotemporal dementia with parkinsonism.

Other causes include toxins (Chapter 19: MPTP, CO poisoning, methanol and manganese) and drugs (dopamine receptor blockers, presynaptic dopamine depletors). Parkinsonism occurs after Japanese encephalitis and encephalitis lethargica. Post-traumatic encephalopathy in boxers and hydrocephalus can cause parkinsonism and occasionally a brain tumour appears to bring on features of PD.

Coexistence of parkinsonism and dystonia should prompt investigation – imaging, genetic and heavy metal studies.

## Tremor

Tremor a feature of many movement disorders is rhythmic sinusoidal alternating movement, divided descriptively into rest tremor, postural tremor, terminal/action/intention tremor, dystonic, neuropathic, physiological and functional tremor.

### Benign Essential Tremor (ET)

ET is a common postural tremor, seen typically in the outstretched arm/hand and can be AD inherited. Most have little disability and never see a neurologist. No gene has been identified. ET often worsens slowly over years, but rarely causes much functional impairment. ET frequently improves with alcohol, even in small doses and may be helped by β-blockers, primidone, gabapentin and topiramate. Disorders mistaken as ET include dystonic tremor and enhanced physiological tremor. To confuse matters, some ET cases have rest tremor and others cerebellar features.

### Dystonic Tremor and Tremor Associated with Dystonia

DT is tremor in a body part that is also dystonic, such as tremulous torticollis. Tremor associated with dystonia describes the situation when a case of spasmodic torticollis also has a tremor of one or both arms, without overt dystonia in those limbs. Such an arm tremor usually has odd characteristics – unilateral or asymmetrical, slow, coming in flurries, jerky, position-specific or markedly worsened by certain tasks. In some, there is AD inheritance. Drugs are disappointing, but levodopa and anticholinergics are worth trying.

DT (and occasionally ET) can sometimes be helped by botulinum toxin or, rarely, thalamic or pallidal DBS.

### Neuropathic Tremor and Fragile X Tremor Ataxia Syndrome (FXTAS)

Some neuropathies, particularly IgM paraprotein neuropathy can cause a postural or resting tremor. Tremor severity does not correlate with the neuropathy. With FXTAS there can be late progressive ataxia and cognitive decline (Chapter 17).

### Cerebellar (Pathway) Tremor and Holmes Tremor

Intention tremor is caused by brainstem or cerebellar outflow lesions. A common cause is MS. The tremor is action/terminal and worsens steadily throughout a movement. Drugs are unhelpful. DBS may help but in MS its benefits are usually minor.

Holmes tremor a.k.a. midbrain tremor or rubral (red nuclear) tremor is a rare three part tremor – tremor at rest, postural tremor and intention tremor. It follows damage to the cerebello-rubrothalamic and nigro-striatal pathways and is sometimes seen in Wilson's disease.

### Palatal Tremor

Rhythmic (1–2 Hz) contractions of the soft palate, follow dysfunction between dentate nucleus, red nucleus and inferior olivary nuclei, a.k.a. the Guillain–Mollaret triangle.

- Essential palatal myoclonus (EPM) consists of contractions of the *tensor veli palatini* (Vth nerve), typically associated with a clicking noise.
- In symptomatic palatal myoclonus (SPM), the main tremulous muscle is *tensor palatini*, SPM may be associated with vertical ocular movements, a.k.a. oculopalatal myoclonus and/or or rhythmic and tremulous limb movements. Causes include Wilson's, and Alexander's disease (Chapter 19) and rarely a stroke.
- Oculomasticatory myorhythmia a.k.a. oculo-facial-skeletal myorhythmia is usually pathognomonic of Whipple's disease (Chapter 26).

### Orthostatic Tremor

This rarity causes people to feel unsteady, and tremulous while standing still, but not on walking. They either sit down or keep moving. There is tremor of leg muscles, easily recorded on surface EMG, and often felt or auscultated. Some cases have parkinsonism or restless legs. Clonazepam sometimes helps.

### Drug, Metabolic, Toxin-Induced Tremors and Functional Tremor

Tremor can be caused by many drugs and toxins: dopamine-depleting or receptor-blocking drugs – cinnarazine, some calcium-channel blockers, diltiazem, valproate and beta-agonists – theophylline, caffeine, nicotine, lithium, amiodarone, SSRIs, tricyclics, ciclosporin, thyroxine excess, chronic alcoholism, and with marijuana, cocaine, amphetamines and mercury intoxication. Functional tremor: see functional disorders, below.

## Dystonia

Dystonia describes involuntary muscle spasms that lead to an abnormal posture of part of the body. Typically, these spasms tend to move around – a slow writhing movements, known as athetosis. Contraction of both agonist and antagonist muscles causes the abnormal posturing. Dystonia varies: in some it is slow, in others jerks predominate. The abnormal posture can be subtle, or task or position-specific, such as only on writing (writer's cramp) or playing an instrument. Another feature, seen in focal dystonia, is a sensory manoevre, a trick to help the posture resolve, a.k.a. *une geste antagoniste*. For example, with torticollis, a light touch in a particular place on the neck, known to the patient, helps muscles relax.

**Classification**

Clinically, I try to divide cases into one of these categories:

- primary dystonia – where dystonia is the only feature, either focal (such as writer's cramp) or generalised, and +/− tremor,
- secondary – hereditary or degenerative dystonia – conditions such as Wilson's, and symptomatic – following TBI or stroke
- dystonia-plus – rare dopa-responsive dystonia (DRD) and myoclonus-dystonia (MD)
- paroxysmal dyskinesias, with dystonia
- psychogenic dystonia.

Age of onset, below about 30, and whether it is focal, segmental, generalised can be useful to decide whether a case fits into a category. A young-onset focal dystonia, such as a torticollis is likely to be primary. A 35-year-old with generalised dystonia and progressive cognitive decline is probably secondary.

## Primary Generalised Dystonia

Generalised dystonia, before 30 years commonly begins in one limb, followed by gradual generalisation. *Dystonia musculorum deformans*, a.k.a. Oppenheim's dystonia describes many cases. About 70% carry a single GAG deletion in the *DYT1* gene on chromosome 9 – AD, with low penetrance.

There are over 25 genetic associations (DYT1–DYT25), divided into young and adult onset groups. One condition causing primary cranio-cervical dystonia with onset in young adults is *DYT6*, follows mutation in the *THAP1* gene on chromosome 8. Laryngeal, cervical and/or oromandibular dystonia spread to the limbs.

**Primary Focal Dystonia**

When dystonia appears in later adult life, focal dystonia is common. Cervical dystonia, a.k.a. spasmodic torticollis, cranial dystonias, such as blepharospasm, Meige syndrome [blepharospasm with oromandibular dystonia], writer's cramp, laryngeal dystonia and other task-specific dystonias are examples. Cranio-cervical dystonia is commoner in women, while task-specific dystonias, such as writer's cramp are commoner in males.

**Secondary Heredo-Degenerative Dystonias**

Dystonia can feature in many neurodegenerative conditions: Wilson's disease, neurodegeneration with brain iron accumulation (NBIA, *PANK2* mutations), neuro-acanthocytosis, Huntington's, Niemann–Pick type C, metachromatic leuco-dystrophy, GM1/GM2 gangliosidosis, glutaric acidaemia, SCA2 or SCA3.

**Wilson's Disease**

Wilson's disease (WD) is a treatable AR disorder of copper metabolism. It occurs worldwide with prevalence of 1–3/100 000. More than 300 mutations have been identified in the gene *ATP7B* on chromosome 13 that encodes a copper-dependent transmembrane protein P type ATPase. The commonest mutation is H1069Q in Europe.

### Presentations

Most neurological WD presents before 20, with slurred speech, a movement and behavioural disorder – and almost always before 40. The pseudo-MS form is commonest, with a wing-beating tremor, a.k.a. Holmes tremor, ataxia and dysarthria. Dystonia or an akinetic-rigid syndrome may predominate, with *risus sardonicus* and/or pseudobulbar palsy. Chorea occurs in about 10%. Cognitive dysfunction develops, seizures, myoclonus and pyramidal signs. Virtually everyone with WD with neurological dysfunction has brown or greenish Kayser–Fleischer (K-F) rings – copper deposition on the cornea in Descemet's membrane.

WD can also present with acute liver failure, hepatitis or cirrhosis and with haemolytic anaemia. Other features include a blue-ish nail discolouration, aminoaciduria and cardiomyopathy.

### Diagnosis

Any emerging movement disorder should raise the question of WD. Possible cases should also be seen by an ophthalmologist.

Low serum caeruloplasmin is diagnostic when K-F rings are present. A few WD patients with decompensated liver disease have normal levels. In females, the contraceptive pill can raise a low level to normal. Some heterozygotes have a reduced caeruloplasmin level. Urinary copper is elevated. Liver biopsy shows cirrhosis and high hepatic copper. Genetic testing is available. MRI: T2W and T1W changes in the putamen, globus pallidus, thalamus, midbrain, pons and cerebellum, white matter abnormalities and cortical atrophy. Screening of first degree relatives is essential following diagnosis.

### Treatment

All cases should be treated in a specialist unit. The first treatments were British anti-Lewisite (BAL) in 1951 and penicillamine in 1956. Over 50 years penicillamine's value has been confirmed. Trientene is an alternative. Chocolate, liver, nuts, mushrooms and shellfish contain copper and are best avoided. Anticholinergics may help dystonia. Some with an akinetic-rigid syndrome improve with levodopa. There is an elevated risk of liver cancer. With liver disease, transplantation can be life-saving.

## Secondary Symptomatic Dystonia

Dystonia follows basal ganglia damage. Dystonia can develop following TBI, cerebral palsy – such as kernicterus following haemolytic disease of the newborn – and following stroke. A static deficit is usual. Onset can be delayed for years following injury.

## Dopa-Responsive Dystonia (DRD)

Dopa-responsive dystonia (DRD; *DYT5*), a.k.a. Segawa disease, typically presents in childhood with lower limb dystonia. Parkinsonism may develop, typically when onset is in a young adult. DRD is an AD condition with poor penetrance, caused by mutations in the GTP cyclohydrolase 1 gene (*GTPCH1*; *DYT5*), a rate-limiting step in dopamine production from tyrosine. Although rare, DRD is important because it is treatable with small doses of levodopa. This typically leads to resolution, without levodopa complications seen in PD.

DRD can present with unusual phenotypes, such as spastic diplegia, writer's cramp, cervical dystonia and even ataxia. Thus, a trial of levodopa is essential in all with young onset dystonia. It is important to differentiate DRD patients from those with young onset PD and foot dystonia. DaT imaging can help – normal in DRD.

### Myoclonus-Dystonia (MD)

Patients with myoclonus-dystonia (MD; *DYT11*), caused by AD mutations in the ε-sarcoglycan gene on chromosome 7q21, have early onset dystonia with sudden, lightning jerks. The myoclonus responds dramatically to alcohol, in small amounts. *DYT11* MD typically starts in childhood. Movements affect mainly the head, neck and arm. Myoclonus worsens during movement (action myoclonus). Anxiety, depression and OCDs are also common. Some cases are mutation-negative.

### Paroxysmal Dyskinesias

Paroxysmal dyskinesias are attacks of involuntary movements, usually dystonia, chorea or ballism, with normal neurological examination between attacks. The duration can be seconds to hours. Episodes are typically induced by triggers:

- sudden movements (paroxysmal kinesigenic dyskinesia; PKD)
- prolonged exercise (paroxysmal exercise-induced dyskinesia; PED)
- alcohol and coffee (paroxysmal non-kinesigenic dyskinesia; PNKD) and
- sleep (paroxysmal nocturnal dyskinesia; PND).

Mutations in these primary paroxysmal dyskinesias have been identified:

- PRRT2 gene mutations underlie most sporadic and familial PKD cases.
- Mutations of the myofibrillogenesis regulator gene (*MR-1*) have been identified in PNKD.
- Mutations in the glucose transporter 1 gene (Glut1) can lead to PED.
- In PND, nicotinic acetylcholine receptor gene mutations occur – an example of a ligand-gated channelopathy.

Secondary paroxysmal dyskinesias also occur in MS, and rarely in vascular disease, HIV, cytomegalovirus, following TBI, in many neurodegenerative diseases, cancers and cerebral palsy.

Anticonvulsants – carbamazepine in PKD, benzodiazepines, barbiturates or acetazolamide may help. PED related to Glut1 gene mutations may benefit by ketogenic diet. Trigger factors should be avoided, obviously.

### Management of Secondary Dystonia

Investigation depends on the setting. Exclusion of Wilson's is essential. Drug treatment is disappointing. Anticholinergics such as trihexyphenidyl are used. Clonazepam can help tremor, jerks and pain. Other drugs include tetrabenazine and baclofen. Botulinum toxin has revolutionised focal dystonias – injected by a doctor with experience of movement disorders, not cosmetics. DBS can sometimes help.

# Chorea

Chorea is derived from Greek (a dance) and describes excessive movements, irregular, random and abrupt. Severity ranges from restlessness with exaggeration of normal gestures, fidgeting and/or dancing gait to continuous violent movements.

Acquired causes: stroke, hyperglycaemia, mass lesion, neuro-acanthocytosis, drugs, thyrotoxicosis, hypocalcaemia/hypoparathyroidism, SLE/antiphospholipid syndrome, Sydenham's chorea, paediatric autoimmune neurological disorder associated with streptococci (PANDAS), HSV, *chorea gravidarum, polycythaemia rubra vera*, HIV, nvCJD.

Genetic causes: Huntington's disease and phenocopies, Macleod syndrome, dentato-rubro-pallido-luysian atrophy, benign hereditary chorea (BHC), SCAS 1, 2, 3 and 17, mitochondrial disorders, inherited prion disease, Wilson's, Friedreich's, NBIA type 1, ataxia telangiectasia, neuroferritinopathy, lysosomal storage disorders, amino acid disorders, tuberous sclerosis.

Most choreas have a slow onset, usually noticed by others. Whilst many are associated with cognitive and/or behavioural changes, do not make the error that the person whose movements make them appear unusual have either cognitive decline or a non-organic condition. There is also a tendency to overdiagnose Huntington's in an adult presenting with chorea, before investigation for diseases mentioned above.

## Huntington's Disease

Huntington's disease (HD) is a worldwide progressive AD neurodegeneration – the commonest inherited chorea, described in 1872. Onset is around 40 years, though juvenile and elderly cases occur. HD progresses inexorably with death usually within 20 years. Prevalence is around 10/100 000 in most populations.

In 1993, the gene defect was identified as a CAG repeat expansion, encoding polyglutamine repeats within a novel protein, *huntingtin*. This highly polymorphic CAG repeat is located in exon 1 of chromosome 4. Adult onset patients usually have 40–55 repeats, and juvenile cases over 60. CAG repeats above 40 are fully penetrant.

CAG repeat lengths vary from generation to generation but there is a tendency for repeat lengths to increase. This tendency to expand underlies anticipation – increase in severity and earlier onset during transmission between generations.

There is good correlation between CAG repeat size and age of onset, and progression: the larger the repeat, the earlier the onset. Most individuals with more than 50 repeats develop HD before the age of 30.

In the early stages, the brain can look macroscopically and radiologically normal. Later there is cortical atrophy, and atrophy of the caudate, *putamen, globus pallidus* and *substantia nigra*.

### Features and Diagnosis

HD has a varied phenotype and as the disease progresses, signs change: disease duration can modify features. Huntington's may not be obvious in the family history, or may have been concealed. Onset is difficult to discern. Many report psychiatric or mild cognitive symptoms before motor problems. However, the diagnosis is usually made when motor abnormalities appear. Subtle abnormalities include restlessness, darting eye movements, hyper-reflexia, impaired finger tapping, and fidgety finger, hand and toe movements during stress. Oculomotor abnormalities develop: gaze impersistence, distractibility and delayed initiation or slowing of voluntary saccades – vertical worse than horizontal.

As HD progresses, obvious signs develop. Chorea is seen in 90% of adult onset patients but may decrease if dystonia, rigidity and parkinsonism develop. In the limbs there is impaired voluntary function with clumsiness and impairment in fine motor control and speed. Gait disturbance develops with postural reflex changes and falls. Dysarthria and dysphagia are common. Adult-onset HD can occasionally present with parkinsonian features.

Cognitive abnormalities are universal. Key abnormalities are impaired executive function, poor planning and judgement, impulsive behaviour, disorganised actions and difficulty coping with multiple tasks. Many patients exhibit psychomotor slowing with apathy, lack of self-care and loss of initiative. Patients often complain early on of visual and verbal memory problems.Psychiatric and cognitive features often cause the greatest distress. Depression and anxiety, irritability and aggression are common. As the disease progresses, obsessions and compulsions emerge. The suicide rate is higher than in the general population.

Genetic testing provides confirmation. Genotype–phenotype studies have documented disorders similar to HD (HD phenocopies) but are HD gene negative.

### Juvenile Huntington's

Juvenile HD cases are those with onset before 20, usually with repeat lengths greater than 60. Typically they have severe disease and a short life expectancy. An akinetic-rigid form (Westphal variant) occurs in juvenile HD – little chorea and mainly rigidity/dystonia.

## Neuro-Acanthocytoses

Neuro-acanthocytoses are rare conditions in which spikey red blood cells (acanthocytes) are seen in peripheral blood films. There are associated movement disorders, including chorea.

AR neuro-acanthocytosis is associated with mutations in the *CHAC* gene leading to production of a truncated protein *chorein*. Onset is typically in the fourth decade with a progressive movement disorder, psychiatric and cognitive changes which mimic HD. Unlike HD, seizures are seen in 50%. A distal amyotrophy and/or axonal neuropathy, with a high CK level can occur. Analysis of fresh blood films for greater than 3% of acanthocytes is diagnostic. Genetic testing is difficult: confirmation relies on finding low erythrocyte membrane *chorein* blood levels.

Macleod's syndrome is an X-linked recessive disorder linked to mutations in the *XK* gene, that encodes a specific Kell system antigen. Disease usually begins around the age of 45 and is slowly progressive, with chorea and facial tics. Dystonia is less common than in AR neuro-acanthocytosis. Dementia and psychiatric features develop. Axonal neuropathy, cardiomyopathy and haemolytic anaemia can occur. CK is often elevated.

Acanthocytes have also been described in pantothenate kinase-associated neurodegeneration (PKAN, PANK2, NBIA type 1) and HDL2.

## Post-Streptococcal Autoimmune Disorders

Sydenham's chorea and PANDAS (Paediatric Autoimmune Neurological Disorders Associated with Streptococcal infection) can both present with chorea and neuropsychiatric problems. Sydenham's chorea is a manifestation of rheumatic fever. It occurs between 5 and 15 years, mainly in girls and is now rare. Widespread chorea, behavioural disturbance and OCD symptoms are common. It is self-limiting, usually within 6 months, though some are recurrent. Antibodies to basal ganglia can be detected in some. The mechanism is thought to be cross-reaction between anti-streptococcal antibodies and basal ganglia neurones, an example of molecular mimicry. PANDAS is discussed under tics.

## Benign Hereditary Chorea

BHC is a rare AD disorder caused by mutations in the gene encoding thyroid transcription factor 1 (*TITF1*), and rarely other mutations such as ADCY5, encoding adenyl cyclase 5. It is usually of early onset, with progressive chorea but without cognitive decline. Some cases have dystonia, myoclonic jerks, dysarthria, gait disturbances or low intelligence. Some also have hypothyroidism and respiratory abnormalities, a.k.a. brain–thyroid–lung syndrome.

## Drug-Induced Chorea

Many drugs can cause chorea – neuroleptics (tardive dyskinesia), levodopa/dopamine agonists/anticholinergics, anti-epileptics (phenytoin, carbamazepine, valproate, gabapentin), CNS stimulants (amphetamines, methylphenidate, cocaine), benzodiazepines, oestrogens (oral contraceptives and rarely, HRT) and lithium.

## Chorea: Drug Management

Chorea can cause distress but some do not notice its severity: their relatives do. No drug is particularly good. Sulpiride, olanzapine, risperidone and tetrabenazine can help to damp down movements but they can worsen speech, swallowing, gait and balance.

# Tics

Tics are brief rapid intermittent stereotyped involuntary movements, or sounds a.k.a. motor tics. Common tics are blinking, shoulder elevation, a grimace, or a sniff – all part of our normal repertoire. Tics can be suppressed, at least temporarily, but at the expense of rising inner tension, often followed by an exacerbation. Most tics are abrupt (clonic). However, they can be slow, sustained, dystonic or tonic – simply with muscle tensioning.

## Gilles de la Tourette Syndrome

Gilles de la Tourette syndrome (GTS) is a widely recognised childhood tic variety. Criteria include multiple motor tics and phonic and/or vocal tics. These must last longer than a year for a GTS diagnosis. Motor and phonic tics need not occur together – they wax and wane, occur in bouts and are suggestible and suppressible. Mean age at onset is 7–11 years. Some disappear by 18, the usual latest age of onset. Behaviours such as OCD (Chapter 22) may well persist.

Tics in GTS can be blinking, eye rolling, head nodding, facial grimacing or complex – touching, squatting. Premonitory sensations can be localised – around the area of the tic – or generalised. Tics usually begin in the head and face. Phonic tics are sniffs, gulps, snorts and coughs. Complex vocal tics include barking, and inappropriate words. New tics can appear, such as a cough persisting after a respiratory infection. Other features include echolalia – copying what others say, and echopraxia – copying what others do, palilalia – repeating part of a sentence. Swearing (coprolalia) – often disguised – is uncommon.

GTS occurs worldwide. M:F 3:1. In some families it seems that males have GTS, whereas females have OCD. Prevalence in individuals with learning difficulties or autistic spectrum disorders is high. Over three quarters with GTS have psychiatric co-morbidity. Among the more common are ADHD and OCD. Checking and counting rituals and compulsions – to touch objects or people can be present. Anger control problems, sleep difficulties, and self-injury are common. Patients with GTS tend to have depression, anxiety and a degree of hostility.

Various causes have been postulated – genetics, neuro-immunological reactions to an infection, prenatal and perinatal problems, and less credibly psychological explanations. Segregation analysis suggests that GTS is genetic, consistent with a single major gene and AD transmission, but with incomplete penetrance. PANDAS was coined for children with post-streptococcal OCD and tics. This mechanism remains controversial, but anti-basal ganglia antibodies occur in some GTS cases. The general view is that streptococcal infection probably does not cause GTS, but individuals inherit susceptibility both to GTS and to the way they react to some infections.

## Other Tic Disorders

Tic disorders, usually motor are much more common than GTS. The most common are:

- Transient tic disorder (TTD) – single or multiple tics, for a month or so
- Chronic motor or vocal tic disorder – motor or vocal tics but not both for more than 1 year

Tics can also be seen in WD, neuro-acanthocytosis, Lesch–Nyhan syndrome, neuroferritinopathy, autism spectrum disorders, following TBI and after neuroleptics.

## Management of Tics

In many cases, explanation, reassurance and education may be all that are required. When a tic is causing problems, CBT and habit reversal training may be useful. The main drugs, when they are really necessary are neuroleptics in small doses. The older neuroleptics such as pimozide, and the newer atypical neuroleptics such as risperidone can help. Clonidine and guanfacine can also help tics and ADHD. Individuals with these benign conditions should be warned of the risk of a tardive movement disorder. Antidepressants may help.

## Myoclonus and Startle Syndromes

Myoclonus is a sudden brief shock-like involuntary movement following muscular contraction or inhibition. Positive myoclonus is a muscle contraction. Inhibition causes negative myoclonus, a.k.a. asterixis – liver flap. Many conditions produce myoclonus, leading to extensive lists but the movements are seldom much help in diagnosis. Myoclonus is common in epilepsy, in many neurodegenerations, following TBI and stroke and in many metabolic disorders such as hepatic failure. Varieties are not discussed further here.

Treatment of myclonus depends upon the underlying disorder. Valproate, piracetam, levetiracetam, clonazepam, lamotrigine and phenobarbital are used. Bilateral pallidal DBS has been used for severe myoclonus-dystonia. Botulinum toxin can help palatal myoclonus and hemifacial spasm.

The startle reflex means the bilateral synchronous shock movements evoked by sudden stimuli. The nucleus *reticularis pontis caudalis* is important. Abnormalities can be grouped into:

- Excessive startle occurs in anxiety, panic and PTSD.
- Hyperekplexia: generalised stiffness is noticed soon after birth, subsiding during infancy, but with excessive startle that persists throughout life. There is generalised stiffness for a few seconds following startle, that can cause a fall. Mutations in the α1 subunit of the glycine receptor gene, *GLRA1* have been found.
- Startle epilepsy is an asymmetric tonic epileptic seizure induced by a sudden stimulus, mostly in children with infantile hemiplegia.
- The Jumping Frenchmen of Maine: a family of nineteenth century lumberjacks with a disorder of unknown origin: an exaggerated startle reflex and an uncontrollable jump.

## Functional Movement Disorders

Functional movement disorders (FMD) can take many forms: dystonia and tremor are the most common. A synopsis of functional neurological problems is in Chapter 22, and illustrates a potential difference between neuropsychiatrists and movement disorder neurologists. In short, in movement disorder neurology, these conditions tend to be labelled as psychogenic, and thus have a potential psychiatric cause. Neuropsychiatry is less dogmatic; frequently, no psychiatric diagnosis emerges. Diagnosis of a FMD is primarily clinical.

Though none is pathognomonic, positive features include:

- fluctuations during examination, distractibility, increase with attention/suggestion
- incongruence with patterns of recognised movement disorders

- non-organic signs, discrepancy between objective signs and disability
- abrupt onset with rapid progression to maximum severity, inconsistency over time
- a history of previous somatisations; substantial response to placebo or psychotherapy.

In some cases investigations can help to exclude a psychogenic cause. In myoclonus, electrophysiology (EEG/EMG) can be helpful. With apparent slowness, a normal DaT SPECT scan points away from Parkinson's.

An FMD diagnosis should not be made simply because a movement is bizarre. Be aware of exaggeration of a typical organic movement disorder, and that many movements labelled initially as non-organic turn out to be true disorders of movement.

The prognosis of any long-standing FMD is generally poor. Exploration of psychiatric disorders may be needed. Avoidance of unnecessary drugs and perpetuating illness beliefs are important.

## Movement Disorders and Dopamine Receptor Blockade

Neuroleptics – dopamine receptor blocking drugs – are widely used. Drug-induced parkinsonism (DIP) occurs frequently. Often mild, it can be asymmetrical. The majority remit within weeks of stopping the drug. DaT SPECT imaging is normal in DIP. These notes summarise problems that neuroleptics can cause.

Acute dystonic reactions arise within hours of starting a drug, predominantly of the head and neck, with oculogyric, jaw and neck dystonia. Attacks subside over hours, but within minutes after a small dose of an IV anticholinergic, such as benzhexol.

Akathisia is a compulsion to move, a restlessness with pacing up and down or shifting from one foot to the other.

Tardive dyskinesia arises after weeks, months or years of treatment, but persists, sometimes permanently. It can even begin, or worsen, after discontinuing a drug. Most cases have rapid, choreiform bucco-linguo-masticatory movements, with lip-smacking and tongue protrusion. These are common with increasing age and in females.

Tardive dystonia, commoner in young males, resembles idiopathic dystonia-torticollis, axial dystonia, retrocollis or opisthotonic trunk movements and pelvic thrusting movements occur.

Newer atypical neuroleptic drugs are safer but there are no entirely safe dopamine receptor blocking drugs and, at least for tardive dystonia, no safe period of use. Metoclopramide is also a rare cause of these movement disorders.

Anticholinergics can worsen choreiform tardive dyskinesia, but can improve tardive dystonia. Tetrabenazine can sometimes help both. Paradoxically, just as tardive dyskinesia can present when the dose of a neuroleptic is reduced, or stopped, an increase in the dose of the drug can improve movements, but only briefly, before aggravating the problem.

Tardive tics, myoclonus and tremor are uncommon.

The neuroleptic malignant syndrome is a potentially fatal reaction to dopamine receptor blocking drugs (Chapter 19).

## Restless Legs Syndrome and Painful Legs and Moving Toes

Restless legs syndrome (RLS, a.k.a. Willis-Ekbom disease) is a common movement disorder over 50. RLS causes unpleasant sensations or an urge to move the legs usually on retiring to bed, and almost instantly, relieved by getting up and walking about. There are associations with iron deficiency, uraemia, pregnancy, peripheral neuropathy and PD. Serum ferritin may be low (Chapter 19). In most no cause is found.

If drugs are needed, dopamine agonists, such as pramipexole or ropinirole are better than levodopa. Second line drugs: gabapentin, carbamazepine and clonazepam. RLS is commonly associated with periodic leg movements of sleep (PLMS). Several gene associations have been found.

Painful legs and moving toes (Chapter 23) describes slow undulating flexion–extension movements of the toes with leg pain, usually unilateral. No cause is usually found and treatment ineffective.

## Stiff Person and Stiff Limb Syndromes Fatal Encephalomyelitis with Rigidity

Stiff person syndrome is characterised by axial rigidity at rest mainly of the trunk, causing hyperlordosis, and sometimes stiff proximal lower limb muscles. Continuous motor activity persists even when trying to relax: EMG electrical silence cannot be obtained. Rigidity and continuous motor unit activity lessens or disappears, during sleep, and after spinal or general anaesthesia. Deep tendon reflexes are enhanced and spread, to produce spasms. Some cases have anti-GAD and/or glycine receptor antibodies. There is a limited response to baclofen and to diazepam.

Stiff limb syndrome is rarer – rigidity, spasms and abnormal postures of a distal limb. Autoimmune markers are infrequent. The condition responds poorly to treatment.

An even rarer disorder is a rapidly fatal inflammatory encephalomyelitis with rigidity, sometimes paraneoplastic. Anti-GAD and glycine receptor antibodies may be found and also sometimes amphiphysin and DPPX antibodies.

## Acknowledgements

I am most grateful to Kailash Bhatia, Carla Cordivari, Mark Edwards, Thomas Foltynie, Marwan Hariz, Prasad Korlipara, Patricia Limousin, Niall Quinn, Sarah Tabrizi and Thomas Warner for their contribution to *Neurology A Queen Square Textbook* Second Edition on which this chapter is based. I am also most grateful to Dr Eoin Mulroy, Edmond J. Safra Movement Disorder Clinical & Research Fellow, Department of Clinical & Movement Neurosciences, UCL Queen Square Institute of Neurology who assembled the videos of movement disorders for this chapter. These are available via https://www.drcharlesclarke.com.

## Further Reading

Bhatia K, Cordivari C, Edwards M, Foltynie T, Hariz M, Korlipara P, Limousin P, Quinn N, Tabrizi S, Warner T. Movement disorders. In *Neurology A Queen Square Textbook*, 2nd edn. Clarke C, Howard R, Rossor M, and Shorvon S, eds. John Wiley & Sons, 2016. There are numerous references.

## Websites

https://www.nhs.uk/conditions/parkinsons-disease/
https://www.movementdisorders.org/
Videos of movement disorders and updated information: https://www.drcharlesclarke.com.

# 8

# Epilepsy and Related Disorders

An epileptic seizure is the effect of focal or generalised neuronal activity in the cerebral cortex – with abnormal neuronal synchronisation, excessive excitation and/or inadequate inhibition. Epilepsy implies a liability to have recurrent seizures, with cognitive and psychosocial consequences and co-morbidities. Epilepsy is common. Incidence: about 80/100 000/year. Point prevalence: about 4–10 per 1000, higher in lower socio-economic groups. Seizures are commonest in infants and in later life. About 40% develop epilepsy below 16 and 20% over 65. A first and only seizure occurs in 20 persons per 100 000/year. The lifetime risk of a fit is 4%. For established epilepsy, mortality is double that in the general population – either from the cause, such as a tumour, or from accidents, sudden death in epilepsy (SUDEP) or suicide. SUDEP causes one death/100 patients/year amongst those with severe epilepsy. Many with epilepsy have learning disability and are dependent upon others.

## International League Against Epilepsy Classification

Seizure types are divided broadly into partial and generalised. The ILAE detail is outside the scope of this chapter, but the framework is useful:

- Simple partial and complex partial seizures
- Partial seizures evolving to a secondarily generalised seizure
- Generalised seizures – absence, tonic-clonic (*grand mal*) and others

A generalised seizure arises from cortex in both hemispheres – consciousness is lost. A partial (a.k.a. focal) seizure arises from a unilateral focus. Complex partial denotes loss of consciousness, while simple partial seizure implies preservation of consciousness.

A secondarily generalised seizure has a focal (partial) onset that becomes generalised. A partial seizure implies some focal pathology, that may remain occult.

### Simple and Complex Partial Seizures

Features reflect the cortical focus:

*Neurology: A Clinical Handbook*, First Edition. Charles Clarke.
© 2022 John Wiley & Sons Ltd. Published 2022 by John Wiley & Sons Ltd.

- Motor: jerking, spasms or posturing, speech arrest, choking, head turning, hemiparesis (a.k.a. Todd's paralysis)
- Sensory: tingling, numbness or pain.
- Visual: flashing lights and colours.
- Temporal lobe: a rising epigastric sensation.

The aura, the seizure prelude – itself a simple partial attack – may also point to the origin:

- Dysphasia/speech arrest – frontal or temporo-parietal
- Memories – flashbacks, *déjà vu, jamais vu,* memory distortions: mesial temporal
- Cognitive – dreamy states, sensations of unreality, depersonalisation: temporal lobes
- Affective – fear, depression, anger, elation, erotic thoughts, serenity, exhilaration: mesial temporal. Laughter a.k.a. gelastic seizures – fronto-temporal,
- Illusions of size (macropsia, micropsia), shape, weight, or sound – temporal or parieto-occipital
- Hallucinations – visual, auditory, gustatory or olfactory, crude or elaborate – temporal or parieto-occipital association areas
- Tastes, usually unpleasant – frontal or temporal lobes
- Auditory/changes in auditory perception (rare): Heschl's gyrus.

With a complex partial seizure the focus is within one temporal lobe in over half, in a frontal lobe in a third and elsewhere in about 10%. There are three components: aura, absence and automatism. Aura is a simple partial seizure, usually a few seconds; isolated auras are common. Absence: motor and speech arrest – the patient appears vacant. Automatism: involuntary action, with impaired awareness – and amnesia. Automatisms, commonest with temporal and frontal lobe foci, include chewing, lip smacking, swallowing or drooling, fiddling, tidying, undressing, walking, running, humming, whistling. Violent behaviour – usually when confused – is seldom coordinated and rarely remembered.

## Generalised Seizures

These include tonic–clonic seizures, a.k.a. *grand mal* fits, absence seizures, and rarer tonic and atonic seizures. Consciousness is impaired, jerking is bilateral and largely symmetrical.

A tonic–clonic seizure is a generalised convulsion, a *grand mal* fit, sometimes preceded by an ill-defined feeling or myoclonic jerking. If an aura preceded the fit – a partial seizure in the seconds before it - this indicates that the convulsion was secondarily generalised. Loss of consciousness follows, sometimes with a guttural sound, a.k.a. epileptic cry. Stiffening, the tonic phase ensues. The patient may fall, sometimes flexed but then in axial extension, with jaw clamped, limbs stiff, adducted and extended, fists clenched. Respiration ceases, with cyanosis. The eyes remain open with pupils dilated. Tachycardia, bradycardia and even asystole occur. This tonic phase lasts 10–30 seconds.

The clonic phase follows, with convulsions, usually of all four limbs and face. Breathing is stertorous. Saliva froths from the mouth. Tongue biting occurs – typically unilaterally. Convulsive movements cease, usually within two minutes followed by flaccidity. Consciousness slowly returns, but the patient remains confused, headachy, dazed and sleepy. During a seizure periorbital petechiae can form; vertebral crush fractures and posterior shoulder dislocation can occur, rather than the common anterior dislocation. All these features do not occur in every *grand mal,* but the phases are important. For example, a sudden apparent convulsion, without any prelude or tonic phase should raise the question of NEAD. Less common variants such as tonic (stiffness alone) and atonic seizures (drop attacks) tend to occur with diffuse damage, usually with other seizure types.

### Typical and Atypical Absence Seizures, and Myoclonic Seizures

These are also generalised epilepsies. *Petit mal* (a typical absence seizure) develops in an otherwise normal child. In *petit mal* there is abrupt loss of consciousness and cessation of motor activity. The patient looks vacant. The attack ends abruptly and activity is resumed as if nothing had happened. Most last less than 10 seconds. Blinking, jerks, alterations in tone and/or brief automatisms can occur, many times a day. Absences may follow flashing lights, hyperventilation, or exhaustion. EEG is diagnostic: high voltage, symmetrically synchronous 3 Hz spike-waves.

An atypical absence, usually associated with learning disability and/or multiple seizure types tends to be longer than a *petit mal*; loss of awareness is often incomplete. Jerks can be prominent and onset and cessation less abrupt. Ictal EEG: diffuse, asymmetric spike-wave bursts at 2–2.5 Hz. In a myoclonic seizure there are brief muscle contractions following a cortical discharge. These seizures vary, from almost imperceptible twitches to severe repetitive jerking with falling or propulsion of objects. Myoclonic seizures occur in idiopathic generalised epilepsy, in epileptic encephalopathies, such as Lennox–Gastaut and in progressive myoclonic epilepsies. Focal myoclonus can also occur in epilepsy of frontal or occipital origin.

## Classification and Causes of Epilepsy

One problem is that classification varies in authoritive texts. Another issue is that subdivisions are not absolute, for example a neurocutaneous syndrome such as tuberous sclerosis is both genetic and structural. Broadly: in childhood, genetic and congenital conditions are common. In adults, acquired causes are more frequent. In some regions, infections – such as neurocysticercosis – are important. The main question with new onset epilepsy in an adult neurology clinic is typically whether there could be an underlying cause such as a tumour. Many conditions in Table 8.1 will not be discussed further here – and there are many more.

Symptomatic epilepsy means seizures caused by any known or suspected CNS disorder – many brain diseases can cause epilepsy. An epilepsy syndrome (ILAE framework) implies features that occur together, such as in West and Lennox-Gastaut syndromes.

### Single-Gene and Other Disorders

Childhood Absence Epilepsy: seen mainly below 10 – about 10% of childhood epilepsies. Absence attacks occur and tonic-clonic seizures. Prognosis: generally good response to therapy.

**Table 8.1**  Epilepsy: by aetiology

| ILAE category/cause | Subcategory | Examples |
| --- | --- | --- |
| Mainly genetic and/or metabolic | Single-gene and other disorders | Childhood absence epilepsy, juvenile myoclonic epilepsy, Benign Partial Epilepsy with Centrotemporal Spikes (BECTS) |
| | Neurocutaneous | Tuberous sclerosis, NF1 and 2, Sturge–Weber |
| | Chromosomal | Down syndrome |
| Structural | Developmental | Focal cortical dysplasia |
| Structural – acquired | Hippocampal | Hippocampal sclerosis |
| | Perinatal | Cerebral palsy, vaccination |
| | Trauma | TBI, neurosurgery |
| | Cerebral tumour | Glioma, DNET, meningioma, metastasis |
| | Infection | Meningitis, encephalitis, brain abscess, neurocysticercosis, TB, HIV, syphilis, malaria |
| | Cerebrovascular | Stroke, AVM, cavernoma, cortical venous thrombosis, eclampsia, hypertensive encephalopathy |
| | Degenerative &c | Alzheimer's and other dementias, MS |
| Immune | Various | SLE, vasculitis, Rasmussen's encephalitis |
| Largely unknown | Provoked and reflex epilepsies | Febrile seizures, drugs, alcohol, toxins |

*Source:* Modified from ILAE Commission Report (1989).

Juvenile Myoclonic Epilepsy: brief jerks, typically after waking, mainly of shoulders and arms develop between 12–18 years. Generalised tonic–clonic and absence seizures also occur. Some are photosensitive, or precipitated by lack of sleep or hunger. Treatment succeeds in most.

Benign Partial Epilepsy with Centrotemporal Spikes (BECTS or rolandic epilepsy) is a common partial childhood (4–10 years) epilepsy. EEG: high-amplitude spikes. Seizures are infrequent: 50% have less than 5 attacks, and often only at night, usually with clonic unilateral facial jerking, speech arrest and/or generalised attacks. Intellect is normal. Attacks typically cease by the age of 12.

West and Lennox–Gastaut syndromes: West syndrome is characterised by severe infantile spasms and chaotic EEG changes (hypsarrhythmia). Tuberous sclerosis is one cause. Others are neonatal brain damage, malformations and Down syndrome. Spasms are sudden, symmetrical and can occur many times a day. In one type – salaam attacks – arms and legs suddenly held in flexion/adduction. Prognosis: poor. About 5% die during attacks. Lennox–Gastaut denotes a childhood encephalopathy with marked learning disability. This can develop from West syndrome. Seizures are frequent – atypical absence, atonic, myoclonic, tonic and tonic–clonic seizures. Non-convulsive status can last hours to days. Prognosis: poor.

## Hippocampal Sclerosis and Perinatal Disorders

Hippocampal sclerosis is a common cause of mesial temporal lobe epilepsy found in about a fifth with refractory complex partial epilepsy. Cerebral palsy is strongly associated with epilepsy.

## Trauma

TBI is an important cause. Post-traumatic epilepsy is defined as immediate when a seizure occurs within 24 hours of injury, early – within the first week, and late thereafter. There is no increased epilepsy risk following mild/minor head injury – without skull fracture and less than 30 minutes post-traumatic amnesia. Following moderate TBI – skull fracture and/ or post-traumatic amnesia more than 24 hours – there is a slightly increased (4%) cumulative probability of a seizure at 30 years. Following severe TBI – post-traumatic amnesia more than 24 hours, intracranial haematoma/contusion, there is a 15% epilepsy cumulative probability at 30 years. Following a penetrating cortical injury, if early epilepsy develops, late epilepsy follows in about 25%.

## Tumours and Neurosurgery

With new-onset adult epilepsy, about 5% are caused by a tumour (Chapter 21). Seizures occur in about 50% of cortical tumours. Frontal and temporal tumours are more likely to generate epilepsy than others. Gliomas are the commonest cause: low grade gliomas are more epileptogenic than high grade. Oligodendrogliomas, DNETs, astrocytomas, gangliogliomas and hamartomas can all present with fits. Seizure activity, typically arises in the cortex, not in tumour tissue. With meningiomas, tumours that compress cortex – parasagittal/falx and sphenoid ridge are those likely to cause epilepsy. Following neurosurgery, there is a variable risk – from less than 3% following focal stereotaxis to around 80% following cerebral abscess surgery. Surgery for an unruptured aneurysm, a glioma, meningioma or cerebral haemorrhage carries risks of 5–10%.

## Infection

CNS infections are substantial risk factors. Fits are a common effect of a tuberculoma and a brain abscess. Neuro-cysticercosis is a major cause of epilepsy in Latin America, Asia and West Africa. Solitary or multiple parenchymal cysts cause seizures. Malaria carries an increased risk: a seizure, or a TIA-like event can be a presenting symptom.

## Cerebrovascular

Stroke is a common precursor of epilepsy in those over 50. An occult stroke explains some cryptogenic seizures. Both cerebral haemorrhage and infarction can be followed by epilepsy. Epilepsy develops in more than 15% of aneurysmal SAH survivors. With arteriovenous malformations around one quarter of cortical AVMs present with seizures. A cavernous haemangioma (cavernoma) can present with seizures. Cortical venous infarcts are epileptogenic. Epilepsy occurs in eclampsia, hypertensive encephalopathy and following anoxia after cardiac arrest. An unruptured aneurysm can cause epilepsy.

### Degenerative

Epilepsy is common in degenerative brain disease. Alzheimer's and frontotemporal dementia cases are more likely to develop epilepsy than age-matched controls. Huntington's cases can have epilepsy, more common in the juvenile type. Epilepsy can be a presenting feature of MS, and if rarely, of sporadic CJD.

### Immune-Mediated

While all are rare, the commonest is SLE. Seizures also occur in cerebral vasculitides, and Kawasaki disease (mucocutaneous lymph node syndrome in children, a complication of Covid-19). Limbic encephalitis (Chapters 19 and 26) either associated with neoplasms, or idiopathic and associated with many different autoantibodies can present with seizures. Rasmussen encephalitis is a rare, presumed autoimmune inflammation in one hemisphere begins in childhood, progresses for a decade or more, and then stabilises. Focal and/or secondarily generalised seizures develop, with *epilepsia partialis continua* (EPC), progressive loss of motor and cognitive skills, and hemiparesis/hemianopia. Imaging shows progressive hemisphere atrophy. Antiepileptics and immune suppression rarely help. Hemispherectomy can sometimes arrest progression.

### Provoked and Reflex Epilepsies

These include febrile seizures of childhood and various provoked seizures, such as alcohol-induced and alcohol-withdrawal, hypoglycaemia, non-ketotic hyperglycaemia, hypocalcaemia and with drugs – for example cocaine. Toxins: chemical weapons (e.g. sarin) and pesticides such as parathion can cause a seizure. Photosensitivity occurs with many epilepsies. Startle-induced, reading and auditory-induced, eating-induced and hot-water seizures are other rarities.

## Differential Diagnosis

There are many transient phenomena where epilepsy needs consideration. The key is a detailed history and observation. Misdiagnosis is rife: many with a possible fit do not have epilepsy. Loss of awareness, generalised and focal movements, drop attacks, focal sensory, visual and vestibular symptoms, psychological experiences, aggressive outbursts, sleep phenomena and prolonged confusional and fugue states are mentioned briefly here.

### Loss of Awareness

Syncope, seizures, non-epileptic attack disorder and cardiac dysrhythmias are common. Transient cerebral ischaemia rarely causes loss of awareness. Microsleeps can occur with a severe sleep deprivation. Hypoglycaemia and panic attacks occasionally cause loss of awareness.

### Generalised Movements - Epilepsy and Non-Epileptic Attack Disorder (NEAD)

A generalised convulsion is usually clear from a witnessed account. If possible, ascertain how each phase of a *grand mal* seizure is described. In NEAD, semi-purposeful limb thrashing, over many minutes, with pelvic thrusting and back arching are typical. The non-epileptic attack rarely evolves through the stages of a tonic–clonic seizure. However, complex frontal lobe partial seizures can produce bizarre motor features, often thought to be NEADs. A simple faint is often accompanied by twitches. Occasionally a true hypoxic convulsion occurs, a.k.a. an anoxic seizure, with urinary incontinence and tongue biting.

### Focal Seizures, Tics, TIAs, MS, Movement Disorders

Focal motor seizures involve jerking and posturing of one extremity, with progression, a.k.a – the epilepsy march. *Epilepsy partialis continua* (EPC) can produce focal jerking for hours or days, and in sleep. Movements in EPC can also be slow, resembling dystonia. Hemifacial spasm is usually obvious.

Tics are stereotyped and unlike myoclonus can be suppressed voluntarily. TIAs usually cause negative phenomena, such as hemiparesis or aphasia, but jerking and paraesthesiae can occur, lasting for a few minutes only. There is rarely loss of awareness. Tonic spasms in MS last typically for several seconds.

Paroxysmal kinesiogenic choreoathetosis can cause focal motor attacks. Tremor is sufficiently persistent and rhythmical to make its nature clear. Myoclonus or spinal myoclonus should be evident from its focal distribution. Tetany can cause localised spasms – for example of an arm.

Paroxysmal dystonias tend to last for hours. Idiopathic torsion dystonia in an acute exacerbation can cause jerky movements, but there is preserved consciousness. Head banging and rocking movements can resemble seizures. Hyperekplectic attacks, usually genetic, are an excessive startle – a jerk of all four limbs, to unexpected stimuli, typically noise. Hyperekplexia can resemble frontal lobe seizures.

### Drop Attacks

- Idiopathic drop attacks are the commonest. In middle-aged women, there is a sudden fall – the legs give way. The patient remembers falling. Recovery is instantaneous.
- In epilepsy drop attacks occur with learning disability and secondary generalised epilepsies. Falls – tonic or atonic – cause injuries.
- Cerebral hypoperfusion can be sufficiently severe for a drop attack to occur.
- Movement disorders that cause drop attacks have features that make the diagnosis clear – such as Parkinson's and PSP. Paroxysmal kinesiogenic choreoathetosis can present as drop attacks.
- A third ventricle tumour such as a colloid cyst, or a cord AVM can present with abrupt episodes of lower limb weakness.

- Cataplexy usually occurs with narcolepsy. Attacks can be precipitated by emotion, especially laughter. Often there is slumping of the head/trunk, rather than falls.
- Periodic paralyses with changes in plasma potassium are possibilities.
- Vertebrobasilar ischaemia: typically in the elderly with vascular disease and cervical spondylosis.

### Focal Sensory, Visual and Vestibular Symptoms

In focal epilepsy, a seizure arising from the sensory cortex can cause spreading paraesthesia. Transient sensory phenomena can also occur with peripheral nerve compression, with tetany, and with TIAs. Hyperventilation, panic and migraine can cause paraesthesia, such as in one arm. In migraine this usually evolves into a migraine attack.

Transient visual symptoms are frequently migrainous. Evolution of visual symptoms is usually gradual, over several minutes: fortification spectra are diagnostic and do not occur in epilepsy. Epileptic visual phenomena are usually sudden, evolving over seconds, with coloured blobs rather than the jagged lines of a fortification. Exceptionally, a migraine can bring on a seizure – a.k.a. migralepsy.

Vertigo: peripheral vestibular disease is much the commonest cause. Migraine can also cause transient vestibular symptoms. Acute vertigo can if rarely be part of a partial seizure.

### Transient Psychological Experiences

These can be difficult to differentiate from epilepsy, especially if brief, and do occur in some seizures.

Epilepsy: a partial temporal lobe seizure can cause fear, *déjà vu*, flashbacks, visual, olfactory or auditory hallucinations. Altered perception of the environment can occur – distancing from reality, change in size or shape of objects, altered language, sadness, laughter, elation and occasionally sexual arousal. *Déjà vu* in epilepsy is intense – not a vague recollection. A rising epigastric sensation can occur with déjà *vu*.

Migraine: psychological phenomena sometimes involve an initial heightening of awareness, with visual illusions, such as change in the size of objects, or self. A migraine usually follows.

Panic attacks: intense anxiety, hyperventilation, dizziness and unpleasant abdominal sensations. The increase in heart rate and respiration usually make a panic attack obvious, but occasionally a temporal lobe seizure can cause a similar attack.

Drug-induced phenomena: these can share some of the qualities of a temporal lobe seizure.

Hallucinations/illusions with loss of a sensory modality: odd sensations and pain follow limb amputation. Similarly, people who lose sight either in the whole or part field can experience visual phenomena in the blind field.

Hallucinations and delusions: these tend to be hallmarks of psychoses. A psychiatric basis is suggested by their complexity, with an evolving or argued theme, auditory nature, paranoia/thought disorder and/or instructions from a third person.

A psychotic episode is usually more prolonged than a seizure. Pseudo-hallucinations, usually visual with retained insight can also occur in affective disorders and confusional states.

NEAD: hallucinations and illusions may seem plausible, but should be suspected if they are florid, multiple in type – auditory, olfactory and visual at different times, with evolving stories and with emotional outbursts.

## Aggressive Outbursts and Criminal Activity

Rage is rarely epileptic. Exceptionally, a frontal lobe seizure can lead to aggressive behaviour.

Criminal activity is also exceptional in a seizure. A complex epileptic automatism is a distinct rarity. Pointers against epilepsy are:

- Planning, preparation and directed violence without previous automatisms
- Complex/organised activity, witness accounts of no impaired consciousness
- Attempts to conceal evidence, motive, and/or prolonged aggression.

## Sleep Phenomena

Attacks during sleep are often poorly witnessed. Unless there is good evidence of a fit, most sleep phenomena are not epileptic.

Normal sleep movements: whole body jerks occur in normal people as they fall asleep. Fragmentary physiological myoclonus usually involves the hands, feet or face during stages 1 and 2 and REM sleep. Periodic movements in sleep (nocturnal myoclonus) occur occasionally in young adults, and in about half of those over 65, in whom nocturnal cramps are also common.

Epilepsies and other phenonomena: generalised tonic–clonic seizures can be confined to sleep and/or occur on awakening. Complex automatisms in TLE – the patient gets out of bed and wanders around – can mimic parasomnias. Frontal lobe seizures, though rare, can be brief, bizarre and occasionally be confined to sleep.

Restless legs (Chapter 7) is an urge to move the legs, especially in the evening, when lying or sitting. Periodic movements in sleep are also typical – they can be severe and occur when awake.

Non-REM parasomnias (Chapter 20) occur typically in childhood, and are often familial. Night terrors and sleep walking occur about 4 hours after going to sleep, and arise from slow wave sleep. Usually a single attack occurs in one night. Sleep walking can involve complex tasks. Brief episodes are also common – sitting up and fidgeting, sometimes resembling a partial seizure. These non-REM parasomnias can lead to injury, but rarely to aggression. Enuresis is common, especially in boys and typically of no consequence.

REM parasomnias usually arise in middle-aged males. During REM sleep, there are episodes of thrashing about, even violence, and/or acting out dreams. Episodes last from seconds to minutes. These can occur in normal people, but they are also seen with tricyclics, alcohol and PD and multi-system atrophy.

Sleep apnoea and other movements in sleep: these cases usually have daytime hypersomnolence, but at night the apnoea can produce grunting, or flailing about that can resemble a fit. Exceptionally, hypoxia causes a seizure. Body rocking during sleep occurs in learning disability, or rarely following TBI.

## Prolonged Confusional and Fugue States

A fit usually lasts for seconds or minutes. After a generalised tonic–clonic seizure or, less frequently, a complex partial seizure there may be confusion for around an hour.

Non-convulsive status epilepticus: complex partial seizures, typical or atypical absences in status can cause a prolonged confusional state.

Transient global amnesia commences acutely, and lasts for minutes or hours (Chapter 6). Patients are able to perform complex activities, but afterwards have no recall. There are no other neurological signs. Consciousness is preserved.

Acute encephalopathy: metabolic disturbances can cause loss of awareness – diabetic ketoacidosis, hypoglycaemia, respiratory, renal or hepatic failure, porphyria and urea cycle enzyme defects, drugs, hyperpyrexia, and infection.

## Intermittent Psychosis and Fugues

Patients with schizophrenia, for example, can have abrupt episodes of delusions, hallucinations and/or apparent confusion, lasting for hours or days.

A fugue is usually a psychiatric conversion phenomenon. These dreamy episodes may be brief or prolonged – for days or even weeks. Inconsistencies in the mental state examination are often evident. Usually there is a previous psychiatric illness, alcohol or drug abuse. In some, the question of malingering arises, commonly when someone professes amnesia for an important event.

# Investigation

This addresses two questions:

- Is the diagnosis epilepsy? If so, what type?
- What is the cause of epilepsy?

The first question is determined largely from the history. EEG and MRI are the two definitive tests. A faint does not usually require investigation. Most others should have routine bloods and ECG. Other tests depend on context.

## EEG in Epilepsy Diagnosis – Epileptiform and Normal Phenomena

EEG is valuable but has limitations – it is our only view of cortical electrical activity – the sum of inhibitory and excitatory post-synaptic potentials, amplified more than 100000. EEG is vulnerable to artefacts, such as eye and tongue movement.

Abnormal EEGs can be divided broadly into:

- specific – either epileptiform or, rarely, in disorders such as CJD or SSPE
- non-specific – of unclear significance.

Epilepsy diagnosis is essentially clinical. Epileptiform features are multiple spike/polyspike and wave complexes. These reflect hyperexcitability of a cortical area. About 6–10 cm$^2$ of cortex must be activated for an epileptiform discharge to be visible on a scalp EEG.

Some phenomena – 3/second spike-wave complexes, chaotic activity (hypsarrthymia) and generalised photo-paroxysmal responses – are strongly correlated with epilepsy. Centro-temporal sharp waves are poorly correlated. Isolated spikes are normal variants that have no link with epilepsy in most people.

Epileptiform discharges occur exceptionally in the normal population. They also occur rarely, without a seizure with a tumour, following TBI or cranial surgery. Thus, an isolated epileptiform EEG does not indicate that someone must have had a fit.

EEG has a high false negative rate, that is a normal EEG does not exclude epilepsy, and, as above a low false positive rate. EEGs are frequently misinterpretated because of insufficient knowledge of normality – especially spikes and sharp waves. An EEG should be performed if the history really suggests a seizure – a NICE recommendation. The distinction between simple partial and complex partial seizures is clinical. However the EEG can complement and help define a seizure. There is no absolute EEG classification – some important abnormalities are mentioned below.

### Idiopathic Generalised Epilepsy and Asbsence seizures

Typical interictal EEG findings are generalised spike/polyspike and slow wave complexes at 3–5 Hz with a normal background and sometimes photosensitivity (Figure 8.1).

### Some Specific Epilepsies

These notes mention conditions largely in childhood with EEG changes:

- In Benign Childhood Epilepsy with Centro-Temporal Spikes, defining features are high-amplitude focal sharp waves – central and temporal – potentiated by sleep.
- Lennox–Gastaut syndrome: typically slow 1–2.5 Hz spike-wave complexes, generalised or lateralised, with disorganised slow background.

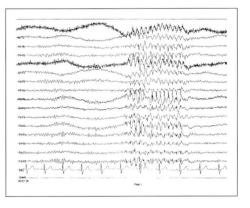

**Figure 8.1** Spike-wave discharge with typical absence epilepsy.

Electrical status epilepticus in sleep: in this rarity continuous spike-wave discharges occur in non-REM sleep, with few abnormalities when awake and in REM sleep. Most children have regression of cognition.

Progressive myoclonic epilepsies: generalised spike-wave discharges, photosensitivity and slow background.

### Partial Epilepsies

Localised EEG changes are common in TLE and likely when a focus is superficial. However, even prolonged interictal EEGs can be normal if an epileptogenic region is remote from scalp electrodes such as in the mesial frontal lobe, if the focus involves too small a neuronal aggregate, and sometimes inexplicably even when extensive. Mesial TLE with hippocampal sclerosis shows temporal interictal spikes in more than 80%, of value in assessment for epilepsy surgery (Figure 8.2).

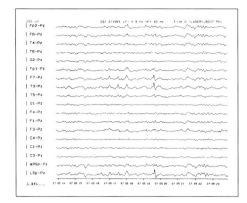

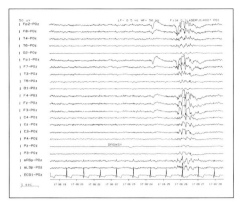

**Figure 8.2** Interictal EEG: left mesial TLE. Focal spikes: F7, T3 and LSp.

**Figure 8.3** Widespread bilateral spike-wave discharge with a frontal complex partial seizure.

In frontal seizures (Figure 8.3), focal interictal EEG abnormalities are the exception: many patients show widespread abnormalities.

EEG localisation in seizures of parietal and occipital lobe origin can also be unhelpful – a wide variety of changes occur. With sensory partial seizures, many have negative interictal and ictal EEGs.

### Prediction of Seizure Recurrence and Drug Effects

When an EEG shows an epileptiform discharge in a first unprovoked fit, seizure recurrence follows in about two-thirds at two years, but in those with a normal EEG in around one quarter. Generally, the EEG is of limited value for defining response to treatment. However, in childhood absence epilepsy with valproate, which suppresses the spike-wave complexes, the EEG can help monitor progress. Spike-wave discharges with IGE point to high recurrence rates. Clinical patterns are generally more important when considering medication and its withdrawal.

### EEG Monitoring

EEG monitoring with video can be most valuable. The usual aim is to document attacks in the differential diagnosis of non-epileptic seizures, in the characterisation of seizure type, in the quantification of epileptiform discharges and their frequency and in epilepsy surgery evaluation. Monitoring is of particular value in status epilepticus – convulsive, non-convulsive and pseudo-status – and can help in nocturnal epilepsy and parasomnias.

In ICU, monitoring can also help to distinguish coma from diminished responsiveness, for example in psychiatric or deliberate settings, in sedation, neuromuscular blockade or locked-in, and an encephalopathy. In the determination of brain death, the EEG is not essential.

## Imaging

MRI is essential. The fine detail of MR and specialised MR (fMRI, tractography, single-photon emission CT, PET, magnetoen-cephalography) is outside the scope of this chapter. Whilst normal MR imaging occurs in more than 50%, hippocampal sclerosis (Figure 8.4), malformations of cortical development, a brain tumour, vascular malformation, previous trauma, stroke or infection may be found. CT is useful in an emergency, and also shows focal cortical calcification, blood, and bone changes.

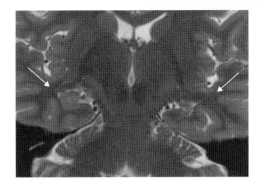

**Figure 8.4**  Left hippocampal sclerosis. Coronal T2-W: atrophy in left hippocampus.

## Management: Newly Diagnosed Cases

Firm diagnosis and a first-hand account are essential. Misdiagnosis is common. Pitfalls include accepting a previous diagnosis, statements by inexperienced people and self-assessment. Do not be overconfident: we have all been wrong.

Risk of recurrence: about three quarters of adults with a first unprovoked seizure have further attacks – nearly 50% by 6 months, a third in the next 6 months and less than a quarter in the second year. If more than one seizure has occurred, the risk of further attacks without treatment is over 80% – the more the seizures, the greater the risk. We generally treat such levels of risk in clinical practice.

In an adult recurrence risks are influenced by age, EEG, seizure type and aetiology. Risks are greater in those over 60, when the EEG shows spike-wave discharges, when there is a cortical lesion and with a partial as opposed to generalised seizure.

Treatment with antiepileptics has implications. The object is obvious, but therapy confers a stigma, the epilepsy label and affects self-esteem, relationships and employment. Benefits include lower seizure risk, security and less chance of injury and even death. Drawbacks include drug side-effects, and inconvenience. Subtle effects may not be obvious – learning difficulties are one reason why paediatricians tend to initiate therapy less readily than adult neurologists. Some seizure types have less impact than others on the quality of life, for example simple partial seizures, absence or sleep attacks. Benefits of treating such seizures can be few and if frequency is low, disadvantages can be unacceptable. It would be unusual to treat someone with less than one seizure/year, if confined to sleep, minor or partial.

Initial treatment aims are complete control without adverse effects. Principles include: monotherapy, titration towards a low maintenance dose, an alternative if the first drug fails and polytherapy only if three individual drugs have failed. Counselling is essential – about goals, risks, driving, outcome, logistics and support. A written treatment plan, its goals, risks and limitations should be agreed.

## Management: Established Epilepsy

Resist nihilism and inertia – fresh approaches can revolutionise a patient's life.There are over 10 first line antiepileptics, and thus many combinations, so one needs to press on for several years, though drugs fail in about 15%. Reassess: diagnosis, classification and previous drugs. Consider reinvestigation to exclude a progressive lesion. Explore: possibilities of poor compliance. Agree a treatment plan. Consider NEAD: some attacks may not have an epileptic basis. Refer: for specialist advice, a second opinion and/or specialist nursing support.

The question of stopping drugs arises, usually following a long remission – meaning no attacks for 2–5 years; there is no absolute definition. Drug doses should be minimised beforehand.

### Antiepileptic Drugs

The choice of a drug is based on seizure type and syndrome – a single drug will provide optimal seizure control in about 70%. Advantages are better tolerance, fewer side-effects, less intrusive regime, better compliance and no potential for drug interactions. Combination therapy is needed in about 20%, and prognosis for control less good. Nevertheless, combination therapy can sometimes optimise control – possibly because drugs with differing modes of action have synergistic effects. Serum levels of some antiepileptics are helpful. In chronic refractory patients advantages include assessment of optimal doses, toxicity, side effects, drug interactions and compliance. Levels of phenytoin should be measured regularly – it has non-linear kinetics.

Currently available drugs are listed alphabetically.

#### Acetazolamide
This carbonic anhydrase inhibitor used for glaucoma can also be used as an adjunct in epilepsy.

#### Benzodiazepines
Benzodiazepines: emergency medication for serial seizures and for long-term treatment. Clobazam is used as an add-on for patients with refractory seizures. Clonazepam can also be used, particularly in myoclonic seizures. Diazepam, midazolam or lorazepam are used in *status epilepticus.*

#### Carbamazepine
Carbamazepine is a first line drug for partial and tonic–clonic seizures. Some experience diplopia, nausea, dizziness or headache on initiation of therapy, usually transiently. Common side effects include drowsiness, ataxia, confusion/agitation, hyponatraemia, neutropenia and skin rashes. Controlled release preparations are preferable. Carbamazepine, an enzyme inducer reduces levels of oral contraceptives, steroids, haloperidol, antineoplastic and antihypertensive drugs, tricyclics, antipsychotics and warfarin. Conversely, some drugs inhibit its metabolism, and can cause neurotoxicity: cimetidine, clarithromycin, dextropropoxyphene, diltiazem, erythromycin, antifungal drugs, isoniazid, tricyclics, antipsychotics, verapamil and viloxazine.

**Cenobamate**
Cenobamate has recently (2020) been licenced for partial seizures.

**Eslicarbazepine Acetate**
Licensed as an add-on medication for focal epilepsy, it is the pro-drug of eslicarbazepine, the major active metabolite of oxcarbazepine.

**Ethosuximide**
First line drug for generalised absence seizures in children and young adults, but not generally effective for other seizures types.

**Felbamate**
Felbamate is effective in partial and in generalised seizures, and used in refractory partial epilepsy. Its use is restricted – high rates of hypersensitivity, aplastic anaemia and hepatotoxicity.

**Gabapentin**
Gabapentin is occasionally useful as add-on treatment of partial seizures.

**Lacosamide**
Licensed as an add-on for focal epilepsy in adults.

**Lamotrigine**
Lamotrigine is a first line drug for partial and generalised seizures. Initiation should be with low doses and slow titration to decrease the risk of rashes, common side effects. Elimination is accelerated by enzyme-inducing antiepileptics, such as carbamazepine, phenytoin and phenobarbital and inhibited by valproate. As an add-on, drug doses may need adjustment.

Lamotrigine levels may be reduced, occasionally dramatically, by the combined contraceptive pill or during pregnancy.

**Levetiracetam**
Levetiracetam is a broad-spectrum first line medication for partial and generalised seizures, well tolerated overall. Side effects are lethargy, irritability, drowsiness, dizziness, headache, emotional lability, insomnia and anxiety.

**Oxcarbazepine**
A variant of carbamazepine with similar efficacy. An add-on drug for refractory partial seizures, and a first line agent in previously untreated patients with tonic–clonic and partial seizures.

**Perampanel**
Licensed for the adjunctive treatment of refractory partial epilepsy.

**Phenobarbital**
The oldest barbiturate is an effective antiepileptic against most seizure types, IV and orally. Phenobarbital is now hardly used orally, though still used IV in emergencies.

**Phenytoin**

Phenytoin is an effective oral treatment of partial seizures and tonic–clonic seizures and is also useful IV in status epilepticus. Because of its chronic side effects, it is now not used as first line therapy. Common side effects include cosmetic changes – gingival hyperplasia, acne, hirsutism, facial coarsening – and neuropsychiatric disturbance, particularly depression, fatigue and cognitive slowing. Other side effects include nausea, tremor, paraesthesiae, dizziness, headache, anorexia and rashes. Rarely, it may cause hepatotoxicity, peripheral neuropathy, Dupuytren's contracture, lymphadenopathy, osteomalacia, megaloblastic anaemia, leucopenia, thrombocytopenia, lupus erythematosus and Stevens–Johnson syndrome. As with phenobarbital, it can cause megaloblastic changes: folic acid supplementation is recommended.

Large increases in plasma concentrations can occur with small dose increments – it has non-linear pharmacokinetics – and levels may fall abruptly with modest dose reduction. Phenytoin is the only antiepileptic for which blood level monitoring is essential. Phenytoin is a potent enzyme inducer. Conversely, its metabolism can be inhibited by enzyme inducers such as allopurinol, chloramphenicol, cimetidine, isoniazid, metronidazol, phenothiazine and sulphonamides.

**Piracetam**

Piracetam was licensed first as a memory enhancer but has a remarkable effect against some myoclonic seizures and is useful in progressive myoclonic epilepsy.

**Pregabalin**

Pregabalin, a gabapentin analogue, is a second line antiepileptic for partial seizures. Pregabalin is also used for anxiety and neuropathic pain. Weight gain, drowsiness and fatique are side effects.

**Primidone**

Primidone is largely metabolised to phenobarbital, and rarely used.

**Retigabine**

Retigabine is licenced as add-on therapy in partial epilepsy. A side effect is a blue skin discoloration, around the eyes and the nails, and pigmentary changes in the retina. It is now rarely prescribed.

**Rufinamide**

Rufinamide was licenced in the Lennox–Gastaut spectrum; it has modest effects on drop attacks.

**Stiripentol**

Stiripentol is licensed for use in Dravet's syndrome with sodium valproate and clobazam. Its effects are modest.

**Tiagabine**

Tiagabine, a GABAergic drug, has a moderate efficacy in the control of partial seizures. It has no indication in other seizure types and can exacerbate generalised seizures. It is now rarely prescribed.

### Topiramate

Topiramate is effective against partial and secondarily generalised seizures. However, it has a difficult side effect profile at high doses. These can be avoided by using low doses and titrating upwards slowly. Adverse effects include headache, sedation, impaired memory, speech disturbance, asthenia, anxiety, depression, sleep disorders, visual disturbances and confusion. Weight loss and paraesthesia are common. Rarely, topiramate may cause acute myopia with angle-closure glaucoma. Enzyme inducers tend to accelerate the clearance of topiramate and higher doses may be required if they are used concomitantly. Topiramate does not affect clearance of other antiepileptics significantly.

### Valproate

Valproate is the most effective drug in idiopathic generalised epilepsy – in controlling absences, myoclonus and generalised tonic–clonic seizures and also partial seizures. Common side effects include weight gain, tremor, behavioural disturbances, menstrual disturbances, ankle swelling and loss or curling of hair. Cognitive impairment is sometimes seen and encephalopathy has been reported. Rare cases of fatal hepatotoxicity, have occurred, typically in infants during polytherapy. Valproate is effective in controlling anxiety. Valproate should be used rarely, if at all in pregnancy: there is a risk of teratogenicity and later learning disability.

Valproate has a complex interaction profile. It mildly inhibits metabolism of other antiepileptic drugs – rarely of clinical relevance except when with lamotrigine, plasma levels of which are greatly elevated on co-medication with valproate. Interactions with phenytoin and carbamazepine can also be significant. Carbapenem antibiotics cause a profound lowering of valproate levels. Valproate concentrations are also lowered by some antineoplastic drugs. Valproate concentrations can be greatly elevated with co-medication with some antidepressants. Serum level monitoring is not recommended routinely.

### Vigabatrin

Use is limited by irreversible visual field defects in over half on long-term therapy. Vigabatrin has a niche indication in West syndrome – an alternative to ACTH or steroids.

### Zonisamide

Zonisamide is a sulphonamide with some action against a wide variety of seizure types.

## Emergencies: Prolonged Convulsions, Serial Seizures, Status Epilepticus

If a tonic–clonic seizure continues for 5 minutes, this is potentially hazardous. Give a benzodiazepine IV, by mouth or rectally – usually IV diazepam, lorazepam or clobazam. Buccal midazolam is an alternative. Status epilepticus is continuous seizure activity for longer than 30 minutes. Serial seizures without full recovery typically progress to status. Status can occur without a history of epilepsy: *de novo* status can follow cerebral anoxia (myoclonic status in coma), alcohol, cerebral tumour, encephalitis – including with NMDA receptor antibodies, stroke, TBI, febrile status in children, drugs, toxins and genetic/metabolic disorders such as mitochondrial disease. In epilepsy cases, status can follow reduction of antiepileptics and intercurrent illness. If tonic–clonic status persists for more than 2 hours, there is a substantial risk of cerebral damage – over 10% of these cases die.

### Treatment

- Early status: first 30 minutes. Immediate IV lorazepam. Admission to ICU, respiratory support and EEG monitoring.
- Established status: if lorazepam fails, add IV phenytoin (or fosphenytoin), valproate or levetiracetam.
- Refractory status: consider anaesthesia – propofol, thiopentone/pentobarbital or midazolam.
- Super-refractory status is refractory status despite anaesthesia for 24 hours. Antiepileptics should always be continued. Hypothermia, magnesium infusion, pyridoxine infusion (in children), steroids and or IVIg or plasma exchange are sometimes tried.

In non-convulsive status, generally IV benzodiapines are effective, such as in typical absence status and complex partial status. In the elderly IV valproate or levetiracetam may be better tolerated. Non-convulsive status that progresses to coma has a poor prognosis.

## Epilepsy Surgery

The aim is to stop or ameliorate seizures. In UK, about 500 patients annually are deemed suitable and in some this is highly successful. Temporal lobe resection for hippocampal sclerosis is the most frequent operation. Resections in other areas are performed less frequently – mainly for frontal lesions. Suitability criteria include a secure diagnosis (multiple seizure types are usually excluded), drug resistance and concordance of seizure type, MRI and ictal EEG findings.

Resective surgery is the main technique, sometimes via stereotactic radiosurgery. Patients with discrete lesions tend to have a good outcome. A case with a dysembryoplastic neu-roepithelial tumour or discrete AVM has a greater than 50% chance of seizure freedom. Mortality is less than 0.5%. Memory loss depends upon baseline memory, age and hemisphere (dominant>non-dominant). Visual field defects occur in 10%. Depression is common; psychosis occasionally occurs. There are potential risks of cognitive decline. Resections in other areas are performed less frequently – mainly for frontal lesions. Other techniques include hemispherectomy, corpus callosotomy, multiple subpial transections and vagal nerve stimulation.

## Driving Regulations: UK

The patient must notify the DVLA if epilepsy is diagnosed. https://www.gov.uk/epilepsy-and-driving: *You must tell DVLA if you've had any epileptic attack, seizure, fit or blackout.* A single epileptic attack results in withdrawal of a Group 1 Licence – for a car and motor-cycle – for 6 months from the seizure date. With a high recurrence risk, withdrawal will be for longer. Rules are stricter for Group 2 licences – lorries, heavy goods vehicles, taxis and buses. A doctor should clarify with the patient their legal duty to inform the DVLA. If driving continues, the doctor should disclose relevant information to the DVLA and inform the patient. For electric wheelchairs and mobility scooters a licence is not needed.

## Acknowledgements

I am most grateful to Simon Shorvon, Beate Diehl, John Duncan, Fergus Rugg-Gunn, Matthias Koepp, Josemir Sander, Matthew Walker and Tim Wehner for their contribution to *Neurology A Queen Square Textbook* Second Edition on which this chapter is based.

## Further Reading

Shorvon S, Diehl B, Duncan J, Rugg-Gunn F, Koepp M, Sander J, Matthew W, Tim W. Epilepsy and related disorders. In *Neurology A Queen Square Textbook*, 2nd edn. Clarke C, Howard R, Rossor M and Shorvon S, eds. John Wiley & Sons 2016. There are numerous references.
ILAE Commission Report. Commission on Classification and Terminology of the International League Against Epilepsy. Proposal for revised classification of epilepsies and epileptic syndromes. *Epilepsia* 1989; 30: 389–399.
Scheffer IE, Samuel B, Giuseppe C, Mary BC, Jacqueline F, Laura G, Edouard H, Satish J, Gary WM, Solomon LM, Douglas RN, Emilio P, Torbjörn T, Samuel W, Yue-Hua Z, Sameer MZ. Position paper: ILAE commission for classification & terminology. *Epilepsia* 2017; 58(4): 512–521.
Hopkins, AP, Garman A, Clarke CRA. The first seizure in adult life. Value of clinical features, EEG and CT scanning in prediction of seizure recurrence. *Lancet* 1988; 1: 721–726.

Also, please visit https://www.drcharlesclarke.com for free updated notes, potential links and references as these become available. You will be asked to log in, in a secure fashion, with your name and institution.

## Websites

https://www.nhs.uk/conditions/epilepsy/
https://www.epilepsy.org.uk/
https://epilepsysociety.org.uk/

# 9

# Infections

For the general neurologist infections are important because correct diagnosis can make the difference between life and death – a situation that pertains with few other conditions.

My own approach has four tenets:

One is obvious: acute bacterial meningitis is fatal unless treated immediately.

A second, also evident is that many febrile illnesses cause symptoms such as headache that require no specialist attention.

Third, a corollary: serious infections can present similarly. Thus, particular demands are placed upon physicians and others to recognise them.

Finally, CNS infections can progress slowly with few features that one expects of sepsis. A brain or spinal abscess can be indolent.

It may appear simple in print to distinguish intracranial sepsis from a viral infection, but this is by no means so at the bedside – the meningitic syndrome can be caused by bacterial infection that demands immediate attention, by viral infection, or by conditions such as TB meningitis, an abscess, malaria or blood in the CSF. My focus here is largely on infections in Britain. Worldwide there are obvious regional differences.

## Acute Bacterial Meningitis

Pyogenic bacteria infect the subarachnoid space. UK adult incidence: 1.5/100 000/year. Fatalities remain at 20%. Meningococcal disease is most common between 16–25 and has declined in the United Kingdom, following the meningococcus Group C vaccine. Immunisation has reduced greatly *Haemophilus influenzae* type B, and *Streptococcus pneumoniae* meningitis. Other bacteria include *Listeria monocytogenes* (mostly in the over 50s and immunocompromised), *Streptococcus pyogenes*, Enterococci, Group B streptococcus, non-type B Haemophilus, Klebsiella, Pseudomonas and Enterobacter. TBM is mentioned later.

In community-acquired meningitis, direct invasion occurs via respiratory droplets. Bacteria colonise the nasopharynx, reach the blood where they multiply and then the CSF via choroid plexus or capillaries. There is little antibody response. Bacterial cell wall components induce the CSF polymorph response. Purulent exudate develops within the subarachnoid space. Cerebral blood flow increases, autoregulation fails: intracranial pressure

*Neurology: A Clinical Handbook*, First Edition. Charles Clarke.
© 2022 John Wiley & Sons Ltd. Published 2022 by John Wiley & Sons Ltd.

rises. Exudates infiltrate vessels to produce cerebral ischaemia. Systemic shock causes hypotension. Cerebral venous thrombosis can follow. Exudate can obstruct CSF resorption, leading to hydrocephalus, or a subdural abscess can develop. Bacteria can also reach the brain either by direct invasion, via the bloodstream or infected thrombi.

## The Meningitic Syndrome

The meningitic syndrome means fever, headache and neck stiffness. There is usually intense malaise, nausea, vomiting and photophobia. Lethargy, stupor or coma follow. Seizures can occur, and rarely opisthotonus – fixed spasm with legs and head arched back. A rash – sometimes subtle – suggests meningococcus. In practice, assume any rash is meningococcal. Kernig's sign is frequently positive. Hold one leg firmly: flex hip and knee to 90°, and then try to extend the knee – this is painful and restricted. Brudzinski's sign: passive neck flexion causes hip and knee flexion – less used than Kernig's.

Acute bacterial meningitis evolves typically over a few hours. Fulminating disease can be faster, resembling subarachnoid haemorrhage, but the meningitic syndrome is variable and even with acute bacterial meningitis there can be a subacute (progressive) course over several days, particularly in the elderly or immunosuppressed. Neck stiffness can be absent. Cranial nerve lesions, especially hearing loss can present early. Seizures occur in 40%. Acute bacterial meningitis can cause brain and/or cord infarction, and hydrocephalus.

Without exaggeration, assessment of any febrile illness should include the thought: 'could this be bacterial meningitis?' Viral meningitis, typically milder and self-limiting is an untenable spot diagnosis. TBM is also less dramatic.

## Management

Minutes matter: in hospital liaise closely with the laboratory and an infectious disease expert. Protocols vary, depending upon local epidemics and antibiotic resistance. The 2016 Guidelines of the British Infection Association are summarised:

### Antbiotics in the Community?
YES. In suspected meningococcal meningitis, give benzylpenicillin 1200 mg IM or IV, cefotaxime 2 g or ceftriaxone 2 g IM or IV, before immediate transfer to hospital.

### Immediate Hospital Management?
In hospital, for all suspected meningitis: stabilise airway, circulation, establish IV access, fluids &c.

Involve a senior physician and/or ITU physician promptly. Take a travel history. Document and monitor GCS. Blood cultures: immediately. LP: provided this is safe, within one hour. Commence antibiotics immediately after LP. If LP cannot be done within one hour commence antibiotics immediately after blood cultures (Table 9.1).

Usually avoid LP with: impaired consciousness, focal signs, papilloedema, seizures, shock, extensive purpura or petechial rash, coagulopathy/anticoagulants/clopidogrel, infection at LP site.

Table 9.1   CSF in meningitis.

|  | Normal | Bacterial | Viral | TBM | Fungal |
|---|---|---|---|---|---|
| Appearance | 'Gin' clear | Turbid | Clear/opalescent | Clear/ opalescent | Clear/ opalescent |
| Pressure | <180 mm $H_2O$ | Increased | Normal/high | High | Normal/ high |
| White cells/ mm$^3$) | 0–5 | 100–50 000 | 5–500 | 5–500 | 20–500 |
| Neutrophils | None | >80% | <50% | <50% | <50% |
| Glucose (% of blood) | >3.5 mmol/L (75%) | Low (<50%) | Normal | Low (<50%) | Low-ish (50–75%) |
| Protein (g/L) | <0.4 | >0.9 | 0.6–0.9 | 0.6–5 | 0.6–5 |

All suspected bacterial meniningitis should be treated with cefotaxime 2 g or ceftriaxone 2 g IV 6 hourly. Over 60, immunocompromised and/or diabetic: 2 g IV ampicillin/amoxicillin 4-hourly + cephalosporin. Dexamethasone (10 mg 6 hourly) for 4 days.

### Should CT (Brain) Precede LP and Antibiotics?

Guidelines favour early LP and antibiotics – the meningitic syndrome is rarely caused by pathology whose outcome will be harmed by LP. Waiting delays antibiotics.

Additional routine tests: high blood polymorph count and raised inflammatory markers – invariable. Platelet consumption: common. Blood (multiple) cultures. Throat swab, PCR of blood/CSF. Appropriate Gram and other CSF stains. Hypocalcaemia, hyponatraemia. Multi-organ failure may develop.

### Outcome

With prompt treatment, complete resolution of bacterial meningitis can be expected in more than 50%.

## Neisseria Meningitidis

In Britain, this remains a leading infective cause of death in childhood. Asymptomatic nasopharyngeal carriers are common.Infection can develop within minutes. Everyone should know 'an acute febrile meningitic syndrome + spots = mengingococcus until proved otherwise'. A red maculo-papular rash develops into (non-blanching) petechiae/ purpura on the trunk, limbs, in mucous membranes and sometimes on the palms and soles, with fever, headache, meningism, nausea, vomiting and photophobia. Signs of septicaemia are a rapidly rising pulse rate and hypotension. Waterhouse–Friderichsen syndrome is fulminating disease – adrenal haemorrhage, DIC, shock coma and death can follow.

Mortality remains around 25%. Survivors: 20% have hearing loss, loss of limbs secondary to vasculitis, and/or disabilities following brain ischaemia.

Close contacts are at risk: screen and treat to eradicate possible nasopharyngeal carriage with rifampicin 600 mg 12-hourly for 22 days, or with a single dose of ciprofloxacin 750 mg. Immunisation in the United Kingdom is carried out in childhood and protects for 3–5 years.

### Streptococcus Pneumoniae

The Gram-positive coccus spreads via respiratory droplets; carriers are common. Also caused by extension from otitis media, or a paranasal sinus, following a skull fracture or dural tear, coexisting pneumonia, alcoholism, diabetes, immunocompromised states.

## Brain Abscess

Focal suppurative infection (Figure 9.1) spreads from paranasal sinuses, mastoiditis, otitis media, osteomyelitis, postoperatively and penetrating brain injuries or via bloodstream spread. No cause is found in around one-fifth. Cerebellar abscesses and multiple abscesses are usually from bloodstream spread.

Onset can be gradual, over weeks or even months, with headache, sometimes with vomiting, seizures and focal signs. Fever can be absent: it is hard to believe that brain suppuration can sometimes produce so few symptoms. There can however be rapid progression, especially with a cerebellar abscess, a prominent cause of acute hydrocephalus. Rupture of an abscess causes a dramatic headache and meningitis.

Routine haematology: almost always raised ESR and white count. Blood cultures: seldom positive. Brain CT: typical thin ring. MR imaging: restricted diffusion within central pus can help distinction from metastases. Early abscesses are frequently diagnosed as gliomas.

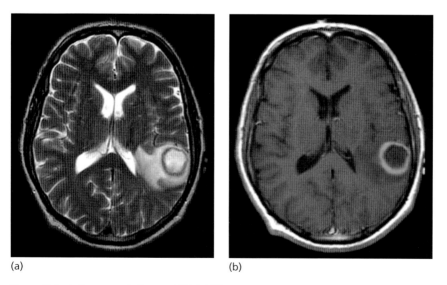

(a)        (b)

**Figure 9.1**  Left temporal abscess MRI: (a) T2-W. (b) T1-W post-contrast.

Management: pus evacuation by image guidance and antibiotics. Steroids for cerebral oedema. Pathogens can be multiple and typically isolated only after pus evacuation. Numerous organisms can cause an abscess: group D streps such as *S. milleri*, anaerobes, fusobacteria, listeria, staph. aureus, aerobic streps, enterobacteriaceae, pseudomonas, nocardia, actinomyces, prevotella, strep. viridans, TB, cryptococcus, candida, aspergillus and toxoplasma. Survival is excellent (80%) when fully alert, but less than 50% if in coma.

## Subdural Empyema

Intracranial suppuration develops between dura and arachnoid usually following ear or paranasal sinus infection, skull osteomyelitis, penetrating head trauma, neurosurgery or infection of a subdural effusion.

Onset is typically acute with pyrexia, headache and rapid progression of mass effect to tentorial herniation. A more gradual meningitis-like picture may evolve over several weeks. Seizures occur in more than 50%. Venous extension can lead to meningitis, brain abscess or septic intracranial venous thrombosis. Imaging: see radiopaedia.org. Management: immediate decompression and antibiotics.

## Intracranial Epidural Abscess

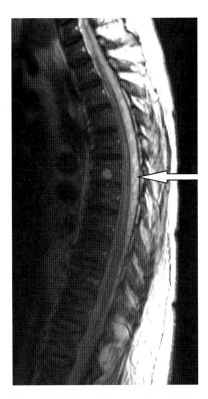

These rare abscesses follow cranial osteomyelitis or complicate ear, sinus or orbital infection. Onset is typically insidious with localised headache, sometimes with evident local infection. An epidural abscess near the petrous bone can lead to V and VI cranial nerve lesions, with spread along the epidural space to produce sequential cranial nerve lesions, both upwards (V-I) and downwards (VI-XII). CT imaging may be normal – surprising for such extensive cranial nerve palsies, but usually these abscesses are visble on MRI. Extension can lead to subdural empyema, meningitis, brain abscess and/or venous sinus thrombosis. Management: drainage and antibiotics.

## Spinal Epidural, Subdural and Intramedullary Abscess

Such abscesses (Figure 9.2) usually develop after spinal osteomyelitis, soft tissue wounds or septicaemia, but they can follow spinal surgery, lumbar puncture or an epidural/spinal anaesthetic.

**Figure 9.2**  Extensive posterior spinal epidural abscess: T2-W sagittal MRI.

Fever, back pain and rapidly progressive spinal cord compression are features of this rare neurosurgical emergency. There may however be an indolent onset of several months, with a history suggesting a cord tumour or TB. *Staphylococcus aureus* is the commonest cause. Urgent decompression is needed and prolonged antibiotics. Cord infarction can follow. An intramedullary abscess can present with a syringomyelia-like picture.

## Infective Endocarditis: Neurology

Most native valve endocarditis is caused by *Strep. viridans* or *Enterococci* spp. – that typically infect left heart valves. *Staph. aureus* is common in IV drug abusers; right heart valves tend to be infected.

Presentation: weight loss and anorexia, indolent malaise over weeks/months, new/changing murmurs, petechiae, splinters, Osler nodes. Neurological presentations are frequent – meningitis, cerebritis, parameningeal foci or infected emboli, with TIAs or cerebral infarction that lead to mycotic aneurysms. Cerebral abscesses tend to be multiple. Retinal haemorrhages, central retinal artery occlusion, III, IV, VI nerve lesions or infarction follow. Treatment: British Society of Antimicrobial Chemotherapy guidelines. Prognosis: with CNS infection mortality remains over 50%.

## Tuberculosis

TB infects via inhaled droplets, multiplies in the lungs and spreads via the bloodstream. Brain and cord lesions develop from caseating foci (Rich foci). These can rupture to cause meningitis (TBM), or enlarge into tuberculomas. TBM and tuberculomas can develop without pulmonary TB.

In TBM a sticky meningeal exudate and vasculitis develop. A prodrome of days/weeks – malaise, anorexia, fever, myalgia, photophobia and headache is typical. Neck stiffness is usually absent initially. TBM can also be acute, with headache, vomiting, seizures and stupor. Cranial nerve palsies, typically IIIrd, or VIth or other cranial nerve lesions can follow, with papilloedema and choroidal tubercles. Sinister complications are hydrocephalus, hemiparesis and coma. Tremor and other movement disorders can occur.

Diagnosis can be difficult. CSF: see Table 9.1. CSF culture takes up to 6 weeks: yield less than 50%. Nucleic acid amplification techniques (NAATs) are positive in CSF in 50%. Biopsy of meninges, lung, lymph nodes, liver or marrow should be considered. CXR: previous or active TB in 50%; 10% miliary TB. Imaging: exudates in basal cisterns, hydrocephalus, parenchymal lesions, infarction, oedema, tuberculoma(s). Test all possible TBM for HIV.

TBM was invariably fatal before anti-TB drugs and remains sinister. Treat promptly if suspected clinically. Follow WHO guidelines; seek expert advice. Mortality remains 20% and sequelae are common. In some, shunting for hydrocephalus may be needed.

## Tuberculoma, TB Brain Abscess and Spinal TB

A tuberculoma (TB granuloma) forms in the cortex, brainstem, cerebellum, cord, sub-arachnoid or epidural space. A TB abscess can also develop. Tuberculomas are often multiple and/or incidental findings on imaging. They can present as expanding mass lesions. Tuberculomas usually become quiescent with drugs but occasionally need resection.

TB can also infect vertebral bodies to form a paravertebral (Pott's) abscess. Spinal collapse leads to gibbus and cord compression. TBM can also be restricted to the cord and cause cord infarction. An intramedullary abscess or tuberculoma may develop.

# Leprosy (Hansen's Disease)

*Mycobacterium leprae* an intracellular AFB has a prolonged incubation of 2–10 years. Leprosy occurs in warm climates – for example in India, Indonesia, Brazil and Nigeria. Prevalence: over 5.5 million. Transmission is via inhaled droplets and/or prolonged close contact and also exceptionally from armadillos in the southern United States of America. There is bloodstream spread to the skin, peripheral nerves, respiratory tract, eye and testes with granuloma formation. Widely feared, leprosy is not highly contagious. The pattern is determined by the host's immune response:

- Tuberculoid (WHO paucibacillary) leprosy develops in peripheral nerves when there is an active immune reasponse.
- Lepromatous leprosy (WHO multibacillary) follows when there is a poor immune response and proliferation of bacilli.

Detailed classification describes various disease stages, only recognisable with experience.

The first skin lesion is usually a hypopigmented, numb patch that evolves into the tuberculoid, lepromatous or borderline form. In tuberculoid leprosy, there are numb skin patches and/or minor, painless red lumps. Lepromatous leprosy causes extensive hypopigmented, nodular or maculopapular infiltration of the trunk, face and earlobes. Facial coarsening develops, a.k.a. leonine facies. The larynx and testes may become involved. Facial weakness and anaesthesia can lead to exposure keratitis.

In tuberculoid leprosy, superficial nerves become thickened – a.k.a nerves of predeliction – ulnar, median, superficial radial, posterior tibial, sural, common peroneal, facial, trigeminal, greater auricular and supraorbital. Lepromatous leprosy can cause a mononeuritis multiplex or a polyneuropathy. Anaesthesia leads to clawed hands and feet.

Diagnosis is initially clinical: numb patches and skin lesions are easily recognised – and feared. A skin smear can assess AFB density – AFBs are always found in multi-bacillary leprosy.Skin and nerve biopsy can be helpful. The Lepromin skin test is strongly positive in tuberculoid but negative in lepromatous leprosy – and can be positive following BCG or TB. PCR amplification can detect AFBs.

Drugs: a rifampicin, dapsone and clofazimine combination is effective. In the United Kingdom, involve a specialist centre.

## Syphilis and Neurosyphilis *(Treponema pallidum pallidum)*

Neurosyphilis was once common. In the United Kingdom and elsewhere it develops mainly in HIV+ve populations. In addition to sexual contact, transmission can occur from mother to fetus and exceptionally from blood products.

Primary syphilis: a painless ulcer a.k.a. a chancre forms at the inoculation site, usually penis or vagina with local lymphadenopathy and bloodstream spread. A chancre, though infectious heals spontaneously.

Secondary syphilis, also infectious, follows in 6–12 weeks. A maculopapular rash involves palms, soles and mucosa, with generalised lymphadenopathy, and fever. Meningitis, proctitis, hepatitis, gastritis, nephrotic syndrome and iridocyclitis can develop. Secondary syphilis also resolves spontaneously to become latent. About one-third of untreated patients develop late disease.

All varieties of late neurosyphilis are non-infectious:

- Asymptomatic – latent, for many years
- Meningeal and meningovascular – subacute/chronic meningitis and/or arteritis
- General paresis (dementia), tabes dorsalis, intracerebral gummas, diffuse hyperplastic pachymeningitis.

Meningeal and meningo-vascular syphilis, a.k.a. early symptomatic neurosyphilis develop within 1–10 years – headache, confusion and meningism. Cranial nerves lesions particularly VII and VIII, stroke, epilepsy, uveitis, retinitis and optic neuritis may develop.

General paralysis (a.k.a. GPI – general paralysis of the insane) develops 3–30 years after infection. Features: cognitive impairment, disintegration of behaviour, paranoia, delusions of grandeur and hallucinations occur, with coarse tremor of the tongue and limbs, pyramidal signs and Argyll Robertson pupils.

Tabes dorsalis has the longest latency, possibly 50 years. Posterior columns and root entry zones become atrophic. Proprioceptive loss leads to ataxia, stamping gait, impaired lower limb pain sensation, bladder, bowel and sexual dysfunction. Neuropathic (Charcot) joints develop. Optic atrophy and Argyll Robertson pupils can occur and lightning leg pains – intensely painful, sharp shooting paraesthesiae. Abdominal pain, known as tabetic crisis can occur – included historically in differential diagnosis of the acute abdomen.

Syphilitic gummas are granulomas in liver, skin, bone and the brain. Diffuse hyperplastic pachymeningitis is a doubtful entity – a motor neurone disease-like condition.

Spirochaetes cannot be cultured. In primary and secondary syphilis, organisms can be seen on dark field microscopy, in skin and mucous membrane samples.

Non-specific antigen tests include the Venereal Disease Research Laboratory (VDRL) and rapid plasma reagin (RPR). Specific tests for IgG and IgM antibodies include the fluorescent treponemal antibody absorption test (FTA-AbS), *T. pallidum* particle agglutination assay (TPPA) and the syphilis enzyme-linked immunosorbent assay. False positive VDRL and RPRs occur with previous yaws. VDRL and RPR can be negative in late syphilis. TPPA, FTA, SELISA remain reactive for life regardless of treatment.

In latent syphilis, CSF shows a lymphocytic pleocytosis (typically 5–100 cells/mm$^3$), protein less than 1 g/dL and a reactive VDRL. In meningovascular syphilis and general paralysis, CSF cell counts are 25–400 lymphocytes/mm$^3$ with protein 1–2 g/dL and reactive VDRL. In tabes, CSF can be entirely normal.

Penicillin remains the main treatment. Pretreatment with prednisolone avoids the Jarisch–Herxheimer reaction – fever, chills, headache and tachycardia. Penicillin prevents progression of late neurosyphilis.

## Lyme Disease and Neuroborreliosis

*Borrelia burgdorferi* causes Lyme disease. The spirochaete reservoir is in mammals – deer, field mice – and birds. Transmission is via an *Ixodes* tick bite that causes a skin lesion – *erythema migrans*. Erythema, neither painful nor pruritic enlarges, with malaise, fever, headache, meningism, arthritis and lymphadenopathy. Bloodstream spread causes meningo-encephalitis, cranial neuropathy, painful radiculoneuropathy and cardiac conduction abnormalities. Facial palsy is common and can be bilateral. Consider Lyme disease when systemic symptoms accompany a Bell's palsy. CSF pleocytosis seen typically in Lyme polyneuropathy makes GBS unlikely. Treatment: IV ceftriaxone for 4 weeks.

A few with untreated Lyme disease develop late neuroborreliosis. Problems include: chronic axonal neuropathy, chronic meningitis, progressive myeloradiculopathy, subacute chronic progressive encephalomyelitis and *acrodermatitis chronica atrophicans*. Chronic fatigue can follow Lyme disease.

## Leptospirosis (Weil's Disease)

*Leptospira interrogans* is carried in urine of domestic animals and rodents. Presentation: flu-like illness, vomiting, myalgia. Aseptic meningitis can develop, encephalopathy and seizures. Conjunctival injection, optic neuropathy, uveitis, cranial neuropathy, radiculopathy, and polyneuropathy can occur. The spirochaete is sensitive to benzylpenicillin, ceftriaxone and doxycycline.

## Brucellosis (Malta Fever, Undulant Fever)

Gram-negative *Brucella* coccobacilli infect sheep, cattle, camels, pigs and others. Usual transmission: infected/unpasteurised milk. Brucellosis is a febrile granulomatous disease, sometimes with a rising and falling (undulant) pyrexia, that can progress to meningo-encephalitis, complicated by hydrocephalus, brain and cord abscesses, granulomatous vasculitis (stroke/cord) and polyneuropathy. Treatment: prolonged doxycycline + streptomycin or rifampicin, with steroids.

## Psitticosis and Cat Scratch Disease

*Chlamydophila psittaci* is transmitted from birds via faecally infected dust to cause pneumonia and can cause brainstem encephalitis, a cerebellar syndrome, uveomeningitis or Guillain–Barré. Diagnosis: serology. Treatment: doxycycline, tetracycline or erythromycin.

Cat scratch: *Bartonella henselae* infects via cat scratches or fleas. There is a local lymphadenopathy. Conjunctivitis with granulomas (Parinaud's oculoglandular syndrome), neuroretinitis (Chapter 14), optic neuropathy, macular exudates, encephalopathy, transverse myelitis, radiculopathy and ataxia can follow. Treatment: azithromycin, clarithromycin or rifampicin.

## Anthrax

*Bacillus anthracis*, a Gram-positive rod survives as a spore in soil. Spores penetrate the skin or are inhaled; bacteria multiply. Exotoxin causes tissue necrosis and brawny oedema. Bloodstream spread leads to mediastinitis and toxaemia. Haemorrhagic meningitis can also develop. Diagnosis: clinical, isolation of *B. anthracis,* immunohistochemistry. Treatment: IV ciprofloxacin with rifampicin, vancomycin, ampicillin and/or meropenem.

## Diphtheria

*Corynebacterium diphtheriae (*and *C. ulcerans)*, aerobic Gram-positive bacteria produce a thick inflammatory pseudomembrane. Immunisation (1942) has almost eliminated the disease in the United Kingdom – there were once 3500 deaths annually, mostly in children. Incubation: 1–7 days, followed by sore throat with pseudomembrane or skin lesions. Toxin leads to myocarditis, palatal/pharyngeal paralysis and bulbar weakness. A severe sensorimotor demyelinating neuropathy can develop, even months later. Diagnosis: clinical, nose/throat swabs, sampling for *C. diphtheriae* and toxin. Treatment: diphtheria antitoxin, penicillin; support for complications.

## Botulism

*Clostridium botulinum*, an anaerobic Gram-positive rod whose spores survive in soil produces a neurotoxin. Toxin can contaminate food and absorbed from the gut to bind irreversibly to presynaptic membranes of neuromuscular and autonomic junctions. Toxin inhibits acetylcholine release. Paralysis follows. After 12–36 hours, nausea, vomiting and abdominal pain are followed by paralysis – blurred vision, diplopia, dysarthria, dysphagia, facial weakness, ptosis, external ophthalmoplegia, limb and respiratory weakenss. Patients remain afebrile, with normal sensation.

Wound botulism has an incubation of 4–14 days and similar features. Injection of black tar heroin contaminated with spores is the usual cause today.

Diagnosis: clinical recognition. CSF and routine bloods: normal. *C. botulinum* can be cultured from wounds, stool or food. Toxin detection: serum, stool and food. Electrophysiology may be helpful. Monitor, in ITU. Immediate antitoxin; debride wounds; penicillin and metronidazole. Mortality remains over 10%.

## Tetanus

Tetanus is preventable by immunisation, rare in the United Kingdom but common world-wide. Tetanospasmin is made by the anaerobic Gram-positive rod *Clostridium tetani*. a ubiquitous organism in soil and elsewhere whose spores are resistant to disinfectants and boiling for 20 minutes. Under anaerobic conditions spores germinate. Toxin produced in a wound binds initially to motor nerve terminals and then via axonal transport to the cord and brainstem. Toxin inhibits release of GABA and glycine, important inhibitory neuro-transmitters. Motor neurones then fire rapidly to produce muscle spasms and rigidity. Preganglionic sympathetic neurones are also affected. Tetanospasmin can also produce weakness through blockade of acetylcholine release.

Tetanus develops following infected wounds, contaminated injections and occasionally after abdominal surgery, and in neonates with umbilical stump infection. Incubation is from several days to several weeks. Localised spasm develops near the wound, and then back pain. Increased tone in the masseters leads to trismus (lockjaw) and rigidity of facial muscles to *risus sardonicus*. Sustained rigidity develops – of the neck, back and abdomen with spasms and opisthotonus. Contractions follow trivial stimuli and can cause fractures, tendon avulsion and rhabdomyolysis. Respiratory muscle spasm lead to asphyxia. Autonomic features develop – sweating, hypersalivation and hyperpyrexia. Circulatory and renal failure can follow.

Diagnosis is predominantly clinical. Culture of *C. tetani* is confirmatory. Serological tests for toxin and tetanus toxin antibody are helpful. Differential diagnosis includes strychnine poisoning, dystonic drug reactions and autoimmune limbic encephalitis. Non-organic rigidity may be mistaken for tetanus.

ICU support is essential but there remains a mortality. Give antitoxin (tetanus immune globulin) and penicillin, or an alternative. Rigidity may last for weeks, but recovery is usual.

## Whipple's Disease

Whipple's is a rare multisystem disorder caused by a Gram-positive bacillus *Tropheryma whipplei*. CNS involvement occurs in 40% after many months or years. Slowly progressive cognitive change evolves into dementia – and rarely coma. Retinitis and/or uveitis can develop, papilloedema and optic atrophy. Supranuclear vertical gaze palsy and an oculo-masticatory myorhythmia can occur – repetitive movements that persist during sleep and can involve the neck. Seizures, myoclonus and ataxia can develop. Patients typically lose weight with abdominal pain and steatorrhoea. An arthropathy, low grade pyrexia, lymphadenopa-thy, splenomegaly, hyperpigmentation, endocarditis and constrictive pericarditis occur.

*T. whipplei* is identified on jejunal biopsy. PAS+ve staining is seen in mucosa, lymph nodes, heart valves, brain and CSF. CSF: pleocytosis, elevated protein, +ve PCR. MRI: white matter changes.

Outlook for resolution of neurological features: poor. Penicillin, ceftriaxone (or meropenem) and prolonged cyclical therapy with co-trimoxazole, doxycycline and cefixime are used.

## Tick-Borne Diseases

Ticks feed on blood of mammals and amphibia. They can themselves produce toxins (e.g. tick paralysis) and are vectors for:

- *bacteria* – Lyme disease, relapsing fever (other species of borrelia), ehrlichiosis and tularemia
- *rickettsiae* – Rocky Mountain spotted fever, Q fever
- *viruses* – tick-borne meningoencephalitis, Colorado tick fever, Crimean–Congo haemorrhagic fever
- *protozoa* – babesosis.

These are not discussed further here.

## Other Infections

Neurological complications typically meningo-encephalitis or polyneuropathy have been described in many other situations. Two are mentioned briefly here.

Mycoplasma, that lack cell walls grow in both aerobic and anaerobic conditions. Antibodies against glycolipid mycoplasma antigens act as autoantibodies as they cross-react with brain and erythrocyte antigens. Atypical pneumonia, rashes, arthritis, glomerulonephritis, uveitis can follow. Aseptic meningitis, polyneuropathy, brainstem encephalitis, cranial nerve palsies, ataxia and transverse myelitis are also described. Encephalitis occurs, mostly in children. Investigations: haemolytic anaemia with positive Coombs test; mycoplasma PCR. Treatment: doxycycline, erythromycin, azithromycin or a fluoroquinolone.

Melioidosis caused by the Gram-negative *Burkholderia pseudomallei* occurs in South Asia and Australia. Infection is via contaminated water through the skin. Cavitating, nodular pneumonia develops and encephalomyelitis, occasionally with abscesses. Treatment: ceftazidime or meropenem.

## Viral Infections

Viruses cause many neurological illnesses – from shingles to self-limiting viral meningitis, to HSV encephalitis, HIV and rabies.

### Varicella Zoster Virus: Chickenpox and Shingles

The herpes virus (VZV) causes chickenpox. VZV reactivation leads to shingles or rarely generalised zoster. Chickenpox (varicella) is typically a self-limiting childhood rash, but can cause encephalitis, meningitis, myelitis and ataxia.

Shingles follows VZV reactivation in sensory ganglia long after chickenpox. Shingles tends to be severe with reduced cell-mediated immunity and in the elderly. Tingling pain develops in one or more dermatomes several days before a vesicular rash. Thoracic or lumbar dermatomes are commonly affected. Red papules evolve into vesicles (bullae). Vesicles become pustular or haemorrhagic after 3–4 days. Zoster can spread to an adjacent dermatome. Occasionally scattered lesions occur or generalised zoster develops. Pain is often severe with allodynia. Occasionally, shingles occurs with no rash (*herpes zoster sine herpete*).

*Herpes zoster ophthalmicus* (Chapter 13) is shingles in the trigeminal ophthalmic division. Conjunctivitis, episcleritis, iritis and keratitis can follow. Nasal vesicles (Hutchinson's sign) indicate involvement of the trigeminal nasociliary branch.

*Herpes zoster ophthalmicus* (Ramsey-Hunt syndrome) is VZV reactivation in the geniculate ganglion. There is ipsilateral facial paralysis, ocular pain and vesicles in the auditory canal and auricle. Taste, hearing and lacrimation may be affected. Other cranial nerves can be involved – V, IX and X. Facial paralysis tends to have a worse prognosis than in Bell's palsy.

Post-herpetic neuralgia (Chapter 23) tends to occur with increasing age – in about one-fifth over 80. Resolution is usual after two years.

Complications include aseptic meningitis, Guillain–Barré, transverse myelitis, radiculopathy and encephalitis may occur, sometimes months later or even in the absence of evident infection. All tend to be associated with extensive zoster in the immunocompromised, especially with HIV. VZV can cause stroke from a granulomatous vasculitis and acute retinal necrosis.

Prompt antiviral therapy lessens severity and reduces post-herpetic neuralgia. Valacyclovir, famciclovir and acyclovir are used. Shingles vaccination is recommended for all between 70 and 80.

### Viral Meningitis

Many viruses cause an aseptic meningitis with meningo-encephalitic features.

A flu-like prodrome is typical, frontal headache, fever, neck stiffness, photophobia, malaise, myalgia, nausea and vomiting ± a pruritic rash, pleurodynia or even myocarditis. Meningeal irritation signs are usual, but these patients are generally less unwell than those with bacterial meningitis. Be aware that the clinical diagnosis of viral meningitis is not secure – errors occur, when infection has been pyogenic or TB. I have never made a firm initial bedside diagnosis of a viral meningitis.

Brain imaging: typically normal. CSF: cell count typically less than 300 lymphocytes/$mm^3$. Polymorphs may be present initially. Glucose: normal. Protein: normal or less than 100 mg/L (Table 9.2).

Frequently no virus is isolated – diagnosis is one of exclusion of pyogenic bacteria and TB. Throat, urine, stool and CSF samples should be cultured and serum/CSF PCR tested.

**Table 9.2** Main causes of viral meningitis.

Enterovirus: echovirus, Coxsackie A, B, enterovirus 70, 71
Mumps, measles, parvovirus B19
Herpesviruses
Varicella-zoster virus
Epstein–Barr virus
Cytomegalovirus
Arboviruses, for example West Nile virus, influenza, parainfluenza, adenoviruses
Acute HIV and seroconversion
COVID-19 – possibly

HSV-2: treat with aciclovir (famciclovir, valaciclovir, ganciclovir and foscarnet are alternatives).

Prognosis: spontaneous recovery within two weeks. There may be residua – mainly fatigue and headaches.

Mollaret's meningitis describes recurrent pyrexia and lymphocytic meningitis separated by weeks, months or years, a rarity caused by HSV-2. Attacks usually cease within a few years.

## Viral Encephalitis

Encephalitis is inflammation of brain parenchyma caused by many viruses. Encephalopathy means disruption of brain activity without brain inflammation, for example Wernicke's. Acute disseminated encephalomyelitis (ADEM) is an allergic phenomenon following infection or vaccination. Parainfectious and autoimmune encephalitides are mentioned in Chapter 26.

Worldwide, arboviruses are commonest (e.g. Japanese encephalitis (JE) and West Nile virus), but these are very rare in Europe. In the United Kingdom, herpes simplex (HSV-1) is commonest, followed by VZV. The reason why viruses cause encephalitis in some but not in others remains unknown. Over 100 viruses are known to cause encephalitis. Sometimes the cause is not found.

### Herpes Simplex Encephalitis

Herpes simplex encephalitis (HSE) is the commonest sporadic fatal viral encephalitis in the United Kingdom (90% HSV-1, 10% HSV-2). Infection from oropharyngeal mucosa spreads transneuronally, usually via the trigeminal nerve or olfactory bulb. Labial herpes is of no diagnostic relevance. In the temporal lobes, orbital frontal cortex and limbic system, there is necrotising inflammation.

Fever, seizures with stupor are typical, developing over several hours, with personality change, dysphasia, behavioural disturbance and occasionally psychosis. Hemiparesis, field defects and coma can follow. Seizures can occur with olfactory or gustatory auras.

CT brain: often normal initially. MR: high signal intensity on T2W, DWI and FLAIR:(see Radiopaedia.org for the spectrum of imaging changes).

CSF: increased pressure; 5–500 lymphocytes/mm$^3$; high protein; glucose – normal or low. CSF can be normal. PCR: CSF and blood. EEG: usually abnormal – lateralised sharp/slow wave complexes.

Brain biopsy is now rarely undertaken. Full supportive care is necessary. Aciclovir has reduced mortality substantially but about two thirds are left with residual deficits.

## Japanese Encephalitis and Viral Haemorrhagic Fevers

Cause: Culex mosquito-borne arbovirus. Prevalent throughout SE Asia and Far East. Only about 1% of infections cause symptoms. Usual features: febrile prodrome, encephalitis, seizures, coma. Unusual features: parkinsonism, tremor, choreo-athetotic head nodding, axial rigidity; flaccid paralysis.

Imaging: T2W high signal in brain and cord. Serology, culture &c: helpful. Treatment: supportive. Antivirals unhelpful. Mortality: 50%. Residual sequelae: common – deafness, focal deficits, cognitive impairment.Vaccination available; recommendations vary.

Haemorrhagic fevers include Ebola, Rift valley fever; Crimean–Congo haemorrhagic fever; Lassa fever; Yellow fever; dengue; Marburg. Features: coagulation deficits, capillary leak and shock.

## Poliomyelitis

The last polio epidemic in the United Kingdom was in the 1950s. Pockets of polio still exist worldwide, because of failure of immunisation. Incubation: 7–14 days. Cause: enterovirus – entry via gut. Features: flu-like illness, a self-limiting meningitic phase, followed by muscle pain and asymmetrical, predominantly lower limb flaccid weakness, maximal after 48 hours. Bulbar form, with minimal limb weakness. Permanent weakness is common.

Diagnosis: clinical features; virus isolation from nasopharynx or stool. Serology: helpful. Treatment: supportive. Vaccination: oral (Sabin) polio vaccine has largely eradicated polio.

Differential diagnosis: other casues of a flaccid paralysis – enterovirus 71, bacterial and viral infections, acute motor axonal neuropathy (AMAN), transverse myelitis, infarction and cord compression, and non-organic weakness.

Post-polio syndrome: some patients develop new disabilities after long periods of stability – muscle atrophy, weakness, pain and fatigue, caused by degeneration of motor units, age, overuse, arthritis or disuse.

## Subacute Sclerosing Panencephalitis (SSPE)

Subacute sclerosing panencephalitis (SSPE) is a rare fatal disease associated with measles. Onset: in children under 10 years; males:females 3:1. Seldom seen in adults.Features: intellectual regression, withdrawal or hyperactivity. Dysarthria, incoordination and tremor ensue. Stereotyped myoclonic jerks and seizures. Sometimes choroido-retinitis and optic atrophy. Progession: usually to death within 1–3 years.

Diagnosis: clinical features; EEG bilateral synchronous periodic discharges every 4–12 seconds. Measles antibody – serum/CSF. MRI: cortical white matter lesions. Treatment: supportive only.

## Rabies

Rabies, a mammalian zoonosis, fatal in man is endemic in all continents, but absent in the United Kingdom. The lyssa virus is usually inoculated via a dog bite. There is massive viral replication in brain neurones – Negri bodies are seen at autopsy.

- Incubation: 1–3 months, or more after the bite.
- Onset: malaise, fatigue, pain, pruritus, paraesthesiae and fasciculation close to the bite.
- Progression: encephalitis – furious (80%) or paralytic rabies.
- Furious rabies: hyper-excitability and periods of lucidity. Aggression, confusion and hallucinations. Hypersalivation, sweating and piloerection. Muscle spasms – throat, trunk and respiratory muscles triggered by sight or sound of water, attempts to drink (hydrophobia), or a draft (aerophobia).
- Death: usually within a week.
- Paralytic rabies is an ascending paralysis with urinary retention, bulbar and respiratory muscle involvement. Hydrophobic spasms may also occur. Cases tend to survive longer than furious rabies.

Clinical features are usually obvious. CSF: mononuclear pleocytosis. Viral isolation from saliva, throat, trachea, CSF. PCR – blood/CSF. Skin biopsy (neck): rabies antigen in cutaneous nerves in hair follicles.

Rabies is almost invariably fatal. Management: supportive. Prevention: eradicate rabies from dogs by immunisation, border controls. Pre-exposure immunisation: highly effective. Consider when travelling to an endemic area. Post-exposure immunisation: effective – protocols where rabies is endemic.

## HTLV-1

HTLV-1, an RNA retrovirus causes adult T-cell lymphoma/leukaemia and tropical spastic paraparesis (TSP) and rarely myositis. A small proportion of seropositive people develop disease. HTLV-1 is endemic in the Caribbean, South America, sub-Saharan Africa and Japan. Transmission: sexual contact, blood products and mother to child.

TSP is an inflammatory myelopathy, more common in females. Onset: typically around 45, with progressive paraparesis, predominantly proximal. Upper limb and sphincter problems follow; bulbar muscles are not involved. Burning back pain, leg dysaesthesiae and occasionally cerebellar ataxia.

Diagnosis: clinical suspicion, antibodies in blood and CSF. CSF: lymphocytosis <50/mm$^3$, elevated protein, specific oligoclonal bands. MRI: cervical and/or thoracic cord atrophy; brain – periventricular high signal. TSP is slowly progressive. Treatment: palliative.

HTLV-1 myositis, neuropathies and uveitis are all rare.

### Epstein–Barr Virus (EBV)

This lymphotropic herpes virus causes infectious mononucleosis, Burkitt's and Hodgkin's lymphomas, hairy cell leukaemia, lymphocytic lymphoma, nasopharyngeal carcinoma, and primary CNS lymphoma in HIV cases. Neurological complications of primary infection: rare – aseptic meningitis, encephalitis, cerebellar ataxia, transverse myelitis, polyneuropathy, brachial plexopathy, VIIth nerve and other cranial nerve lesions.

### COVID-19

Many different neurological complications have been reported such as confusion, headache, encephalopathy, stroke, venous sinus thrombosis and polyneuropathy. *Status epilepticus* and hippocampal sclerosis have been questioned. Loss of the sense of smell as a presenting complaint will be common knowledge. Guillain-Barre has been considered as a sequel and also myelitis. Chronic fatigue a.k.a. long Covid, is also well described.

## Fungal Infections

Fungal yeasts multiply by budding. Filamentous fungi grow by extension of hyphae, liberate spores and lead to brain parenchyma lesions. Fungi cause granulomatous meningitis, subacute cranial nerve lesions, arteritis/infarction and abscess formation. All fungal infections are potentially fatal and hard to treat.

Primary pathogens: cryptococcus, coccidioides, histoplasmosis and blastomycosis. Secondary opportunistic pathogens: candida, aspergillus and mucormycosis.

Cancer, chemotherapy, non-HIV immune compromise predispose particularly to candida and aspergillus. HIV predisposes to cryptococcus, histoplasmosis and coccidiomycosis. Fungal infection can follow penetrating skull trauma or neurosurgery. Actinomycosis is a rare cause of a cerebral abscess.

Diagnosis: CSF pleocytosis (20–500 cells/mm$^3$). India ink staining, culture and serology. Imaging: meningeal enhancement, mass lesions, and/or hydrocephalus.

Treatment: amphotericin B, flucytosine, other antifungals – sometimes unsuccessful.

## Parasitic Worms

All are rare in the United Kingdom except *Toxocara canis* in children – not discussed further here.

Neurocysticercosis (NCC) is a common cause of acquired epilepsy in many countries and should be considered from the travel history, if blood eosinophil count is more than $0.4 \times 10^9$ cells/L or any CSF eosinophils are seen, and from imaging. In the United Kingdom, specialist advice will usually be needed. NCC is caused by the larval form of *Taenia solium,* the pork tapeworm – the pig is an intermediate host. The adult tapeworm resides in the human small intestine. Humans develop cysticercosis if they eat *T. solium* eggs, shed in human faeces, from contaminated food, from food handlers, family members, themselves (auto-infection) and others. A pig can also eat eggs, from human stool. Eggs develop into larvae in pig muscle (cysticerci) that humans ingest in undercooked infected pork. Larvae emerge from cysts in the human gut and develop there into adult tapeworms, to complete this alternative life cycle.

NCC in man develops when ingested eggs hatch in the gut and embryos become larvae, that cross the gut wall. They then travel in the bloodstream to the CNS, and elsewhere. Larvae develop into cysticerci after 2–3 months. Main target organs are brain parenchyma, the subarachnoid space, ventricular system or cord – and skeletal muscle. Cysticerci provoke a variable inflammatory response, but can remain viable for years before they degenerate and calcify.

Initial CNS infection is often symptomless. Epilepsy – generalised or partial – is one common presentation. In the meninges, cysticerci can induce an intense inflammatory response, with hydrocephalus, and/or arterial occlusion. Massive infection of striated muscle leads to muscle enlargement and weakness. Cysticerci can occur elsewhere: intrasellar cysticerci cause visual field defects and pituitary involvement. Ocular cysticerci cause visual impairment. Cord and root lesions can occur.

Plain films show cigar-shaped calcification, usually less than 1 cm long, in brain, in the eye, and in skeletal muscles. Where the disease is prevalent, small brain lesions are often taken to be NCC, and almost as incidental findings. On MRI, the initial vesicle appears as a cyst with the scolex as a central dot. Oedema and ring-enhancement develop as this degenerates, eventually into a small calcified nodule. Differential diagnosis includes TB and glioma (Figure 9.3).

Serum and CSF serology can be either positive or negative. Cysticerci can be found on muscle biopsy. Stool examination; tapeworm eggs, in T. solium carriers.

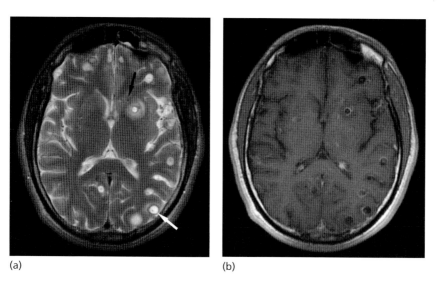

(a)  (b)

**Figure 9.3** Neurocysticercosis MR: (a) T2-W (b) T1-W post-contrast – lesions in different states of maturity. Scolex: hypointense dot (white arrow). Calcified lesions – hypointense foci.

Measures to manage raised intracranial pressure, hydrocephalus or mass effect, and/or surgery to remove a large cyst may be needed. Albendazole and praziquantel are cysticidal antihelminthics. Treatment-related exacerbations may occur. Antihelminthics are not indicated for old, calcified NCC.

## Schistosomiasis (Bilharzia) and Other Parasitic Worms

Schistosome infection is believed to cause about 200 000 deaths a year. CNS involvement occurs with *Schistosoma mansoni*, (Africa, Middle East, South America), *Schistosoma haematobium* (Africa, Middle East) and *Schistosoma japonicum* (SE Asia).

Eggs in human urine and faeces hatch in water; larvae penetrate freshwater snail hosts where they grow and multiply to become cercariae. These penetrate human skin and migrate into lungs and liver where they mature into adult worms that liberate eggs. Schistosomiasis commonly causes urinary tract and liver disease. CNS disease is unusual. *S. japonicum* causes 60% of brain infections. *S. mansoni* tends to be confined to the cord. *S. haematobium* can involve brain or cord.

CNS involvement develops after weeks or months. Mass lesions are produced by expanding granulomas leading to raised intracranial pressure or intracranial haemorrhage. Spinal cord involvement causes transverse myelitis, cauda equina and conus lesions.

Diagnosis: blood eosinophilia, serology, egg identification in urine and/or faeces. Imaging: multiple 1–2 cm enhancing lesions. There is usually a CSF eosinophilia.

Praziquantel, is effective against all schistosome species and curative in >90%. Alternatives include niridazole or artemether. Steroids are usually used. Large granulomas may need excision. Most recover if treatment is prompt.

Other parasitic worms include paragonimiasis, trichinois, angio-strongyliasis, sparganosis and gnathostomiasis can all rarely cause CNS disease – cysts, enhancing granulomas and eosinophilic meningoencephalitis.

## African Trypanosomiasis (Sleeping Sickness)

Sleeping sickness is caused either by *Trypanosoma brucei gambiense* (90%) or *Trypanosoma brucei rhodensiense* (uncommon) and is widespread in Africa. The vector is the tsetse fly. A chancre forms at the bite site; larvae migrate via the bloodstream. There is spread to lymph nodes, spleen, liver, heart, endocrine system, eye.

*Trypanosoma brucei gambiense* trypanosomiasis (West and Central Africa) is a chronic infection, indolent in onset, with a rash, intermittent fever and lymphadenopathy.

*Trypanosoma brucei rhodensiense* trypanosomiasis (Central and South Afrcia) can affect the CNS. There is meningo-encephalitis, with anxiety and uncontrolled behaviour. Urges to sleep and day–night reversal occur. Progression follows: ataxia, rigidity, akinesis and progressive pyramidal signs, coma and death. Optic neuritis can develop.

Management: trypanosomes can be seen in wet preparations of stained blood, CSF or biopsy. MR imaging: deep white matter and other abnormalities. Drugs: pentamidine, suramin and others.

### American Trypanosomiasis (Chagas Disease)

Chagas is caused by *Trypanosoma cruzi* – endemic in Latin America. Contact with triatomine bugs, guinea pig excreta, blood transfusion (rarely), transplacental infection, and organ transplantation (exceptionally) leads to infection. Parasites multiply inside red cells, that then rupture. Chagas causes malaise, myalgia, headache, anorexia and periorbital oedema (Romana's sign). Cardiac failure and autonomic gut problems (megacolon, Chapter 24) occur. Meningo-encephalitis occurs occasionally. MR: ring enhancing lesions. Trypanosomes may be seen in CSF. Treatment: acute Chagas is eradicated with benznidazole or nifurtimox. Chronic infection is difficult to clear.

### Malaria

Malaria is caused by *Plasmodium vivax, Plasmodium falciparum, P. ovale, P. malariae* and *P. knowlesi*. It is predominantly *P. falciparum* that causes death and in particular cerebral malaria in Africa. Malaria causes over half a million deaths annually. Protozoa are transmitted by the female *Anopheles* mosquito that bites at night. Rarely, transmission can be transplacental, from blood or contaminated needles.

In falciparum malaria – more than 90% of African cases and around 50% elsewhere – red cells become distorted and adherent to endothelial cells, to cause vascular obstruction. Suppression of haemopoiesis leads to anaemia, thrombocytopenia and there is hepatosplenomegaly.

With *P. falciparum* onset is with headache, fever and muscle aches, rigors and even occasionally hypothermia. Cerebral (falciparum) malaria is heralded by TIA-like events or stroke, seizures, followed by coma. Retinal haemorrhages are characteristic.

A fever on return from a holiday from any malarial zone is sufficient for a presumptive clinical diagnosis. A TIA-like episode with a fever also raises the question of malaria. Children and pregnant women are at particular risk.

Falciparum malaria can cause respiratory distress, circulatory collapse, renal failure with haemoglobinuria (blackwater fever), jaundice, DIC, anaemia and hypoglycaemia.

Management: thick blood films – and rapid diagnostic tests (RDTs). Drugs: cinchona alkaloids (quinine, primaquine, chloroquine and quinidine) and artemisinin derivatives (artesunate, artemether, artemotil). In the United Kingdon seek immediate specialist advice whenever malaria is suspected.

Prevention: clothing, repellants and nets. Prophylactic drug recommendations vary, in part depending upon drug resistance. Mosquito eradication remains a challenge.

### Toxoplasmosis

*Toxoplasma gondii* is a protozoa transmitted via infected meat and/or exposure to cat faeces. In most adults, infection causes a minor self-limiting illness. Severe disease, with encephalitis can develop in the immunocompromised, especially with HIV.

# HIV

Many HIV cases present with neurological complications. A working knowledge of transmission, primary infection, seroconversion, latent infection, symptomatic HIV infection and AIDS is assumed. These notes outline the complexity of the effects of this infection, and the immune response. Most neurological conditions can be a presenting feature of HIV.

Primary HIV infection: aseptic meningitis can accompany the fever, lymphadenopathy, rash, myalgia, arthralgia, headache and mucocutaneous ulceration. At seroconversion a glandular fever-like illness develops with aseptic meningo-encephalitis in a minority. ADEM, transverse myelitis, polymyositis-like illness, brachial neuropathy, a cauda equina syndrome and Guillain–Barré are described.

Early symptomatic HIV infection a.k.a. AIDS-related complex (ARC) can present with various neuropathies, including mononeuritis multiplex and dorsal root ganglionopathy – in addition to thrush, leukoplakia, shingles, persistent pyrexia and diarrhoea. Neurological conditions defining AIDS include:

- HIV-associated dementia (HAD), a.k.a AIDs-dementia complex (ADC), HIV encephalopathy (HIVE), asymptomatic neurocognitive impairment (ANI).
- Opportunistic multiple brain and lung infection (e.g toxoplasmosis, CMV, TB, fungi)
- HIV-associated wasting, vacuolar myelopathy
- Cerebral lymphoma
- Progressive multifocal leucoencephalopathy (PML)
- Stroke – vasculitis and/or anticardiolipin antibody and lupus anticoagulant can occur; endocarditis
- Neurosyphilis
- Polymyositis/myopathy.

Other AIDS defining conditions include pneumocysitis pneumonia, oesophageal candidiasis, uterine carcinoma, Kaposi's sarcoma and histoplasmosis. There are also neurological complications of HAART – especially polyneuropthies. Other conditions require consideration such as immune reconstitution inflammatory syndrome (IRIS) – paradoxical worsening of pre-existing infectious processes following HAART and diffuse inflammatory lymphocytosis syndrome (DILS) – salivary gland enlargement, xerostomia, keratoconjunctivitis sicca, uveitis, lymphocytic pulmonary, gut/renal involvement and occasionally a neuropathy.

# Acknowledgements

I am most grateful to Robin Howard, Carmel Curtis and Hadi Manji for their contribution to *Neurology A Queen Square Textbook* Second Edition on which this chapter was based.

## Further Reading

Davies N, Thwaites G. Infection of the nervous system. https://pn.bmj.com/content/11/2/121

Howard R, Curtis C, Manji H. Infection and the nervous system. In *Neurology A Queen Square Textbook*, 2nd edn. Clarke C, Howard R, Rossor M, Shorvon S, eds. John Wiley & Sons, 2016. There are numerous references.

Also, please visit https://www.drcharlesclarke.com for free updated notes, potential links and references as these become available. You will be asked to log in, in a secure fashion, with your name and institution.

# 10

## Nerve, Anterior Horn Cell and Muscle Disease

### Peripheral Nerve Anatomy

Peripheral nerves (Figure 10.1) are bundles of axons, Schwann cells, myelin and vessels, connective tissue and immune systems such as macrophages and mast cells. Their purpose is to deliver impulses back and forth between the central nervous system (CNS) and peripheral sensory or effector structures. The peripheral nervous system (PNS) functions via reflex arcs and by direct conduction to and from the spinal cord and brain. The PNS consists of 10 of the 12 cranial nerves, the spinal roots and peripheral nerves. A neurone-axon–Schwann cell unit is a nerve fibre. A fascicle is a group of nerve fibres and endoneurial elements within the perineurium. A nerve is a collection of fascicles surrounded by epineurium. Protective layers enable nerves to resist physical and immunological attack.

Epineurium: this is loosely packed tissue – fibroblasts, collagen, adipocytes and mast cells. Perineurium is a tight sleeve of flattened fibroblasts, with tight junctions

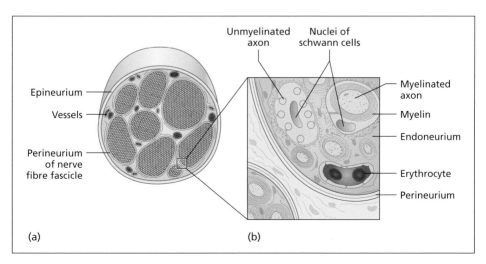

**Figure 10.1** Nerve trunk, transverse section diagram. (a) Light microscopy. (b) Electron microscopy.

*Neurology: A Clinical Handbook*, First Edition. Charles Clarke.
© 2022 John Wiley & Sons Ltd. Published 2022 by John Wiley & Sons Ltd.

that surround each fascicle, a molecular barrier between epineurium and endoneurium. Endoneurium: this space contains axon–Schwann cell units, pericytes, fibroblasts, macrophages, mast cells and vessels whose endothelium also has tight junctions. The endoneurial space is bathed in fluid – electrolytes are those of extracellular fluid, but protein (and immunoglobulin) is low. The perineurium and endoneurial endothelium form the blood–nerve barrier (BNB), relatively impenetrable to cells and macromolecules. Active traffic from perineurium and into the endoneurium occurs via pinocytosis.

The BNB protects and isolates peripheral nerves. The endoneurium is physically shielded and protected from immune attack but relatively unable to mount an immune response. Restricted access/egress of cells and molecules and raised endoneurial pressure contribute to this relative BNB.

PNS axons are ensheathed by Schwann cells. Schwann cells surround small (0.5–1.5 μm) axons – one Schwann cell surrounds several unmyelinated fibres (a Remak bundle). Schwann cells that ensheath larger axons (1–20 μm) wrap around a single axon. Myelin is the lipid-rich extension of the Schwann cell membrane. PNS myelin differs from CNS oligodendrocyte myelin.

Mechanisms that cause peripheral neuropathies are diverse. However, patterns of damage at microscopic level are limited:

- *Axonal degeneration* occurs distal to nerve transection – physical, inflammatory or vascular, focal, multi-focal or diffuse. Axonal degeneration also occurs as a dying-back phenomenon – for example in some toxic and hereditary neuropathies.
- *Demyelination* is the pathology in many hereditary neuropathies. Segmental demyelination occurs in some inflammatory neuropathies.
- *Repair*: remyelination restores some nerve function. Axonal regeneration also occurs less consistently.

Peripheral nerve diseases are either inherited or acquired.

## Inherited Neuropathies

These divide into those where neuropathy is the primary feature and those with a widespread disorder.

- Neuropathy as primary feature: Charcot–Marie–Tooth diseases (CMT), hereditary neuropathy with liability to pressure palsies (HNPP), hereditary sensory neuropathy (HSN) and hereditary sensory and autonomic neuropathy (HSAN), distal hereditary motor neuropathies (dHMN), hereditary neuralgic amyotrophy and familial amyloid polyneuropathy. Only the common CMT1A is outlined here.
- Neuropathy with widespread disorder: examples include lipidoses, such as leucodystrophies, porphyrias, disorders with defective DNA such as ataxia telangiectasia or with other ataxias such as Friedreich's and mitochondrial diseases.

Autosomal spinal muscular atrophies (SMA) and inherited motor neurone diseases (MNDs) are covered elsewhere.

## Charcot–Marie–Tooth Disease(s) and Related Disorders

CMT a.k.a. hereditary motor and sensory neuropathies (HMSN) are characterised by gradual distal muscle wasting and weakness, reduced reflexes, impaired distal sensation and foot deformity. There is wide variation and over 60 varieties, with all modes of inheritance. CMT is classified as demyelinating (CMT1) if the median MCV is less than 38 m/s and axonal (CMT2) when greater than 38 m/s.

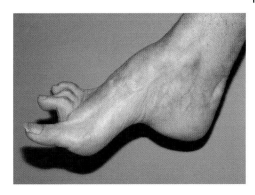

**Figure 10.2** *Pes cavus*, clawed toes in CMT1A.

In the United Kingdom over 90% of CMT cases are either AD CMT1 or X-linked.

AD CMT1 is now divided into six subtypes. The so-called classic CMT1 is the commonest (AD CMT1A). There is difficulty in walking, pes cavus (Figure 10.2), distal wasting, weakness and areflexia/hyporeflexia largely in the lower limbs, from the age of 10 or earlier. Distal sensory loss is typical. Median MCVs are <38 m/s and SAPs reduced or absent. Nerve biopsy is usually unnecessary – demyelination with onion bulbs (Figure 10.3).

With AD inheritance, or if the case is apparently sporadic, then the likely cause is CMT1A secondary to a duplication of the peripheral myelin protein 22 gene (PMP22).

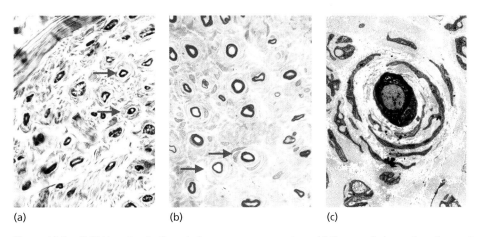

(a)  (b)  (c)

**Figure 10.3** CMT1A: onion bulb pathology transverse sections: (a) Concentric formations (arrows), reduction in fibre density. (b) Onion bulb appearance and wide interstitial spaces. (c) Electron microscopy: Schwann cell, concentrically around axon.

## Inflammatory and Acquired Neuropathies

Acquired neuropathies are primary or secondary to other conditions. These are demyelinating, axonal or mixed. Some are primary, that is diseases of peripheral nerve alone. Others are associated with diseases. Inflammatory neuropathies are linked by immune-mediated pathogenesis, with inflammatory infiltration and destruction of myelin and/or axons.

- Guillain-Barré, a.k.a. acute inflammatory demyelinating polyradiculoneuropathy (GBS, AIDP) and GBS variants
- Chronic inflammatory demyelinating polyradiculoneuropathy (CIDP) and variants
- Focal compressive neuropathies
- Neuropathies with paraproteinaemias
- Vasculitic neuropathies (Chapter 26)
- Other acquired disorders
- Small fibre neuropathies (SFNs)
- Diabetes, malignancy, paraneoplastic (anti-Hu), endocrine (Chapter 26), toxins, drugs, porphyria, vitamin deficiencies (Chapter 19), leprosy (Chapter 9), critical illness neuropathy/neuromyopathy (Chapter 20).

## Guillain–Barré Syndrome and GBS Variants

GBS, the commonest acute neuropathy a.k.a. acute inflammatory demyelinating polyradiculoneuropathy (AIDP) is a post-infectious neuropathy. Annual incidence: c. 1–2/100 000; GBS affects all ages. Axonal variants are common in China, Japan and Latin America. Infections known to predispose to GBS are *Campylobacter jejuni*, cytomegalovirus, mycoplasma, EB virus, HIV, *Haemophilus influenzae* and if rarely, zika virus. Covid-19 has also been implicated.

There is progressive ascending sensorimotor limb paralysis – numbness and weakness – that progresses for up to 4 weeks. Pain, cranial nerve involvement, dysrhythmias and labile BP are also features. Papilloedema can occur. A GBS diagnosis should be questioned if there is persistent asymmetrical weakness, bladder involvement or a sensory level. In the first few days examination can remain near normal with retained reflexes – and an organic illness disregarded. By contrast, some progress to tetraparesis and need ventilation within 48 hours. Regional variants, confined to the cranial nerves, and functional variants – pure autonomic failure, pure sensory neuropathy and pure ataxic neuropathy – all occur.

Pathogenesis: microorganisms associated with GBS have surface ganglioside-like epitopes. Humoral and cellular immune responses to these cross-react with nerve gangliosides. The hallmark of GBS is macrophage-mediated attack on the Schwann cell and/or the axolemma, with demyelination and/or axonal degeneration. The BNB becomes leaky, allowing entry of activated T cells, IgG and complement. Inflammation stimulates upregulation of MHC Class II receptors and promotes endoneurial damage.

Routine bloods are unhelpful. However, they exclude biochemical disturbances or may point to conditions that cause a neuropathy such as SLE and HIV. Hyponatraemia can occur. Nerve conduction: patchy demyelination is typical; studies can be normal in the first week. Slow MCVs, with prolonged distal motor latencies are usual, with conduction block. Lower limb SAPs are initially preserved but reduce and/or disappear. Denervation may develop. Axonal changes, without slow MCVs, can occur. CSF: protein is usually raised for 4–6 weeks but may be normal in the first week and can remain normal, in

Fisher syndrome (see below). There are either no cells or less than $10/mm^3$. Sural nerve biopsy is seldom needed.

Antiganglioside antibodies: IgG anti-GQ1b antibodies are found in most cases of Fisher syndrome and in GBS with ophthalmoplegia. Anti-GD1a and anti-GalNAcGD1a antibodies are associated with acute motor axonal neuropathy (AMAN). Campylobacter and other serology may be helpful. Culture stool for Campylobacter.

Management:
- Respiratory and cardiac monitoring are essential: prompt ventilation can be life-saving.
- Anticoagulation, pressure stockings &c; fluids and nutrition need meticulous attention.
- Physiotherapy: start immediately.
- Pain may be severe – use gabapentin, pregabalin, carbamazepine, amitriptyline, SSRIs, opiates or epidural anaesthesia.

IVIG given over 5 days halves the need for ventilation. There is no additional benefit with plasma exchange. Steroids are not indicated.

GBS remains serious. Advanced age, axonal degeneration and ventilator dependency for more than 3 weeks are poor prognostic features. Even with optimal care, around 7% die. About 25% have disability. The remainder recover, without relapse, once they have begun to improve. Fatigue is common.

AMAN and acute motor axonal and sensory neuropathy (AMSAN) cause less than 5% of GBS in Europe but about 50% in China, Japan and Latin America. Here, GBS tends to occur in seasonal outbreaks associated with Campylobacter infection. Anti-GD1a, GalNAcGD1a and GM1 antibodies occur frequently.

Fisher syndrome – ataxia, areflexia and ophthalmoplegia – is another variant. *C. jejuni* infection is associated; over 75% have anti-GQ1b antibodies. Fisher cases seldom require ventilation but can progress to limb weakness. A pharyngo-cervico-brachial variant involves bulbar and upper limb muscles and is mainly axonal. Anti-GT1a antibodies are often found. Paraparetic variants have pure motor and/or sensory or sensory-ataxic features. Acute dysautonomia can occur, with profound postural hypotension and impaired sweating, impotence and bladder/bowel dysfunction.

## Chronic Inflammatory Demyelinating Polyradiculoneuropathy and CIPD Variants

CIDP is an acquired demyelinating disease – progressive or relapsing proximal/distal limb weakness with sensory loss and areflexia and/or cranial nerve palsies – reaching a nadir in more than 8 weeks. Prevalence: about 3/100000. The cause is unknown.

CIDP can be asymmetrical. Paraesthesiae are common. Limb and back pain occur. Tremor may be prominent. Unusual variants include monomelic (single limb) paralysis, lower limb variants and sensory ataxic forms. Wasting appears late. Bulbar weakness is rare.

There are no specific tests. Exclude secondary causes and CMT. Nerve conduction studies show demyelination in at least two nerves.

CSF: protein raised in 90%; cell count rarely more than $10/mm^3$. MRI: nerve root enlargement (cervical and/or lumbosacral) often seen. Nerve biopsy: reduced numbers of myelinated fibres with active demyelination; macrophage-associated demyelination on EM.

First-line treatment: oral steroids and/or IVIG; if both are ineffectual, consider plasma exchange. Cyclophosphamide is also used. CIDP is a chronic progressive and/or relapsing disease. About 80% respond to steroids/IVIG. If a case fails to respond, an occult paraprotein should be sought, annually. Over half require assistance to walk at some stage.

CIDP variants, all rare include multi-focal motor neuropathy with conduction block (MMNCB), multi-focal acquired demyelinating sensory and motor neuropathy (MADSAM), chronic relapsing axonal neuropathy (CRAN) and chronic ataxic sensory neuronopathy (CASN). Distal acquired demyelinating sensory neuropathy (DADS) is sometimes included – many cases are associated with an IgM paraprotein.

## Focal and Compressive Neuropathies

Focal damage occurs typically because of compression, either as a nerve passes through a tissue tunnel or against a bone, for example the common peroneal nerve against the fibula. At the site of compression, endoneurial fluid, axonal contents and myelin are squeezed down the pressure gradient to produce nerve intussusception and later Wallerian degeneration. In chronic compression, focal demyelination is found. Endoneurial ischaemia can also occur.

### Upper Limb

The common focal neuropathies are summarised in Table 10.1.

**Table 10.1** Some upper limb focal neuropathies.

| Nerve and/or colloquial term | Site | Weakness | Sensory loss |
|---|---|---|---|
| Median – carpal tunnel | Wrist | *Abductor pollicis brevis, opponens pollicis, flexor pollicis brevis,* lumbricals | Palmar skin of thumb, digits II, III and IV |
| Anterior interosseous – motor branch of median | Below elbow | *Flexor pollicis longus, digitorum profundus* impaired pincer: thumb-index finger | None |
| Ulnar (elbow) – cubital tunnel, claw hand | Elbow | As above + *flexor carpi ulnaris, flexor digitorum profundus* (ulnar) | Palm – IV and V |
| Radial, a.k.a. Saturday night palsy | Upper arm/ axilla | Triceps, *brachioradialis*, wrist and finger extensors | Radial – anatomical snuff box |
| Superficial branch radial | Wrist | None | Radial – anatomical snuff box |
| Axillary | Axilla or humeral head | Deltoid | Skin over deltoid |
| Suprascapular | Suprascapular ligament | *Supraspinatus* and *infraspinatus* | None |
| Long thoracic, a.k.a. rucksack palsy | Shoulder/ thoracic wall | *Serratus anterior* | None |

### Median Nerve Compression – Carpal Tunnel Syndrome (CTS)

Median nerve compression between the flexor retinaculum and the carpus is much the commonest – carpal tunnel syndrome (CTS). CTS is more prevalent in women and frequently affects both hands, usually the dominant first. Numbness, paraesthesiae and pain in the hand and in the arm, often at night, are typical. Shaking the hand may relieve it. Tinel's sign: tapping the nerve on the wrist flexor aspect causes tingling in the fingers. Phalen's test: gentle wrist flexion causes tingling. Sensory changes can become permanent. Weakness and, later, wasting of the thenar eminence follow.

Nerve conduction studies are helpful – a prolonged median distal motor latency. A negative study should provoke a search for an alternative, such as a radiculopathy or thoracic outlet syndrome. Causes of CTS should be considered:

- Diabetes, acromegaly, hypothyroidism, HNNP, CIDP, MMNCB, leprosy, rheumatoid, vasculitides, uraemia.
- Pregnancy, repetitive strain, narrow carpal tunnel and/or a ganglion, gouty tophi, osteophytes, wrist fracture, arthritis.
- Amyloid, mucopolysaccharidosis – quite exceptionally.

In practice, if a secondary cause is not reasonably obvious, one is unlikely.

Nocturnal splinting relieves mild symptoms, temporarily. Surgical decompression gives the most satisfactory relief. Results are best if symptoms have been present for less than 2 years. Steroid injection into the carpal tunnel is carried out widely, but the needle can cause median nerve injury.

### Ulnar Nerve Compression

The most common site of damage is at the elbow. Predisposing conditions are unusual. Numbness and tingling in the IV and V digits are the most frequent complaints. Previous elbow trauma may be relevant. A thickened nerve at the elbow may point to a genetic cause or quite exceptionally to leprosy.

Most conditions that might be confused with an ulnar neuropathy should be evident clinically:

- Cord lesions, syringomyelia, thoracic outlet syndrome, C8/T1 root lesions
- Amyotrophic lateral sclerosis (ALS), monomelic atrophy, neuralgic amyotrophy.

Numbness alone usually resolves over weeks with avoidance of pressure at the elbow. Definitive treatment requires surgery – nerve transposition at the elbow, exploration and/ or release.

### Lower Limb

Lower limb focal neuropathies are summarised in Table 10.2. The commonest is probably transient *meralgia paraesthetica* – tingling from compression of the lateral cutaneous nerve of the thigh. Common peroneal neuropathy is discussed briefly here.

Tarsal tunnel syndromes are distinctly rare compared with the common (wrist) carpal tunnel syndrome.

**Table 10.2** Common lower limb focal neuropathies.

| Nerve | Site | Weakness | Sensory loss |
|---|---|---|---|
| Sciatic | Gluteal compression, sciatic notch, trauma, misplaced injections | Hamstrings and all muscles below knee, +/− superior/inferior gluteal nerve | Tibial and common peroneal territories, +/− posterior cutaneous, of thigh |
| Common peroneal – lateral popliteal palsy | Popliteal fossa, lateral fibular head and tunnel | *Tibialis anterior, extensor hallucis longus, extensor digitorum* and *peronei* | Lateral lower leg and dorsum of foot |
| Anterior tibial compartment syndrome (deep fibular nerve branch) | Anterior tibial compartment muscles – over-exertion | *Tibialis anterior, extensor hallucis longus, extensor digitorum* | None or interspace and dorsum of digit I and II |
| Femoral | Pelvis, thigh | Psoas, quadriceps | Anterior thigh and medial aspect calf |
| Lateral cutaneous n. of thigh – *meralgia paraesthetica* | Inguinal ligament – obesity, pregnancy | None | Lateral thigh |

**Common Peroneal Nerve**

This nerve is compressed as it winds around the head of the fibula at the knee. Thence, the nerve passes through the fibular tunnel (fibrous arch of peroneus longus) and divides into superficial and deep peroneal nerves.

There is foot drop – inability to evert the foot or extend the toes – with a high-stepping and slapping gait. Sensory loss involves the lower half of the lateral lower leg and dorsum of the foot. The problem may be clear from the history of squatting or obvious from examination. Neurophysiology studies confirm localisation. MR imaging can help sort out a mass lesion. Most recover spontaneously over several months. Nerve transection and a compartment syndrome are surgical emergencies. Lesions that progress or fail to recover should usually be explored.

**Chronic Neuropathies with Paraproteinaemias**

Prevalence of a serum paraprotein at the age of 50 is about 1%, and 3% at 70. About half with a paraprotein have a neuropathy, most of which are associated with benign paraproteinaemias – monoclonal gammopathies of undetermined significance (MGUS). Acquired amyloid neuropathy: light-chain amyloidosis (ALM) is associated with multiple myeloma, lymphoma or Waldenström's macroglobulinaemia.

POEMS: polyneuropathy, organomegaly, endocrinopathy, M-protein and skin changes constitute this rare paraneoplastic disorder in which the cytokine VEGF is implicated.

A demyelinating and axonal polyneuropathy occurs, with IgA or IgG gammopathy, the light chain being almost always λ.

### Vasculitic Neuropathies

Vasculitic neuropathies including cryoglobulinaemic neuropathy are among the more treatable neuropathies (Chapter 26). Pathology: *vasa nervorum* inflammation, fibrinoid necrosis and occlusion.

### Small Fibre Neuropathies (SFNs)

There is no absolute definition of these neuropathies caused by Aδ or C fibre dysfunction, sometimes with autonomic features:

- *Idiopathic*: idiopathic SFN, burning mouth, burning feet, rectal hypersensitivity, vulvo-dynia and Ross (autonomic) syndromes
- *Metabolic/Toxic/Environmental*: diabetes, hyperlipidaemia, alcohol, metronidazole, HAART, statins, toxins and non-freezing cold injury
- *Infective/Immune*: HIV, EBV, leprosy, Chagas, botulism, MGUS, paraneoplastic, Sjögren's, SLE, sarcoid and AL amyloid
- *Genetic*: SCN9A mutation, Fabry and Tangier diseases, HSAN I, IV and V, familial amy-loid and familial burning feet.

Typically, there is pain first in the feet (burning, pricking and aching), often worse at night and helped by walking or by immersion in cold or warm water. There is an association with restless legs syndrome (Chapters 7, 23 and 26). Reduced temperature and pain sensation with intact deep tendon reflexes is typical, with intact vibration and position sense. Standard nerve conduction tests: normal. Thermal thresholds testing can support a diagnosis. Skin biopsy can quantify intraepidermal nerve fibre density. Treatment is symp-tomatic, with gabapentin and other pain-modulating drugs.

Some 25% of chronic neuropathies remain undiagnosed – mainly slowly progressive axonal neuropathies and SFNs.

# Plexopathies

Brachial or lumbosacral plexus lesions cause post-ganglionic motor and sensory loss in the appropriate distribution. Causes:

- Trauma – direct injury (e.g. painful flail arm – motorcycle trauma), surgery &c and Klumpke paralysis in newborn
- Malignancy and compression – e.g. cancer, neurofibroma, radiotherapy and ruck-sack trauma
- Diabetes, vasculitis and inflammatory, e.g. CIDP and MMNCB
- Genetic – hereditary brachial plexopathy (SEPT9) and HNLPP
- Acute brachial neuritis.

**Acute Brachial Neuritis a.k.a. Neuralgic Amyotrophy**

Neuralgic amyotrophy was described in 1948, unusually late for such a striking condition. Acute pain affects the neck, shoulder and upper arm muscles – for several hours to a fortnight or more. Pain is soon followed by focal wasting (hence amyotrophy, meaning myoatrophy) and weakness, typically from the upper brachial plexus – to deltoid, *serratus anterior, supraspinatus* and *infraspinatus* and biceps. Sensory features occur in about half, typically sensory loss in the axillary nerve territory – over deltoid. Associations with immunisation, infection, trauma, surgery, pregnancy, IV heroin and vasculitides point to an immune mechanism. There is a rare familial form. Strong analgesics (even opiates) are usually necessary. Steroids do not alter the outcome. About 90% recover completely over 3 years. Rarely, the lumbosacral plexus is affected.

# Anterior Horn Cell Diseases

These are either sporadic, for example the typical common MND, or hereditary – SMAs. The wider classification is in Table 10.3, and conditions are either mentioned briefly here or simply listed.

**Table 10.3** Anterior horn cell diseases and related conditions.

| |
|---|
| *Sporadic anterior horn cell diseases* |
| Motor neurone disease – typical MND varieties |
| Facial onset sensory motor neuronopathy (FOSMN) |
| Monomelic amyotrophy (Hirayama's disease) |
| Western Pacific and Madras forms of MND, FTD, MSA, PSP and corticobasal degeneration with MND |
| *Genetic anterior horn cell diseases* |
| Familial ALS |
| Spinal muscular atrophies (SMA, I–IV, etc.) |
| Kennedy's disease – X-linked bulbospinal atrophy |
| Hexosaminidase-A deficiency – form of (adult) Tay-Sachs |
| Brown–Vialetto–Van Laere – bulbar palsy and deafness in females |
| Fazio–Londe – lower cranial nerve MND under the age of 20 |
| Multisystem (spinocerebellar) degeneration with MND |
| *Acquired/other anterior horn cell diseases* |
| HTLV1 myelopathy (tropical spastic paraparesis, TSP) |
| HIV-associated MND |
| Creutzfeldt–Jakob disease |
| Poliomyelitis and post-polio syndrome |
| Paraneoplastic syndrome and PLS |
| MND-like disease with lymphoproliferative disorders |

## Motor Neurone Disease

MND is a common degenerative disease of the neurones within the corticospinal tracts, brainstem and anterior horn cells that leads to disability and death. Varieties:

- Amyotrophic lateral sclerosis (ALS) – UMN and LMN involvement of bulbar, upper and lower limbs
- Progressive bulbar palsy (PBP) – mainly bulbar weakness (UMN and LMN)
- Primary lateral sclerosis (PLS) – UMN involvement alone
- Progressive muscular atrophy (PMA) – LMN features alone.

These patterns overlap, and variants occur. The cause remains unknown, and why, initially, localised groups of anterior horn cells fail. Annual incidence is 2–3/100 000, increasing with age, and prevalence about 4–8/100 000. M:F 1.5:1. Executive impairment develops frequently and frontotemporal dementia in about 10%.

### Amyotrophic Lateral Sclerosis

Onset is usually asymmetrical, with weakness and wasting (amyotrophy, meaning myoatrophy) of contiguous muscles in the upper limbs. There can be initial weakness of one limb, for example a flail arm(s), or a weak leg. A spastic paraparesis (lateral sclerosis) or tetraparesis emerges. Some present with dysarthria and/or dysphagia. Rarely, there is early respiratory weakness. Distal weakness is typical – hand weakness and/or foot drop. There is progression, without remission, of wasting and weakness, with fasciculation, cramps, spasticity and extensor plantars. Sensory and bladder symptoms are distinctly unusual. Ocular muscles tend to be spared.

With bulbar involvement there is tongue wasting and fasciculation, slow palatal movement and a brisk jaw jerk. Aspiration and drooling/dribbling develop. Emotional lability occurs with pseudobulbar palsy. There is increasing difficulty with communication and eventual anarthria, with dysphagia. Respiratory muscle weakness leads to respiratory failure. Selective diaphragm weakness causes breathlessness on lying flat, with paradoxical movements of the abdomen on inspiration. Depression is, obviously, frequent.

### Progressive Bulbar Palsy

In PBP, weakness is initially restricted to bulbar muscles, in about 20%. The pattern is mainly UMN, but wasting, fasciculation and palatal weakness can also be present. Subsequent spread is usual after several months. Occasionally, bulbar weakness remains the main feature for years.

### Primary Lateral Sclerosis

PLS is exclusively UMN and occurs in less than 10%. The spasticity can be slow to progress. Bladder involvement can develop. LMN features develop in a minority.

### Progressive Muscular Atrophy and MND Variants

PMA describes exclusively LMN involvement, at least initially. However, about 30% develop UMN signs within 18 months and progress to ALS. Flail arm/leg cases, with flaccid weakness of an arm or leg are more common in males below the age of 50.

The hemiplegic variant of Mills is rare – mixed UMN and LMN signs on one side of the body. Monomelic MND is disease in one limb, but this tends to progress to generalised disease. Overlap of MND occurs with features of other neurodegenerations, such as parkinsonism and progressive supranuclear gaze palsy.

### Aetiology and Genetics

In sporadic MND it is sometimes said that 'both genetic and environmental factors contribute'. The reality in almost all is that we have little idea about either. The concept that in some way neurones are programmed at conception to perish in later life has a following. About 10% of ALS is familial (FALS), mostly AD. Some apparently sporadic MND cases are genetic forms. Mutations in more than 15 genes are known – e.g. SOD1, C9orf72 and TDP 43.

No environmental factors are known in the vast majority. In the western Pacific there is a high incidence of MND that differs from sporadic ALS – dementia and parkinsonism frequently coexist. Possibly, these are caused by a toxin – cycads (palm-like shrubs/trees) are one suggestion.

### Management

There is little difficulty recognising MND. Routine bloods: normal. CK may be mildly elevated. Neurophysiology: SAPs, normal; MCV, more than 70% normal. EMG: neurogenic changes – denervation and reinnervation. MRI: degenerative changes in pyramidal tracts in severe cases. Gene analysis is not indicated routinely.

The usual natural history is steadily downhill. Occasional periods of stability occur. Patients with PBP have the worst outlook, because of aspiration – usual survival less than 3 years. In ALS, the mean disease duration is 3–4 years In PLS, a survival of 15 years is not uncommon.

There is no specific therapy that alters in any substantive way the course of MND in all its forms. The care of the individual with MND has received attention, perhaps because of past deficiencies. It is germane to outline headings applicable to any disease, particularly one with such a grave prognosis:

- Frankness about diagnosis and prognosis – people generally want to know what is going on and make their wills
- Realities about treatment and multidisciplinary care at home
- Involvement with social services and disability assessments and charities
- Management of respiration – ventilation may be welcomed; sometimes not
- Management of limb dysfunction, musculoskeletal pain, skin and insomnia
- Nutrition – by mouth, NG tube and PEG; communication aids
- Palliative care, end-of-life decisions, carers and their needs.

Riluzole is the only drug shown to prolong survival. It does so by about 3 months and is usually well tolerated. Many look elsewhere to antioxidants, creatine and homeopathy, despite no evidence of their value. Acupuncture, reflexology, chiropractic and massage may help well-being.

### Facial Onset Sensory Motor Neuronopathy

Facial onset sensory motor neuronopathy (FOSMN), a rarity is set apart from MND by prominent facial–onset sensory loss, weakness and slow evolution in a caudal direction – and a better prognosis.

**Monomelic Amyotrophy (Hirayama's Disease)**

Monomelic amyotrophy is an extraordinary sporadic wasting and weakness of an upper limb. M:F 4:1, onset typically between 15 and 25. C7, C8 and T1 myotomes are involved, sparing brachioradialis. There is neither fasciculation nor sensory loss. The condition is separate from the monomelic onset of MND, chronic asymmetrical SMA, brachial neuritis, MMNCB and cervical cord/root lesions. Once established weakness does not usually progress. There is suggestion that cervical cord compression, possibly with venous ischaemia, is the cause. MRI findings include cord flattening against the C5–6 vertebral bodies with the neck flexed and lower cervical cord atrophy.

## Spinal Muscular Atrophies (SMAs)

SMAs are rare and largely AR disorders. There is degeneration of anterior horn cells and bulbar nuclei without corticospinal or sensory involvement. There are four main types and, increasingly, additional varieties:

- *SMA type I:* infantile – Werdnig–Hoffmann: death in early childhood.
- *SMA type II:* intermediate – develops at around 6/12; may survive into adult life.
- *SMA type III:* juvenile – Kugelberg–Welander: onset at around 2 years, fasciculation, cramps and lower limb wasting; variable, may stabilise/survive.
- *SMA type IV:* adult onset – now known to be heterogeneous, with variable patterns and onset in the third to sixth decades. Progressive limb girdle or scapuloperoneal weakness, difficulty with stairs/walking – resembling a limb girdle dystrophy. Respiratory involvement and scoliosis rare.

SMA types I–III and some of type IV (95% of all SMA) are associated with reductions in the product of the *SMNI* (survival motor neurone gene, chromosomes 5q11.2–5q13.3). The *SMNI* gene encodes the SMNI protein, involved in RNA metabolism. Severity of the phenotype correlates with the SMNI protein level. In the majority, the protein is functionally absent; survival depends on expression of the *SMNII* gene. There are no specific treatments.

## Kennedy's Disease (X-Linked Spinobulbar Muscular Atrophy)

Kennedy's is important because the pattern can resemble MND. With a frequency of 1/50000/year, it is not uncommon. Kennedy's affects males from the third decade. It is caused by a CAG trinucleotide repeat expansion in exon 1 of the androgen receptor gene on Xp11–12. There are:

- prominent oral and perioral fasciculations
- progressive dysarthria and dysphagia – LMN bulbar weakness
- shoulder girdle, axial and limb weakness, with cramps.

Upper motor neurone signs are absent. Sensory loss occurs. Other features include diabetes, testicular atrophy and gynaecomastia. Kennedy's progresses more slowly than typical MND – many have a near normal life expectancy. There is no specific treatment.

**Investigation: SMA and Kennedy's**

Serum CK: often normal in SMA types I–III but elevated in Kennedy's and some SMA IVs. Nerve conduction: reduced CMAPs but normal MCVs and SAPs, except in Kennedy's disease where sensory changes occur. EMG: acute denervation and chronic reinnervation. Muscle biopsy: acute denervation and secondary myopathic change – excludes primary muscle disease.

# Neuromuscular Junction Disorders

## Myasthenia Gravis

In myasthenia gravis (MG), autoantibodies interfere with post-synaptic acetylcholine receptors (AChRs) of the skeletal neuromuscular junction (NMJ). In Lambert–Eaton myasthenic syndrome (LEMS), antibody-mediated block of the pre-synaptic calcium channels causes impaired ACh release. MG is caused by antibodies against the AChR in the muscle membrane (Figure 10.4). There is an association with thymus hyperplasia and thymoma.

Anti-acetylcholine receptor IgG antibodies (AChRAb) are detectable in the majority of MG patients. These antibodies have many potential actions but importantly:

- Bind to receptors, leading to NMJ blockade – receptor channels fail to open normally
- Bind complement, leading to destruction of the motor end plate (MEP).

Loss of voltage-gated $Na^+$ channels at the MEP leads to reduced muscle depolarisation and an increased threshold for muscle action potential initiation. Anti-MuSK antibodies are also found (see below).

MG occurs more in women than men in the second and third decades. There is also a second peak in the sixth and seventh decades, more so in males. Prevalence: about 15/100 000. Fatigable weakness is the hallmark, in ocular, cranial nerve, limb, trunk and/or respiratory muscles.

Initial complaints are often difficulty focussing, diplopia and/or unilateral or asymmetrical ptosis that worsens as the day passes. Weakness remains within the ocular muscles in 15%. Jaw and facial muscles, speech/swallowing, neck and respiratory muscles are all commonly affected. Muscles simply feel more tired than normal in the early stages. In many, initial weakness is dismissed as non-organic, especially in young females. MG is usually lifelong though there can be long remissions.

Examination: fatigable weakness can be found in any affected muscle, with repetitive or sustained activity. Ptosis is common. Cogan's lid twitch sign is said to be pathognomonic, but many find it hard to see – when the patient refixates from downgaze to the primary position, there is overshoot of the eyelid before it returns to the position of ptosis. Ophthalmoplegia is fatigable and tends not to fit the pattern of a single oculomotor muscle palsy. Even total external ophthalmoplegia can occur.

Respiratory weakness limits chest wall movement, and accessory muscles come into use. Trunk weakness leads to difficulty sitting up. Limb weakness is fatigable, typically

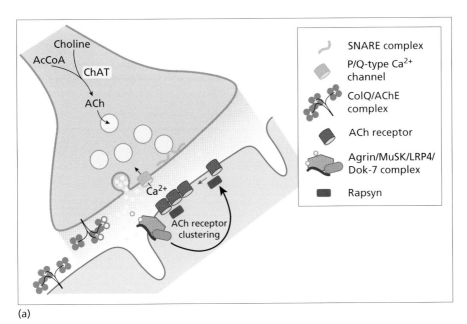

(a)

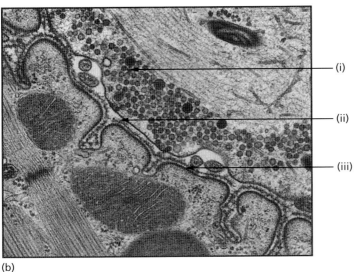

(b)

**Figure 10.4** Neuromuscular junction. (a) Motor end plate: acetylcholine (ACh) synthesis and release. AChE, acetylcholinesterase; AcCoA, acetyl coenzyme A; ChAT, choline acetyltransferase; ColQ, AChE collagen-like tail subunit; Dok-7, downstream of tyrosine kinase 7; LRP4, low-density lipoprotein receptor-related protein 4; MuSK, muscle-specific kinase; SNARE, soluble NSF attachment protein receptor. (b) Electron micrograph: (i) presynaptic vesicle, (ii) synaptic cleft and (iii) post-synaptic membrane.

proximal, sometimes asymmetrical and worsens towards evening or with extreme heat, stress, infection, pregnancy and menstruation. 20% have prominent bulbar symptoms early on.

Anti-MuSK MG often occurs in young women – with facial, bulbar and respiratory muscle weaknesses. MG can coexist with autoimmune diseases such as diabetes, rheumatoid, pernicious anaemia, SLE, vitiligo and thyroiditis.

Drugs can precipitate or exacerbate MG:

- NMJ blocking agents such as succinylcholine
- aminoglycoside antibiotics
- phenytoin
- chloroquine and D-penicillamine
- quinine, lidocaine and β-blockers

Congenital myasthenic syndromes (CMSs) are rare genetic disorders with NMJ abnormalities. Mainly, autosomal recessive, they are classified into over 10 subtypes.

### Management

MG is usually a clinical diagnosis, supported by serology and electrophysiology. Botulism and other causes of a paralytic illness should be considered.

AChRAbs, the most specific marker, are detected in 75% with generalised MG and 50% with pure ocular MG. AChRAb levels fluctuate with disease severity. Anti-MuSK antibodies occur in more than 50% of seronegative myasthenia gravis (SNMG) and are not found in AChRAb-positive MG. Other autoantibodies found include anti-striated muscle, anti-smooth muscle, antinuclear and antithyroid antibodies, rheumatoid factor and antibodies to gastric parietal cells and red cells.

Electrophysiology (Chapter 4): repetitive stimuli at 3 Hz lead to a decrement in the CMAP amplitude of >15%. An increase in jitter, sometimes restricted to ocular or facial muscles, and blocking is also seen. However, single fibre EMG is not specific – jitter develops in other disorders.

Tensilon (IV edrophonium – the Tensilon test) may transiently improve weakness. However, false negatives are common, false positives occur and the test is unsafe in the elderly and with heart disease, because of bradycardia and ventricular fibrillation.

Treatment is with anticholinesterases (symptomatic), disease-modifying drugs (steroids, immunosuppressants, IVIG and/or plasma exchange) and/or thymectomy. Pyridostigmine is the most widely used anticholinesterase. Anti-MuSKAb myasthenia is less responsive to pyridostigmine than AChRAb-positive myasthenia.

Steroids are effective in establishing remission. Prednisolone should be commenced, gradually in hospital because of the risk of deterioration during the first fortnight. Marked improvement follows in more than 50% and remission in 25% within 6 months. 5% do not improve. Azathioprine reduces the dose of prednisolone. Mycophenolate, methotrexate and ciclosporin are sometimes used as alternative immunosuppressants. Rituximab is also used occasionally. Plasma exchange reduces AChRAb titres and is valuable in producing short-term improvement; IVIG is similar in efficacy.

Thymectomy has been used in the treatment of MG for more than 50 years. In most young patients the thymus is hyperplastic. 10% of MG patients have a thymoma. Thymectomy is recommended in seropositive MG from late childhood up to the age of 60. In those over 60, with seronegative or ocular MG, its role is unclear.

Myasthenic crisis means development of ventilatory failure. Less than one-fifth will have a myasthenic crisis, precipitated by infection, surgery, inadequate treatment or rapid tapering of steroid dosage. Ventilation will frequently be needed.

Cholinergic crisis, though rare, should be considered in patients who become weak on high doses of pyridostigmine. Cholinergic side effects include sweating, hypersalivation, profuse bronchial secretion and miosis. Eventually, weakness and respiratory failure develop.

### Lambert–Eaton Myasthenic Syndrome (LEMS)

LEMS is a rare disorder caused by impaired release of ACh at the presynaptic terminal of the NMJ associated with small cell lung cancer and rarely other malignancy or autoimmune disease. The NMJ voltage-gated calcium channel (VGCC) has an $\alpha$1A subunit. Antibodies to this P/Q type VGCC cause aggregation and internalisation of the VGCC, reducing the number of functional P/Q-type VGCCs and ACh release.

There is gradual progressive weakness and fatigue. Malignancy may not become apparent until after the onset of LEMS. Weakness tends to be proximal, in the legs, with aching and stiffness. Autonomic features are common. Ophthalmoplegia, ptosis, bulbar and respiratory weakness can sometimes occur. Reflexes are reduced/absent, but after a short period of sustained effort they can become brisk – post-tetanic potentiation.

Diagnosis: clinical features, anti-VGCC Abs. Tests for underlying malignancy. Electrophysiology: a small CMAP, a decremental response to repetitive stimulation at low frequency (1–5 Hz) but an increment following sustained maximum voluntary contraction or 20–50 Hz repetitive stimulation are typical. SFEMG: increased jitter and block.

Cancer treatment may lead to improvement. 3,4 diaminopyridine (3,4 DAP) is helpful. This blocks presynaptic calcium channels, lengthens depolarisation and increases ACh release. If severe weakness persists, prednisolone, azathioprine and ciclosporin may help. Plasma exchange and IVIG are less helpful than in MG.

## Muscle Diseases

The principal function of the muscle cell is to respond to a motor neurone action potential by contracting, thus transforming electrical and chemical energy into a graded mechanical response – and then relaxing.

The myofibril is the essential element of striated muscle, made up from multi-protein complexes of actin, myosin and titin – to form the sarcomere, the functional unit (Figure 10.5). Thousands of sarcomeres are arranged end to end to give the muscle its

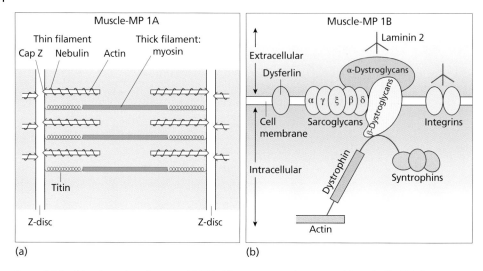

**Figure 10.5**   Muscle action diagram. (a) Thin filaments – actin wrapped in nebulin. Thick filaments – myosin attached by titin. (b) Muscle cell membrane.

striated microscopic appearance. Thin actin filaments and thick myosin filaments are arranged so that they slide over each other, shortening the sarcomere. Myofibrils are enveloped in a mesh – the sarcoplasmic reticulum, a structure central to excitation–contraction coupling. Electrical stimulation of a muscle cell causes release of calcium ions from the sarcoplasmic reticulum. This in turn activates the contractile apparatus, and an energy-dependent interaction occurs between the actin and myosin filaments. As calcium ion levels fall, this interaction between actin and myosin comes to an end: the sarcomere extends again, and the muscle relaxes.

Proteins anchor the contractile apparatus within the sarcomere and link the sarcomere to the sarcolemma and extracellular matrix. Dystrophin is attached at one end to actin and at the other to a complex of glycoproteins – dystroglycans, sarcoglycans and laminin – all associated with the sarcolemma. Ion channels span the cell membrane, controlling the influx and efflux of potassium, sodium, calcium and chloride, crucial to muscle function.

Abnormalities of any of these structures can cause disease. Muscle is metabolically highly active and thus vulnerable to any disturbance of energy generation, such as carbohydrate and lipid metabolism disorders and those of mitochondrial oxidative phosphorylation.

## Assessment and Investigation

Diagnosis can usually be made from pattern recognition in Duchenne muscular dystrophy (DMD), myotonic dystrophy type 1, facioscapulohumoral dystrophy (FSHD) and inclusion body myositis (IBM). However, in many other conditions, genetic, neurophysiological, metabolic tests and histology must also be considered. The details of genetic analysis, neurophysiology, metabolic testing, histology and immunohistochemistry are outside the scope of this chapter.

### Genetic Muscle Diseases

This has become a huge field – only the more common diseases encountered typically by adult neurologists are mentioned here:

- Muscular dystrophies
  - Dystrophinopathies (a.k.a. Xp21 dystrophies) – Duchenne and Becker
  - Limb girdle muscular dystrophies (LGMD), facioscapulohumeral muscular dystrophy (FSHD), oculopharyngeal dystrophy and Bethlem myopathy
  - Emery–Dreifuss muscular dystrophies (EDMD) and congenital dystrophies
- Other genetic myopathies, such as myofibrillar, distal and congenital myopathies
- Myotonic dystrophies (*dystrophia myotonica*)
- Skeletal muscle channelopathies
- Mitochondrial respiratory chain diseases
- Glycogen and lipid storage myopathies, e.g. McArdle's disease and carnitine palmitoyl transferase II deficiency

## Muscular Dystrophies

Pathology in many protein pathways can produce a dystrophy:

- sarcolemmal structural proteins, such as dystrophin, sarcoglycans and dysferlin,
- nuclear envelope proteins – emerin and lamin A/C
- enzymes – calpain and fukutin-related protein
- sarcomeric proteins – myotilin, desmin
- extracellular matrix proteins – laminin and collagen type 6.

### Dystrophinopathies: Xp21 Dystrophies – Duchenne and Becker

Dystrophin is the structural protein that lies just below the sarcolemma. Dystrophin links actin to a complex set of transmembrane proteins, particularly to laminin. The two principal phenotypes are Duchenne and Becker muscular dystrophy (BMD).

DMD is the lethal dystrophy affecting young boys. There is severe reduction in dystrophin. There is no curative treatment, but improved ventilatory support and surgery for kyphoscoliosis have increased life expectancy.

BMD is encountered in adult practice. Severity of the phenotype correlates with the amount of dystrophin protein. BMD presents with limb girdle weakness and pseudohypertrophy of calf muscles. Cardiomyopathy is a complication.

Diagnosis: clinical and multiplex ligation-dependent probe amplification (MLPA) analysis, PCR and analysis of dystrophin mRNA. One third of cases of dystrophinopathy are new mutations. Female carriers can have a mild phenotype, but most are asymptomatic.

Conditions such as limb girdle and other dystrophies, myofibrillar, distal and congenital myopathies are described in more detailed texts.

## Myotonic Dystrophies (*Dystrophia myotonica*, DM1 and DM2)

DM1 is the commonest adult-onset muscular dystrophy. This is a wide-ranging AD disorder – from a severe fatal infantile muscle disease to isolated cataracts that become apparent at the age of 20 or later. Features: facial weakness, ptosis, neck flexion and distal limb weakness – with evident myotonia. Additions include cataracts, hypogonadism, diabetes, arrhythmias, frontal balding, cognitive impairment, daytime somnolence, IBS and respiratory weakness. A pattern recognition diagnosis can usually be made.

DM1 is caused by an expansion in an unstable trinucleotide repeat (CTG) in the region of the myotonin protein kinase (*DMPK*) gene on chromosome 19. DM1 shows genetic anticipation. This correlates with expansion in size of the repeat sequence.

The expanded repeat may exert its effect at RNA level – expression of the voltage-gated chloride channel mRNA is altered in patients with DM1. Mutations in this channel also cause myotonia congenita. See also channelopathies below.

Patients with DM1 should be monitored for cardiac complications. Women should be offered antenatal genetic diagnosis. Life expectancy is around 55. In most patients myotonia does not require treatment. In those with symptomatic myotonia, mexiletene can be helpful. Excessive daytime sleepiness may respond to modafinil.

DM2 is less common, with proximal rather than distal weakness. Muscle pain may be prominent. The defect is a CCTG repeat sequence expansion in intron 1 of a zinc finger protein gene on chromosome 3 (*ZNF9*).

## Skeletal Muscle Channelopathies: Periodic Paralyses and Myotonias

Periodic paralyses were among the first disorders where ion channel dysfunction was identified. In periodic paralyses, episodes of weakness follow changes in skeletal muscle membrane excitability. These AD disorders were originally classified by serum potassium level early in an attack. In hyperkalaemic periodic paralysis, high potassium triggers an attack, ameliorated by eating glucose. Hypokalaemic paralysis improves with potassium but worsens with glucose. In all periodic paralyses, during an attack the muscle fibre becomes inexcitable.

A classification is shown in Table 10.4 – there are mutations in four genes, the voltage-gated sodium ion channel gene *SCN4A*, the calcium ion channel gene *CACNA1S* and two voltage-independent potassium ion channel genes *KCNJ2* and *KCNJ18*. In humans, unlike horses, who can also have these paralyses, death is exceptional.

### *Myotonia Congenita*

Thomsen's disease (AD) and Becker type (AR) are forms of *myotonia congenita*. Patients experience stiffness, myalgia and muscle hypertrophy, with stiffness that wears off, a warm-up phenomenon. Power is usually normal at rest. Muscle hypertrophy and pain may occur in both but is more prominent in the commoner AR form. EMG: myotonia is found in 90%, percussion myotonia in 50%.

Both forms are caused by mutations in a muscle voltage-gated chloride channel (*CLCN1*) located on chromosome 7q35.10. Unlike all other voltage-gated ion channels, this channel has two ion pores through which chloride ions can pass. *CLCN1* mutations cause impaired chloride conductance and thus produce partial membrane depolarisation. This creates

**Table 10.4** Skeletal muscle channelopathies.

| Condition | Channel | Mutations |
|---|---|---|
| Hypokalaemic periodic paralysis | L-type Ca++ channel α-subunit | CACNA1S |
| HypoPP1 | Na+ channel Nav1.4α-subunit | SCN4A |
| HypoPP2 | | |
| Hyperkalaemic periodic paralysis | Na+ channel Nav1.4α-subunit | SCN4A |
| HyperPP | | |
| Thyrotoxic hypokalaemic PP | K+ channel Kir 2.6 | KCNJ18 |
| Andersen–Tawil syndrome (periodic paralysis and cardiac arrhythmia) | K+ channel Kir2.1 | KCNJ2 |
| Myotonias | Cl– channel, ClC1 | CLCN1 |
| | Na+ channel Nav1.4α-subunit | SCN4A |
| *Myotonia congenita* | | |
| *Paramyotonia congenita* | | |
| Malignant hyperthermia (Chapter 19) | Ryanodine receptor | RYR1 |
| Central core disease (AD/AR) | Ca++ release channel | |

increased excitability and repetitive firing after muscle activation that produces myotonia. Mexiletine may help.

**Paramyotonia congenita and Sodium Channel Myotonias (SCMs)**
*Paramyotonia congenita* (PMC) presents as stiffness early in life, with episodes of weakness. Like hyperPP, with which it is allelic, PMC is caused by mutations in the voltage-gated skeletal muscle Na$^+$ channel α-subunit (*SCN4A*). Mutations have been found throughout the gene, although exon 24 appears to be a hotspot. Mexiletene can help. Sodium channel myotonias (SCMs) are a subgroup with pure myotonia without weakness.

# Mitochondrial Respiratory Chain Diseases

Mitochondria are organelles with many functions, especially energy (ATP) generation via the respiratory chain and oxidative phosphorylation (OXPHOS) systems in the inner mitochondrial membrane, calcium homeostasis and neurotransmitter synthesis. Mitochondria are unique – they possess both their own DNA that encodes 13 polypeptides in OXPHOS enzymes and the 24 RNA molecules needed for polypeptide synthesis. A mitochondrial disease was recognised more than 50 years ago – euthyroid hypermetabolism (Luft's disease). Mitochondrial DNA (mtDNA) mutations were discovered in the 1980s and have now been mapped (www.mitomap.org). The mitochondrial proteome contains more than 1000 proteins. Mutations in more than 200 genes have been linked to the disease.

Mitochondrial disorders affect OXPHOS. Birth prevalence is 1 in 5000. Many cause neuromuscular symptoms. They are known by their acronyms (Table 10.5) and divided broadly

**Table 10.5** Principal mitochondrial respiratory chain diseases.

| Acronym | Condition | Features |
|---|---|---|
| PEO | Progressive external ophthalmoplegia | Ptosis, ophthalmoplegia, dysphagia, optic atrophy, cardiomyopathy |
| KSS | Kearns–Sayre syndrome | PEO (<20 yr), pigmentary retinopathy, cerebellar ataxia, heart block |
| NARP | Neurogenic muscle weakness, ataxia, retinitis pigmentosa | Peripheral neuropathy, ataxia, pigmentary retinopathy |
| MNGIE | Mitochondrial neurogastrointestinal encephalomyopathy | Gut motility problems, PEO, myopathy, demyelinating neuropathy |
| MELAS | Mitochondrial encephalomyopathy, lactic acidosis, stroke-like episodes | Stroke-like episodes, migraine, dementia, ataxia, cardiomyopathy, sensorineural deafness, diabetes |
| MERRF | Myoclonus, epilepsy, ragged red fibres | Myoclonus, seizures, ataxia, deafness, dementia, lipomas |
| MIDD | Maternally inherited diabetes and deafness | Diabetes, deafness, maculopathy, cardiomyopathy, renal disease |
| LHON | Leber's hereditary optic neuropathy | Progressive bilateral loss of vision |
| ADOA | Autosomal dominant optic atrophy | Optic atrophy, sensorineural hearing loss, SANDO-like disorder |
| SANDO | Sensory ataxic neuropathy, dysarthria and ophthalmoparesis | Ataxia, neuropathy, dysarthria, PEO |
| MEMSA | Myoclonic epilepsy, myopathy, sensory ataxia | Epilepsy, ataxia, myopathy |
| CMT2A | Charcot–Marie–Tooth disease type 2A | Sensorimotor neuropathy, optic atrophy |

into mitochondrial myopathies, neuropathies, optic neuropathies, encephalomyopathies and multi-system disorders. The details of these rare conditions are not mentioned further here.

## Glycogen and Lipid Storage Myopathies

McArdle's disease: this glycogen storage disorder (GSD V) identified in 1951 is AR myophosphorylase deficiency. Patients complain of muscle pain and cramps soon after commencing exercise. A forearm non-ischaemic lactate test shows blunting of the expected rise in lactate following isometric exercise, because of failure to break down glycogen. Muscle histology: myophosphorylase is absent. The myophosphorylase gene *PYGM*, chromosome 11 is the causative gene.

Carnitine palmitoyl transferase II deficiency is commonest of the rare adult lipid storage disorders. AR CPT-II deficiency presents with muscle pain following prolonged exercise. Post-exercise myoglobinuria is frequent, and rhabdomyolysis can occur. Occasionally, CPT-II deficiency causes a painless proximal myopathy. Blood acylcarnitine profile is useful if any lipid storage disorder is considered. Muscle biopsy: lipid accumulation and enzyme assays. Genetics: *CPT2* gene assay and short arm of chromosome 1.

# Inflammatory Myopathies, Rarities, Drugs and Rhabdomyolysis

## Dermatomyositis

DM is rare and occurs more frequently in non-Caucasians and in females, an autoimmune microvasculopathy. Activated complement is deposited in capillaries. DM produces progressive, proximal symmetrical weakness in lower limbs more than the upper, with myalgia. Face and eye muscles are spared. Dysphagia and respiratory problems can develop. Rarely, an explosive form leads to myoglobinuria. Muscle induration can occur. Skin changes usually precede myopathy – a violet/bluish-purple/reddish rash on the face, eyelids and upper trunk. Knuckles can become thickened (Gottron papules) and skin coarse. Advanced DM can lead to muscle calcinosis. The lungs and heart become involved; adenocarcinomas develop in 20%.

## Polymyositis

PM is a progressive, proximal and symmetrical weakness without skin lesions. PM can be rapidly progressive, but there is usually gradual proximal weakness over months. Myalgia and/or induration is rarely severe. As with DM, the legs are more affected. Distal and facial weakness is rare, but respiratory involvement can occur. PM differs from DM: it is cell mediated. CD8+ve T lymphocytes invade and destroy muscle fibres that express major histocompatibility complex protein (MHC-1). Unlike DM, vessels are spared. Respiratory and cardiac complications can develop.

## Inclusion Body Myositis

IBM is seen more frequently than either DM or PM and occurs mainly in Caucasian men and is painless. Typically, IBM occurs late in life, over many months with wasting and weakness of quadriceps and deep finger flexors. Upright posture and hand grip are affected. Dysphagia develops in 20%. Respiratory weakness is unusual. Aetiology: unknown. There is amyloid deposition in the inclusions and rimmed vacuoles. Antibodies have been found to cytosolic 5′-nucleotidase 1A (CN1A) that has a role in DNA repair.

### Management

CK levels are raised in all three – it can be 50 times normal in PM and DM, but in IBM usually less than 10-fold. Neurophysiology: myopathic features are typical in DM and PM but not always in IBM. Muscle histology is a specialist field. Typical changes are not always present:

- in DM, there is focal infarction and perifascicular atrophy
- in PM, there is invasion by CD8 lymphocytes and macrophages, with expression of MHC-1 on fibre surfaces
- in IBM, there are rimmed vacuoles, inclusions staining for ubiquitin and amyloid and on EM 15–18 nm tubules in nuclei or cytoplasm.

In vessels: in DM, there is capillary necrosis, 'undulating tubules' and/or endothelial changes with immunoglobulin deposition. In PM, vessels are rarely involved. In IBM, vessels can be normal.

Treatment: for DM and PM, immunosuppression. Prednisolone with azathioprine/methotrexate or cyclosporin, IVIG or cyclophosphamide. For IBM, no beneficial effect has been demonstrated.

## Rarities

Granulomatous myopathies cause painful proximal weakness and sometimes muscle hypertrophy. Biopsy shows non-caseating granulomas. The differential is wide: sarcoidosis, rheumatoid, mixed connective tissue disease, granulomatosis with polyangiitis (GPA), TB and fungi.

Three excessively rare conditions are associated with eosinophilic infiltration:

- eosinophilic polymyositis is similar to PM; there is eosinophilic infiltration of muscle and eosinophilia.
- eosinophilic fasciitis: inflammation is limited to fascia – *fascia lata* is the best site for biopsy.
- a dietary L-tryptophan supplement, contaminated with an acetaldehyde derivative, is thought to have led to an eosinophilia–myalgia syndrome – with a scleroderma-like reaction and polyneuropathy.

### Macrophagic Myofasciitis
This rarity is a reaction to the aluminium hydroxide adjuvant in hepatitis B and possibly other vaccines, with PAS positive macrophage infiltration on biopsy and/or associated with previous chloroquine or hydroxychloroquine therapy. Fatigue and raised CK are features. Several years may elapse between the immunisation and onset.

### Malignancy and Endocrine Disorders
Weakness accompanies cachexia, but cancers can cause specific myopathies. A rare necrotising myopathy occurs with lung cancer, gut adenocarcinoma and breast cancer. Waldenström's macroglobulinaemia can provoke IgM antibodies against muscle proteoglycan.

Hypothyroidism, hyperthyroidism, Cushing's, Addison's, hyper- and hypoparathyroidism and acromegaly can cause myopathies.

### Necrotising Autoimmune Myopathy
NAM occurs with autoantibodies specific for SRP or HMGCR (signal recognition particle and 3-hydroxy-3-methylglutaryl-coenzyme A reductase). There is lower limb weakness, dysphagia, respiratory muscle weakness, high CK, fibrillation and myotonic discharges. Statins, connective tissue disorders and malignancy have all been blamed.

## Drugs and Myopathies

Many drugs can cause a myopathy:

- statins, fibrates, nicotinic acid, ezetimibe
- steroids

- alcohol, heroin, cocaine
- amiodarone, perhexiline
- colchicine, chloroquine, hydroxychloroquine
- streptokinase, zidovudine, alpha-interferon, d-penicillamine, ipecac.

Some drugs such as steroids will eventually affect all who take them. Statins affect only few. The spectrum varies from a symptomless raised CK to profound weakness with rhabdomyolysis. Drugs may worsen an existing muscle disease or unmask one.

### Rhabdomyolysis

Rhabdomyolysis means breakdown of striated muscle and results from muscle injury. Myoglobinuria occurs when the brown haem-binding myoglobulin discolours urine. Substance abuse and toxins can cause rhabdomyolysis through a wide variety of mechanisms including prolonged coma, seizures, agitation, hypothermia, metabolic effects and direct myotoxicity. Severity varies from slight muscle pain to severe myalgia and pigmenturia with a CK >100000. Lower limb compartment syndrome, following severe prolonged exercise, can cause extreme pain and neurovascular damage. Renal failure, hyperkalaemia, hypocalcaemia, hypotension, shock and cardiac arrhythmias may develop. Compartment syndrome requires urgent fasciotomy. Management generally is that of any underlying disorder.

## Acknowledgements

I am  most grateful to Michael Lunn, Michael Hanna, Robin Howard, Matthew Parton, Shamima Rahman, Mary Reilly, Katie Sidle and Christopher Turner for their contribution to *Neurology A Queen Square Textbook* Second Edition on which this chapter is based.

Figure 10.1 Source: Fitzgerald (2012). The late Professor MJ Turlough Fitzgerald, Emeritus Professor of Anatomy, National University of Ireland, Galway generously provided all the neuroanatomy illustrations for Neurology A Queen Square Textbook from Fitzgerald MJT, Gruner G, Mtui E. *Clinical Neuroanatomy and Neuroscience.* 6th edn. Elsevier 2012.

Figure 10.4. Source: Spillane J, Beeson DJ, Kullman DM. Myasthenia and related disorders of the neuromuscular junction. *J Neurol Neurosurg Psychiatry* 2010; 81:850–857.

Figure 10.5 Source: original artwork by Matthew Parton.

## Further Reading and Websites

Lunn M, Hanna M, Howard R, Parton M, Rahman S, Reilly M, *et al.* Nerve & muscle disease. In *Neurology: A Queen Square Textbook*, 2nd edn. Clarke C, Howard R, Rossor M, Shorvon S, eds. Chichester: John Wiley & Sons, 2016. There are numerous references.

O'Brien MD. *Aids to the Examination of the Peripheral Nervous System*, 5th edn. London: W.B. Saunders, 2010.

https://www.nhs.uk/conditions/peripheral-neuropathy/

https://www.musculardystrophyuk.org/

Free updated notes, potential links and references as these become available: https://www.drcharlesclarke.com. You will be asked to log in, in a secure fashion, with your name and institution.

# 11

# Multiple Sclerosis, Neuromyelitis Optica (Devic's) and Other Demyelinating Diseases

## Multiple Sclerosis

MS is the principal CNS inflammatory demyelinating disorder and the commonest reason for neurological disability in young adults in Europe, where health care costs are around €25 000/MS case/year. Disseminated sclerosis is an older term for MS.

Incidence varies: generally increasing with increasing latitude, *i.e.* distance from the equator. MS is more common in temperate regions – northern Europe, north America and southern Australasia – than in the tropics. Variations are also seen regionally; for example, MS is more common in Scotland and the Irish west coast than in south-east England. Prevalence in the United Kingdom is c. 150/100 000 population. F:M > 2:1. Possibly MS has been increasing slightly in females.

### Aetiology, Migration, Genetics and Environment

Aetiology remains unknown. MS cannot be ascribed to a single genetic or environmental factor – it appears that interactions between genes and an extraneous factor(s) lead to auto-immune injury. MS is associated, if weakly, with Hashimoto thyroiditis, psoriasis and inflammatory bowel disease, though not with rheumatoid or SLE.

Migration: migrants who arrive in a high-risk MS region when they are children, before adolescence carry the same adult MS risk as that of their destination. Migrants after adolescence carry the MS risk of the region from which they departed. The risk of MS declines, similarly, in migrants from high- to low-risk areas. Migration and genetic susceptibility probably explain the higher-than-expected incidence in Israel and South Africa, given their latitudes.

Genetics: twin studies show higher concordance in monozygotic than dizygotic twins, but not the expected 100% rate if MS was solely genetic. Relatives of MS cases carry a slightly greater risk than the general population. Numerous genes contribute to MS suscep-tibility, but all appear to exert a modest effect.

*Neurology: A Clinical Handbook*, First Edition. Charles Clarke.
© 2022 John Wiley & Sons Ltd. Published 2022 by John Wiley & Sons Ltd.

HLA alleles: five in the HLA region influence MS susceptibility, principally HLA-DRB1*1501. It is likely that there are interactions at the HLA class I and II loci. MS has been associated with more than 100 single-nucleotide polymorphisms. The majority are linked to genes involved in the immune system, supporting the notion that MS has an auto-immune basis or trigger.

The environment has in some way an influence on MS. Migration has been mentioned. The hygiene hypothesis suggests that since MS appears uncommon where sanitation is poor and prevalence of parasitic/other infections high, exposure to childhood infections might protect against it. This has been discredited. Approaches to non-genetic transmissibility have found no evidence of this. The implication is that the environment influences the MS risk in some way, yet unknown. Many factors have been suggested – plant or animal non-infectious agents and/or infections.

### Transmissible Agents

Numerous candidates have been proposed: EBV, human herpes virus type 6 (HHV-6) and human endogenous retroviruses (HERV). EBV-MS data suggest:

- 99% of MS cases have had EBV infection, against 94% of controls.
- People who have had infectious mononucleosis or high titres of anti-EBV antibodies have a higher risk of MS than their counterparts.
- There is some evidence that EBV within B lymphocytes and plasma cells in the brain are reactivated within an acute MS plaque. Whilst this does not establish causation, it does suggest that EBV persistence might have a role. The association might also either be an epiphenomenon or required at the onset of the disease.

### Vitamin D, Sunlight, Tobacco, Diet, Drugs, Infections, Immunisation

Two factors could provide an explanation for a link between geography, latitude and MS: sunlight and vitamin D.

- Some data suggest that high vitamin D levels decrease MS risk.
- Vitamin D supplements possibly reduce the risk of developing MS.
- Inconsistent data suggest that vitamin D supplements decrease MS relapse frequency.
- A lower risk of MS is associated with high serum 25-hydroxy vitamin D levels in Caucasians.

In the northern hemisphere it has been suggested that fewer people with MS were born in November and more were born in May, with a reversal of this in the southern hemisphere. To link birth month and MS risk, a factor could act during or shortly after gestation, such as maternal vitamin D. It has even been proposed that immune system maturation *in utero* might be affected by vitamin D levels: low levels might predispose to autoimmunity, later in life. These proposals are questioned rather than accepted. Tobacco smoking before the onset of MS is a moderate risk factor and increases disease progression.

Diet, supplements, alcohol, recreational and almost all therapeutic drug use, oral contraception, immunisations and infections have not been shown to increase MS risk or outcome.

## Pathology

The characteristic feature of MS is the plaque of demyelination, relative preservation of axons/neurones, gliosis and inflammation (Figure 11.1). However, MS is not confined to white matter; grey matter and neurone loss also follow. Plaques develop throughout the CNS but particularly in the optic nerves, periventricular white matter and corpus callosum, brainstem and cerebellar white matter, and cervical cord. Brain atrophy, ventricular enlargement, cord and optic nerve atrophy follow.

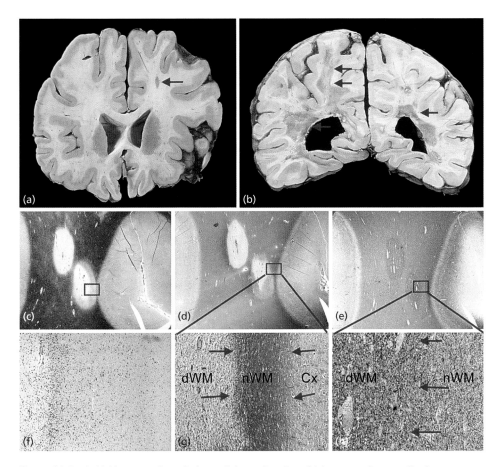

**Figure 11.1**   (a, b) Macroscopic pathology of demyelination.  (a) Arrow to circumscribed demyelination in frontal white matter.  (b) Extensive multifocal and confluent demyelination (arrows). (c, d, e) Two foci of demyelination, one with partial remyelination (red box). (c) Luxol fast blue stains myelinated structures dark blue - defects indicate loss of myelin. (d) Myelin basic product (MBP) immunohistochemistry labels myelinated fibres - shows remyelination. (e) Immunohistochemical staining - axons with  greater density than intact white matter. (f) CD68 immunohistochemistry labels microglia and macrophages. Area corresponds to red rectangle in (c). (g) High  magnification of box in (d). On  left demyelinated white matter [dWM]), a myelinated area in the centre (nWM) and normal cortex (Cx) on right. (h) High magnification of box in (e). Axons in lesion on the left (dWM) and outside it (nWM). Border: arrows. *Source:* courtesy of Sebastian Brandner and Klaus Schmierer.

**Proposed Autoimmune Pathogenesis**

Whilst speculative, this provides a model. The first step is that an environmental agent(s) combined with a genetic predisposition leads to the production of autoreactive T cells. After a latent interval of 5–20 years, a breakdown in immunological tolerance, possibly by a systemic trigger such as a non-specific viral infection or exposure to another antigen, activates these autoreactive T cells and accounts for the clinical onset. A subsequent low-grade inflammatory process follows within the white and grey matter mediated via an innate CNS immune response – activated microglia and perivascular inflammation – that leads to widespread neuronal and axonal loss and a progressive course. This could explain evolution from a relapsing-remitting course to a progressive one. A primary progressive course might be because of a milder initial adaptive immune response phase that is not expressed clinically.

## Types of MS: Clinical Course

MS is characterised by lesions disseminated throughout the CNS that appear, disappear or gradually worsen over time. This is reflected in its variable features, course and unpredictability. There are four main categories.

**Relapsing-Remitting MS (RRMS)**

Over three quarters present with relapses and remissions. The average age of onset is around 30. A relapse means an episode of acute or subacute neurological dysfunction lasting longer than 24 hours. A relapse usually evolves over days or weeks, plateaus and then remits to a variable degree. Further relapses occur, irregularly. The average relapse frequency in RRMS – without disease-modifying treatment is about 1 year.

**Secondary Progressive Multiple Sclerosis (SPMS)**

RRMS can evolve, into secondary progressive MS, with accumulating irreversible deficits. The proportion who develop SPMS increases with time. About half of RRMS cases become progressive within a decade, and over three quarters after 20 years.

**Primary Progressive Multiple Sclerosis (PPMS)**

There is progression from the onset, without relapse or remission. These cases account for less than a fifth of all MS. The average age of onset is about 40. There is no female preponderance. Some initially diagnosed with PPMS have relapses later, after a decade or more.

**Progressive Relapsing Multiple Sclerosis**

PRMS refers to a small group with progressive disease from the onset but with superimposed relapses.

## MS Classifications and Criteria

The majority of experienced neurologists diagnose MS from the clinical features and MR imaging. MS classifications and diagnostic criteria have evolved:

- Schumacher *et al.* (1965) defined definite MS as clinical evidence of two episodes disseminated in space – that is with more than one CNS lesion – and that these were also separated by at least a month or with progression over 6 months – and thus disseminated in time.
- Poser MS criteria (1983) retained this concept but added imaging and CSF findings.
- McDonald 2001, 2005 and 2010 Criteria. Those from 2010 added:
  - Dissemination in space: that lesions could be clinically silent but must involve at least two of four locations characteristic for MS: juxtacortical, periventricular, infratentorial and cord.
  - Dissemination in time: in relation to CIS (clinically isolated syndrome) onset, either a new lesion seen on any follow-up MR imaging, regardless of the timing of the baseline scan, or both gadolinium enhancing and non-enhancing lesions on a single scan.

### Radiological MS and Clinically Isolated Syndrome (CIS)

From time to time, a patient with relevant complaints, for example headaches, is found on routine MR imaging to have lesions typical of MS. About one-third develop clinical MS within 5 years.

CIS describes a first episode suggestive of MS, such as optic neuropathy (MS-ION); an abnormal initial MRI confers a high risk of developing MS – about three-quarters will develop features within a decade.

### Benign, Aggressive Forms and Early-Onset MS

Benign MS refers to a course with minimal or no disability – this is so initially in about 25%. However, even long-standing benign disease may progress.

Aggressive MS describes severe frequent relapses with little recovery. This is uncommon. Early death in MS is rare.

Marburg MS variant refers to a rare fulminating disease, usually monophasic, that can cause death within a few months. MRI shows massive lesions that typically enhance and may have mass effect.

Baló concentric sclerosis refers to a rare neuropathological variant, also evident on MRI – concentric layers of myelin loss alternating with relative preservation.

Early-onset MS: onset occurs in childhood occasionally, usually RRMS.

### Natural History, Prognosis and Mortality

The spectrum ranges from symptomless lesions to an aggressive course. Initial lesion load has some predictive value for disability in the long term. The median time for an MS case to reach a disability level that requires assistance with walking is between 15 and 30 years. Once a person has acquired a moderate disability – when walking becomes impaired – the disability that follows is largely independent of disease type. Accumulation of disability is obviously slower in RRMS than in more aggressive forms. The Kurtzke expanded disability scale (EDSS) is widely used. This runs from 0 to 10 in nonlinear stages. EDSS 0.0 = No disability. EDSS 5.0 = Can walk without aid for 200 m but disability severe enough to impair full daily activities. EDSS 9.0 = Bedbound but can communicate and eat.

Age of onset does not influence long-term prognosis. Factors pointing to a favourable prognosis include single symptom onset, afferent initial symptoms such as sensory complaints and optic neuritis, complete recovery following the first attack, a long interval between the first and second relapses, a low relapse frequency and minimal disability after 5 years. However, such associations are weak. Males may have slightly worse prognosis. Mortality: life expectancy is reduced by about 10 years. The suicide rate is over twice that of the general population.

## Clinical Features

MS can cause many symptoms, mirroring plaques within many CNS regions. The cord, optic nerves and brainstem are commonly involved. At presentation:

- About half present with spinal cord disease
- A quarter present with optic neuritis
- 10% have a brainstem syndrome.

In a quarter, there are features of more than lesion.

In RRMS, the most common symptoms are sensory and visual. In PPMS, the most usual presentation is paraparesis. During the course of MS, many symptoms may develop: weakness, spasticity, numbness, paraesthesia, pain, visual loss, diplopia, ataxia, tremor, vertigo, sphincter and sexual dysfunction, dysphagia, dysarthria, respiratory dysfunction, temperature sensitivity, fatigue, cognitive and psychiatric problems. There are no signs pathognomonic for MS, though the characteristic features are:

- Optic neuropathy (MS-ON) is common and so is diplopia, often caused by a VI nerve palsy or an internuclear ophthalmoplegia (Chapter 14).
- With spinal cord disease, altered sensation starts typically in one foot and spreads to both legs and ascends to the trunk and arms. An Oppenheim hand, a useless hand caused by loss of position sense from a posterior column plaque in the cervical cord, is unusual but characteristic. Focal wasting, flaccidity and loss of tendon reflexes can occur, if rarely; weakness and spasticity with clonus and/or spasms are more typical. Cord disease causes bladder, bowel and sexual dysfunction.
- Cerebellar signs are uncommon initially but become prominent as MS progresses. There is nystagmus, dysarthria, limb ataxia, intention tremor and truncal ataxia. Gait ataxia, with or without spasticity, causes major problems.
- Fatigue can be disabling.
- Heat sensitivity is common, caused by slowing of nerve conduction (Uhthoff's phenomenon). This also refers to transient blurring/diminution of vision on exercise or in a hot bath, when there is optic nerve disease (Chapter 14).
- Cognitive impairment occurs. Attention, information processing, memory and executive functions are affected. Depression occurs frequently, often reactive to both diagnosis and disability. Emotional lability, with involuntary crying or laughing in the absence of mood disorder, can occur. Psychosis is uncommon.

**Paroxysmal Symptoms and Pain**

A characteristic MS feature is attacks – from electrical instability within lesions. Their nature reflects the underlying site of the lesion. MS lesions can cause trigeminal neuralgia, paroxysmal dysarthria and ataxia. Tonic spasms, painful tonic contractions usually involving one or two limbs unilaterally, arise from irritation within the corticospinal tracts. Other sensory disturbances can occur, such as paroxysmal itching. Another positive symptom is Lhermitte's phenomenon, a brief electrical sensation passing from the neck into the arms and/or legs following neck flexion, caused by a plaque in the cervical cord. Phosphenes (sparks and flashes) can follow optic nerve demyelination. Lesions involving the facial nucleus or nerve can cause hemifacial spasm and/or facial myokymia. Epilepsy occurs more commonly than in the general population. Pain is common (Chapter 23), often of cord origin, typically a burning in the legs and hands. Trigeminal neuralgia (Chapter 13) can be a presenting feature. Limb spasms, from spasticity, can cause pain.

## Diagnosis and Investigations

MS is usually a clinical diagnosis, but investigations are usual to exclude other diseases, to confirm the diagnosis with MR imaging and evidence of immunological disturbance in the CSF. Plaques of white matter demyelination are seen readily on MR imaging in the brain and cord (Figures 11.2 and 11.3). Sequences are T2W and FLAIR – that suppresses signal from CSF and increases conspicuity of plaques.

- In clinically definite MS, brain plaques are seen in over 90%, and cord plaques in about 70%. It is distinctly unusual for MRI to be normal in clinically definite MS.
- Location: characteristic sites are periventricular, in the corpus callosum, juxtacortical, in the brainstem, cerebellum and cord. Brainstem and cord plaques usually extend to the surface.

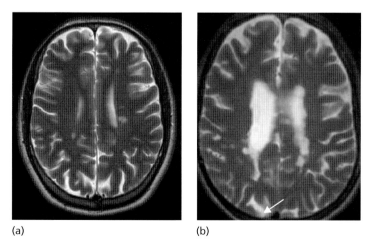

(a)  (b)

**Figure 11.2** MR-T2W. (a) Multiple periventricular MS lesions. (b) Extensive and juxtacortical lesions (white arrow).

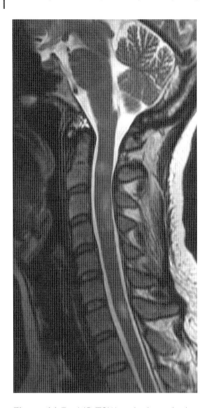

**Figure 11.3**   MR-T2W typical cervical cord MS lesions.

- Size: plaques are usually 3–10 mm, oval or spherical.
- New lesions: gadolinium enhancement, an indication of blood–brain barrier breakdown is typical in a relapse. Lesions can be homogeneous or ring shaped; enhancement persists for 2–6 weeks.
- CIS: silent additional lesions are seen in over half. They indicate the likelihood of clinically definite MS.

One problem with MRI is specificity: brain white matter lesions, often termed small vessel changes, occur in one-third of everyone over 50. These incidental lesions tend to be small, subcortical and also in basal ganglia and pons – but unlike MS, they do not reach the surface. Such lesions in the cord do not occur with ageing.

Imaging features of other multi-focal and inflammatory disorders may be hard to distinguish from MS: sarcoidosis, SLE, Sjögren's, Behçet's and CNS vasculitis. Numerous other white matter disorders can also enter the imaging differential, for example PML, CADASIL, leukodystrophies and metabolic disorders. Rarely, an MS lesion can be single, large and atypical – resembling a tumour or abscess. Acute disseminated encephalomyelitis (ADEM) and neuromyelitis optica (NMO) are discussed later.

CSF: in clinically definite MS cases, intrathecally synthesised oligoclonal IgG is found in about 90%. A parallel blood sample is required. Under one half of MS cases have a raised CSF white cell count (5–50 mononuclears/mm$^3$) and raised protein. When clinical and imaging features are characteristic, many neurologists do not perform a lumbar puncture. Evoked potentials: for the 20 years prior to MR imaging, evoked potentials were measured – typically the visual evoked potential (VEP). They are less used today.

Routine bloods are normal. No autoantibody test is helpful. Frequently, a new test is reported: a potassium channel antibody, anti-Kir4.1, was said to be present in nearly 50% of MS, in 1% with other neurological diseases but in no healthy controls. This has not been reproduced.

### Differential Diagnosis

The differential diagnosis is wide and can be considered in relation to other diseases that cause:

- A single episode of a CNS lesion at a single site, such as in the optic nerve or cord
- A multi-focal neurological condition
- A relapsing neurological condition – focal or multi-focal
- A progressive neurological condition – focal or multi-focal.

## Management

In the United Kingdom, NICE MS guidelines are updated regularly – a model for management and treatments, not only in MS but more generally to provide support, to manage intercurrent problems and in MS, relapses. Guidelines also advise about disease-modifying drugs and rehabilitation.

Some of these are listed here:

- Access to specialist and multi-disciplinary care; lifestyle advice – avoidance of infections and tobacco.
- Pregnancy: relapse rate declines slightly during pregnancy, especially towards term, but increases slightly during the first 3 months postpartum. There is no evidence of any adverse effect of pregnancy in the long term.
- Diet: despite publicity – and an industry dedicated to it – there is no evidence to support any association between diet and disease activity. Vitamin D supplementation has been advocated: the data are inconclusive.
- Immunisations: there is no evidence to support that immunisations cause any problem. However, live vaccines may be contraindicated with immunosuppressants.
- Medication: there is no evidence that the majority of prescribed drugs – or alternative medicines – increases relapse rate or alters disease course. Cannabis, widely used, certainly does not alter either.
- Stress and trauma: suggestions are made that a stressful life event might cause a relapse – a reasonable proposition but wholly unproven. Physical trauma and surgery have been proposed as triggers for a relapse: a detailed systematic review has not supported any such link.

## Relapse Management

A relapse means an episode of acute or subacute neurological dysfunction lasting longer than 24 hours. A relapse usually evolves over days or weeks, plateaus and then remits, completely or to a variable degree. Steroid therapy is the only recommended treatment and should be considered if the ability to perform routine tasks is affected. Any underlying infection must be treated. Practical supportive measures, such as the provision of care, help with children and with animals, may be required.

NICE guidelines recommend oral methylprednisolone. IV methylprednisolone should be considered when oral steroids have failed or have not been tolerated, or for those who need admission for a severe relapse or because of conditions such as diabetes and depression. With steroid therapy potential risks should be discussed. Serious complications, such as avascular necrosis, do occur, if rarely. Plasma exchange may be considered in a catastrophic relapse that has not responded to steroids.

### Disease-Modifying Therapy

Many drugs are now available, licensed and prescribed with varying degrees of enthusiasm and availability. Possible therapeutic strategies include:

- Immunomodulation: to prevent or reduce inflammatory relapses
- Neuroprotection: to prevent or slow disease progression
- Remyelination: to repair and to reverse neurological deficit and prevent disease progression.

Immunomodulation may be useful in early disease. Therapies all help through immunomodulation and thus reduction of relapses: none have been proven to delay progression that is independent of relapses or to have a primary neuroprotective or reparative mechanism. The majority are initiated in a specialist clinic.

### Interferon β

There are three recombinant injectable interferon β drugs: interferon β-1b, which differs slightly in amino-acid sequence from natural interferon β, and two preparations of interferon β-1a that are glycosylated and identical in sequence to interferon β. All have been investigated in randomised placebo-controlled Phase III trials in RRMS and SPMS and in CIS. There is no doubt that these drugs reduce relapse rate; lesion load seen on imaging is also less than in controls. The most common side effect is a transient post-dose flu-like reaction. Abnormalities of liver enzymes and blood count may occur. Rarely, an autoimmune hepatitis or thyroid disease may develop; nephrotic syndrome has been reported. Interferon β is usually contraindicated if there is a history of severe depression. Neutralising antibodies reduce or abolish its efficacy.

### Glatiramer Acetate

Glatiramer acetate is a synthetic polypeptide mixture, also given by injection. A randomised placebo-controlled Phase III trial of subcutaneous glatiramer acetate in RRMS showed >25% reduction in relapse rate in the treated group, and a later MRI/clinical study showed fewer new enhancing lesions, less accumulation of lesion load and a reduction in relapse rate. A transient post-dose reaction – breathlessness and palpitation – may occur. Erythema and lipoatrophy can develop at the injection site.

### Prescribing Guidelines and Other Therapies

Interferon β formulations and glatiramer acetate are licensed in the United Kingdom in RRMS in those who can walk – EDSS less than 6.0. Prescribing in the UK NHS is subject to strict guidelines. Teriflunomide, alemtuzumab, dimethyl fumarate, fingolimod and natalizumab: these immunomodulatory drugs are also available in selected cases.

Many other drugs and procedures have been tried in MS but have either been superseded or discontinued, which include mitoxantrone, azathioprine, cladribine, cyclophosphamide, haematopoietic stem cell transplantation, IVIG, laquinimod, methotrexate, percutaneous venoplasty and rituximab. Many other treatments have been tried, often with much publicity, and again all have failed to show benefit. These include hyperbaric oxygen, various diets, total lymphoid irradiation, sulfasalazine, oral myelin, anti-CD4 antibody, ustekinumab and dirucotide. There have also been drugs that have been thought to increase disease activity, including lenercept (the TNF neutralising agent) and atacicept (a B-cell-targeted therapy), or caused unforeseen serious adverse events, such as roquinimex (cardiovascular toxicity).

Complementary and alternative therapies in MS are a separate industry. Over one-third of UK MS cases have paid for and taken such therapies at some time. Evidence-based information provided by organisations such as the UK MS Society is helpful. Physical therapies such as osteopathic treatment can be most helpful symptomatically.

### Symptomatic Treatments and Rehabilitation

A practical rehabilitative approach is essential; issues are summarised here (Table 11.1, and see Chapter 18).

**Table 11.1** Symptomatic treatments and rehabilitation in MS.

| Complaint | Possible action/advice |
| --- | --- |
| Fatigue | Awareness, graded exercise, weight loss, amantadine, 4-aminopyridine |
| Spasticity | Positioning, physiotherapy, splints, baclofen (oral or pump), gabapentin, tizanidine, dantrolene, benzodiazepines, cannabis and cannabinoids, botox, intrathecal phenol, rhizotomy |
| Weakness | Graded exercise, 4-aminopyridine, weight loss |
| Ataxia/tremor | Difficult to help – arm weights, stereotactic surgery, primidone |
| Bladder, bowel and sexual dysfunction | Aperients, stimulator, catheter, lubricants, sildenafil |
| Pain and paroxysmal symptoms | Amitriptyline, carbamazepine, gabapentin, cannabinoids |
| Cognitive and psychiatric problems | Awareness, treatment of depression, CBT |
| Visual loss (Chapter 14) | Usual good prognosis of visual loss |
| Vertigo | Avoid vestibular sedatives, if possible |
| Bulbar and respiratory dysfunction | Monitor carefully, swallowing advice, PEG |
| Heat sensitivity | Awareness, avoidance |
| Neurological rehabilitation | Multi-disciplinary, career change (?) |
| Palliative care and support | At home if possible and desired |

## Neuromyelitis Optica, Devic's Disease

Neuromyelitis optica (NMO), a.k.a. Devic's disease, is a CNS inflammatory demyelinating disease principally of the optic nerves and cord. NMO is distinct from MS and usually associated with a specific aquaporin-4 antibody (AQP4-IgG). The term NMO spectrum disorder (MNOSD) is also used. Core features include optic neuritis, acute myelitis, *area postrema* syndrome (otherwise unexplained hiccups/vomiting), an acute brainstem syndrome and narcolepsy with MNOSD-typical lesions. Criteria for NMOSD with positive AQP4-IgG include at least one core feature and exclusion of alternative diagnoses. Criteria for cases without AQP4-IgG depend on imaging findings.

### Epidemiology and Pathophysiology

Median age of onset is in the late 30s, but there is a wide age range from childhood onwards. F:M ratio 3:1. NMO is rarer than MS in Europe. It can affect all ethnic groups, but it makes up a greater proportion of demyelinating diseases in non-Caucasians. The so-called MS opticospinal variant common in Japan is associated with the NMO-specific aquaporin-4 antibody. Familial occurrence of NMO occurs in about 3%. HLA associations have been reported.

An autoimmune basis has long been suspected because of association with autoimmune diseases such as SLE, Sjögren's and thyroid disease. In 2004, a new autoantibody, NMO-IgG, was reported to be specific for NMO. The target antigen is aquaporin-4 (AQP4), a cell membrane water channel. AQP4 antibody is over 90% specific for MNO and has a direct pathological role. AQP4 antibody binds to AQP4 in astrocyte foot processes and causes complement-dependent cytotoxicity. Astrocyte destruction leads to demyelination and thence to axonal loss. There is perivascular inflammation with complement and immunoglobulin deposition.

## Clinical Features and Investigations

Hallmarks are episodes of optic neuritis and transverse myelitis (TM). Concurrent ON and TM occur in a minority. ON (Chapter 14) is often rapid, with severe visual loss and recovery less complete than in MS. Bilateral ON may occur either simultaneously or sequentially over a few days. TM also develops rapidly and is often symmetrical and bilateral, with motor and sensory involvement, progressing to severe paraparesis or quadriparesis with loss of bladder and bowel function. High cervical cord involvement may cause respiratory failure. Severe ON or TM should flag up the possibility of NMO. However, NMO can also cause mild episodes of both. With the availability of AQP4 antibody testing, the phenotype has expanded. Other presentations include hiccups (*area postrema*) and vomiting – and somnolence – from hypothalamic involvement and painful tonic spasms. Large cerebral hemisphere lesions and a posterior reversible encephalopathy-like syndrome may also be seen (Chapter 6). Routine bloods are normal.

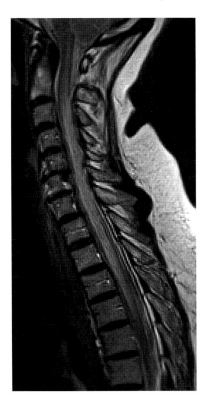

Clinical differences can help distinguish between AQP4 seropositive and seronegative cases. Seronegative patients are more likely to present with bilateral ON or simultaneous ON and TM than seropositive patients, to have less severe attacks, or a monophasic illness, nor is the female predominance seen.

Cord MRI: in TM, cord characteristically shows a lengthy intrinsic cord lesion extending contiguously over three or more vertebral segments. Lesions typically occur in the cervical and thoracic cord (Figure 11.4), and there may be extension into the caudal medulla. Cord lesions are located centrally; acute lesions can occupy most of its cross-sectional area (cf. MS), with cord swelling, T1 hypointensity and enhancement. This contrasts with MS where myelitis is usually associated with small, asymmetrical and often superficial cord lesions that rarely extend over more than a single segment. After the acute phase in NMO, cord atrophy can follow.

**Figure 11.4**  MR T2W: extensive cord lesion in NMO.

Brain MRI: this may be normal initially, but lesions develop later in the majority. Lesions in the hypothalamus and periaqueductal brainstem region are typical of NMO. Non-specific white matter lesions are often seen, and the brain lesions may also fulfil radiological criteria for MS. However, thorough inspection of brain lesions may distinguish MS from NMO. Periventricular and juxtacortical lesions are more characteristic of MS: MNO optic nerve lesions tend to be more extensive than in MS. Posterior ON and chiasmal involvement tend to be more common in NMO.

CSF: often abnormal acutely with pleocytosis greater than $50/mm^3$; usually mononuclears, but neutrophils can be present. CSF protein: usually mildly elevated. Oligoclonal bands are present in less than one-third, and unlike MS, they can be transient. AQP4 serum antibody is an essential investigation in suspected NMO.

### Course, Natural History and Management

The course of NMO is relapsing in 80% and serious. AQP4 seropositivity predicts a high risk of relapse: the majority relapse within a year. Many acquire severe and permanent disability with the initial attack. Before the current era, over 50% were functionally blind in at least one eye or were unable to walk without assistance within 5 years. Mortality rates were about 30% within 5 years. A secondary progressive phase, unlike MS, is uncommon.

Acute attacks need early aggressive treatment. High-dose IV methylprednisolone is followed by maintenance oral prednisolone. With a severe attack unresponsive to high-dose steroids, use plasma exchange. In relapsing NMO and in all AQP4 positive cases, immunosuppression is indicated. Therapies include azathioprine, mycophenolate and methotrexate with oral prednisolone. If patients relapse with these, rituximab is used. Other therapies include mitoxantrone, cyclophosphamide, ciclosporin, pulsed plasma exchange and IVIG. The importance of a correct diagnosis is emphasised because MS disease-modifying therapies – interferon β, natalizumab and fingolimod – may make NMO worse. With a negative AQP4 antibody, a single episode of extensive transverse myelitis, immunosuppression is not recommended unless there is a relapse, but maintenance oral prednisolone should continue for several months. Multi-disciplinary care is essential – principles are the same as for MS. It is important to treat features that occur commonly such as hiccups, vomiting, tonic spasms and pain. The NMO UK advisory service is helpful.

## Acute Parainfectious Inflammatory Encephalopathies

These are monophasic encephalitides characterised by multi-focal CNS lesions. Acute disseminated encephalomyelitis (ADEM) is a post-infective condition; many cases recover. Acute haemorrhagic leukoencephalitis is typically fatal.

### Acute Disseminated Encephalomyelitis

ADEM typically develops in children and young adults and follows a febrile illness or immunisation within 1–4 weeks, after rashes clear and initial fever abates. ADEM is most frequently associated with childhood exanthemata – measles, rubella and varicella. Other infections – mumps, enterovirus, EBV, HSV, cytomegalovirus, HHV-6, HTLV-1, adenovirus, influenza A and B, mycoplasma, chlamydia, borrelia, listeria, leptospira and streptococci – have all been implicated. Post-immunisation ADEM occurs less frequently. The latter has been associated with rabies immunisation and following measles, pertussis, diphtheria, tetanus, rubella, Japanese encephalitis, typhoid and hepatitis B immunisation. The majority improve and resolve. ADEM is immune mediated. Possibly, an infection or vaccine activates an immune reaction to myelin, or this causes activation of pre-existing encephalitogenic T cells. Lesions generally appear to be of the same age. Changes in the unusual fatal cases are within small blood vessels – in both grey and white matter, there is hyperaemia, endothelial swelling, vessel wall invasion by inflammatory cells, perivascular oedema and haemorrhage.

### ADEM: Features and Management

Onset is with a low-grade fever, headache and meningism, drowsiness and encephalopathy that may progress to coma. Deficits are typically multi-focal – seizures, hemiparesis, paraparesis, ataxia, visual loss, sensory disturbance, dysphasia, cranial nerve palsies, choreoathetosis, myoclonus and sphincter disturbance. ADEM usually evolves over hours to days. It is rarely fulminant. In some there is an acute psychosis and hypersomnolence. Characteristic patterns are seen:

- post-measles: myelitis/hemiparesis.
- post-rubella: seizures, coma and pyramidal signs.
- post-varicella: cerebellar ataxia and pyramidal signs.
- post-rabies immunisation: radicular features and polyneuropathy.

Routine bloods are typically normal. CSF: either be normal or at high pressure and/or with a lymphocytosis >50/mm$^3$ occasionally with polymorphs. Protein: usually elevated. Oligoclonal bands: present in about one-third. PCR may show the cause. MRI: this can be normal early in ADEM, but typically on TW2 lesion load is extensive (Figure 11.5) with large multi-focal lesions. An enhancing mass lesion, mimicking a tumour, can occur. Cord lesions extend over several levels, with swelling and mass effect, with a predilection for the thoracic cord. MRI returns normal in over 30%. Appearance of new lesions is inconsistent with ADEM and usually points to MS.

Management includes ICU support. Treatment: high-dose IV methylprednisolone followed by an oral steroid for several weeks. Plasmapheresis or IVIG may be considered. ADEM though serious is usually self-limiting. Improvement takes place over weeks to months with full recovery in over half but sequelae in

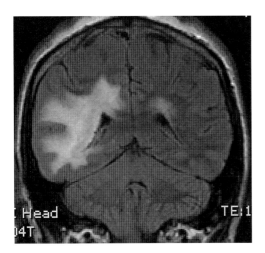

**Figure 11.5** MR FLAIR: acute disseminated encephalomyelitis.

about one-third. Common deficits are hemiparesis, ataxia, visual loss, cognitive dysfunction and epilepsy. Mortality: less than 5%.

### Acute Haemorrhagic Leukoencephalitis

Acute haemorrhagic leukoencephalitis (Hurst's disease, Weston Hurst syndrome) is a rare, fulminant usually fatal encephalopathy of unknown cause typically in the 20–40 age group. An abrupt onset follows a respiratory infection, with fever, headache, photophobia and meningism progressing to coma over several days. Focal signs and seizures are common, cerebral oedema, tentorial herniation with perivascular inflammation, haemorrhage and demyelination. There is a high peripheral white cell count and ESR. CSF pressure is raised with a high protein level, polymorph leucocytosis, red cells and often xanthochromia. Glucose levels can be normal. CT: diffuse oedema +/− haemorrhages. MRI: numerous hyperintense lesions on T2W and haemorrhagic changes. IV steroids, IVIG and cyclophosphamide can be tried. Prognosis: most die within a week. Complete recovery: exceptional.

## Acknowledgements

I am most grateful to Siobhan Leary, Gavin Giovannoni, Robin Howard, David Miller and Alan Thompson for their contribution to Neurology A Queen Square Textbook Second Edition on which this chapter is based.

I am also most grateful to Professor Sebastian Brandner, UCL Institute of Neurology and to Professor Klaus Schmierer, Queen Mary University of London and Barts Health NHS Trust who provided the macroscopic and microscopic images in Figure 11.1.

Figures 11.2, 11.2, 11.3, 11.4 and 11.5 are from *Neurology A Queen Square Textbook Second Edition*. Eds Clarke C, Howard R, Rossor M, Shorvon S. Wiley 2016.

## Further Reading, References and Websites

Leary S, Giovannoni G, Howard R, Miller D, Thompson A. Multiple sclerosis and demyelinating diseases. In *Neurology: A Queen Square Textbook*, 2nd edn. Clarke C, Howard R, Rossor M, Shorvon S, eds. Chichester: John Wiley & Sons, 2016. There are numerous references.
Wiles CM, Clarke CR, Irwin HP, Edgar EF, Swan AV. Hyperbaric oxygen in multiple sclerosis: a double blind trial. *Br Med J* 1986; 292: 367–371.

https://radiopaedia.org
https://www.nhs.uk/conditions/multiple-sclerosis/
https://www.mssociety.org.uk/

Free updated notes, potential links and references as these become available:
https://www.drcharlesclarke.com
You will be asked to log in, in a secure fashion, with your name and institution.

# 12

# Headache

Headache is experienced by almost everyone and thus a common reason to seek advice. Primary headaches meaning those without definable structural cause constitute the majority. Migraine and primary headaches cause disability in all societies. They are not psychologically based nor related to urban life, though stress makes many things worse.

A secondary headache, reflecting underlying pathology, is a relative rarity even to a general neurologist, especially if pain is unaccompanied by specific features or physical signs. Thunderclap headache with subarachnoid haemorrhage (SAH) – see later in this chapter – is a common secondary headache. My purpose is to outline the terminology commonly used by headache specialists and current concepts.

## Classification and Anatomical Concepts

Primary headaches include migraine, tension-type headache (TTH), trigeminal autonomic cephalalgias (TACs), e.g. cluster headache, and other primary headaches with secondary variants.

Secondary headaches cover medication overuse headache (MOH) and withdrawal headache, headache and vascular disorders, headache with high or low intracranial pressure, headache with an intracranial mass lesion, head and/or neck trauma, with infection and other causes.

Nerve plexuses, mainly from the trigeminal nerve (V) and upper cervical roots, surround cerebral and meningeal vessels, venous and paranasal sinuses, dura and arachnoid and the eyes. Fibres project centrally to synapse in V nerve brainstem nuclei. Projections cross to each quintothalamic tract to the periaqueductal grey (PAG), hypothalamus, thalamus and cortex. Connections also exist between the pons and the superior salivatory nucleus – a cranial parasympathetic outflow through the pterygopalatine ganglia, which explains the autonomic features, such as lacrimation and nasal stuffiness of some cephalalgias.

Migraine and cluster are classified as neurovascular or 'endogenous pain-modulating antinociceptive system disorders'. Such primary headaches activate descending systems that facilitate pain and/or as a conjecture do not suppress processing of pain signals. Why some individuals suffer is unknown, but probably reflects how the neurovascular/neurotransmitter system is assembled. Mechanisms are conjectural, but effects evident: central

*Neurology: A Clinical Handbook*, First Edition. Charles Clarke.
© 2022 John Wiley & Sons Ltd. Published 2022 by John Wiley & Sons Ltd.

hyperalgesia/augmentation of central pain perception, *i.e.* headaches and/or facial pain. The postulated neural connections are shown in Figure 12.1.

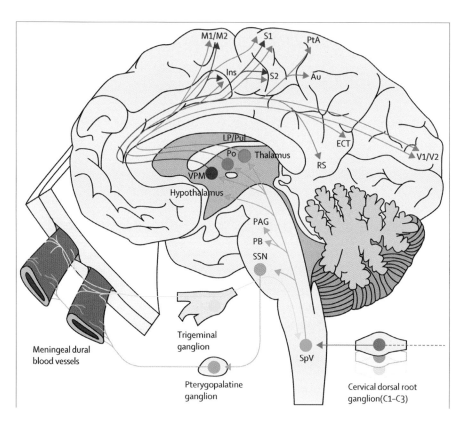

**Figure 12.1** Trigeminovascular system and migraine. Thalamic trigemino-vascular neurones project to a wide array of cortical areas that mediate symptoms associated with migraine, such as transient amnesia and cognitive decline, phonophobia, photophobia and expressive aphasia. Inputs to SpV arise from meningeal dural blood vessels and pial blood vessels (not shown). Green: projections from SpV. Blue: thalamo-cortical projections. Yellow: afferent projections from meningeal blood vessels. Orange: afferent projections from cervical dorsal root ganglions. Peach: efferent projections to meningeal blood vessels. Au, auditory cortex; ECT, ectorhinal cortex; Ins, insular cortex; LP, lateral posterior thalamic nucleus; M1, primary motor cortex; M2, secondary motor cortex; PAG, periaqueductal grey; PB, parabrachial nucleus; Po, posterior; PtA, parietal association cortex; Pul, pulvinar; RS, retrosplenial cortex; S1, primary somatosensory cortex; S2, secondary somatosensory cortex; SpV, spinal trigeminal nucleus; SSN, superior salivatory nucleus; V1, primary visual cortex; V2, secondary visual cortex; VPM, ventral posteromedial. *Source:* Ashina *et al.* (2019).

## Primary Headaches

### Migraine

Migraine affects 20% of any population, is more common in females and usually episodic. Headaches may be occasional, regular and/or frequent. Migraines on 15+ days/month for more than 3 months defines chronic migraine. Migraineurs may have a warning for one or more days before the headache – for example yawning, fatigue, increased micturition or even elation. Relaxation (weekend) migraine occurs. Conversely, worry such as anxiety prior to an examination or an event rarely provokes an attack. Headache is usually unilateral, pulsating and aggravated by movement. Nausea with or without vomiting and photophobia and/or phonophobia are associated.

Auras occur as a prelude in about 30%. Auras are transient focal symptoms that develop over 5–30 minutes and last less than 1 hour. Commonly: visual with flashing lights, zig-zag lines, or negative, with scotomata – holes in vision. Other auras: speech/language disturbance, hemiparetic/hemisensory symptoms, dysarthria, vertigo, tinnitus, hyperacusis, diplopia, ataxia and drowsiness.

Pathophysiology: a wave of cortical depression in the relevant area with initial hyperaemia followed by hypoperfusion. Auras can occur with other primary headaches such as cluster or even without headache at all – they may resemble a TIA.

## Management

A clearly defined migraine requires no investigation, but imaging is often done, if only to reassure. Assess frequency and disability. There are various scales, e.g. the Migraine Disability Assessment Scale (MIDAS).

General: migraineurs are stimulus and change sensitive. Regular eating, hydration, regular sleep and exercise help. Avoid excessive caffeine and alcohol. Cognitive behavioural therapy (CBT) can help allay irrational/catastrophising thoughts.

Acute attacks: commence with analgesics and NSAIDs before moving to a triptan. Claims abound for the triptan of choice.

Limit paracetamol and NSAIDs to a maximum of 15 days/month, to avoid medication overuse pain, and triptans to 10 days/month. Track therapy with a headache diary. Anti-emetics – prochlorperazine, metoclopramide or domperidone can help.

Prevention: widely advertised, various drugs reduce frequency in some, for example topiramate, valproate and pizotifen. Other therapies include calcium channel antagonists (flunarizine), angiotensin modulators (angiotensin-converting enzyme inhibitors and angiotensin receptor inhibitors), nutrients and vitamins (coenzyme Q10, riboflavin and magnesium) and herbal products such as feverfew. Botox and occipital nerve stimulation are also used. Fremanezumab (Ajovy) and galcanezumab (Emgality) are recent additions, monoclonal antibodies which are inhibitors of the biological activity of calcitonin gene-related peptide. They are believed to target the CGRP ligand and block its binding to the receptor. They are on occasion highly effective.

Table 12.1 Acute migraine treatments.

| Simple analgesics and NSAIDS | Triptans |
| --- | --- |
| Aspirin | Sumatriptan |
| Paracetamol | Almotriptan |
| Ibuprofen | Rizatriptan |
| Naproxen | Zolmitriptan |
| Tolfenamic acid | Eletriptan |
| | Frovatriptan |
| | Naratriptan |

## Tension-type Headache

TTH is a relatively featureless headache unlike migraine and is either episodic or chronic. Chronic TTH implies headaches on more than 15 days/month. TTH is more common than migraine, affecting over 60% of the population at some time.

TTHs are pressing or tightening rather than throbbing, typically not associated with photophobia, phonophobia, nausea and motion sensitivity. Cases of episodic TTH with a normal examination do not require routine imaging. Reassurance is important. Medication may be unnecessary. Acupuncture may help. Acute treatment: NSAIDs or paracetamol. Prophylaxis: amitriptyline and/or topiramate.

## Trigeminal Autonomic Cephalalgias (TACS)

TACs are primary headaches with unilateral pain and cranial autonomic features. TACs include cluster headache, paroxysmal hemicrania, the very rare short-lasting unilateral neuralgiform headache with conjunctival injection and tearing (SUNCT) and its variant short-lasting unilateral neuralgiform headache with cranial autonomic symptoms (SUNA) and *hemicrania continua*. These pains respond well to medication. They are important to recognise.

### Cluster Headache

Cluster is the most common TAC and familiar to every general neurologist. Pain is excruciating – cluster is intensely painful. There is striking periodicity – cycles tend to recur each year, in the same season and attacks between 1 a.m. and 4 a.m. are typical, waking the patient and leaving them exhausted.

Prevalence: 2 per 1000. M:F 5:1. Pain is of rapid onset, severe, unilateral and typically around the orbit and temple. Attacks last 15 minutes to 3 hours. Typical features are autonomic: conjunctival injection, lacrimation, miosis, ptosis, eyelid oedema, rhinorrhoea, nasal blockage and forehead/facial sweating or restlessness/agitation. These are usually transient. Partial Horner's – ptosis or miosis – may persist, especially after frequent attacks.

Attack frequency: one every alternate day to three or more daily. Alcohol, volatile odours, exercise and warm ambient temperatures can bring on attacks. Migrainous symptoms – nausea, vomiting, photophobia, phonophobia and even aura are seen occasionally. However, cluster sufferers are usually restless and irritable, preferring to move about, rather than preferring a dark room. Most patients have episodic cluster. Some have chronic cluster with no remission within a year or remissions lasting less than a month.

Diagnosis is clinical. However, it can be difficult to exclude a secondary cause, for example a painful Horner's from primary cluster. Imaging is often carried out.

Acute attacks: oxygen inhalation is highly effective in most – 100% oxygen at 7–12 L/min for about 15 minutes. Injectable sumatriptan is one drug of choice. Oral zolmitriptan also helps.

Prevention: verapamil (check cardiac status) is one drug used in both episodic and chronic cluster. Others include lithium and methysergide. Topiramate, valproate, pizotifen and gabapentin are also used. A short course of steroids can give transient relief. Greater occipital nerve block is also used.

Surgery: pterygopalatine or trigeminal ganglion destruction and trigeminal nerve root section have been tried. Neurostimulation – occipital nerve stimulation, sphenopalatine ganglion stimulation and deep brain stimulation of the posterior hypothalamus are also used.

### Paroxysmal Hemicrania and Hemicrania Continua

Paroxysmal hemicrania is a rare syndrome that responds dramatically to indometacin. Features are characteristic: unilateral, brief (2–30 minutes) and attacks of pain associated with cranial autonomic features 1–40 times/day. Excruciating pain is centred around one orbit and/or temple with ipsilateral cranial autonomic features (see cluster), but no tendency for nocturnal attacks, cf. cluster. A few cases are provoked by head movement, possibly via pressure on cervical transverse processes or the greater occipital nerve.

*Hemicrania continua* is a rare indometacin-responsive continuous headache – persistent unilateral pain with exacerbations and autonomic features/restlessness. A response to indometacin is almost a prerequisite. Diagnosis: clinical. An underlying cause is exceptional.

### Short-lasting Unilateral Neuralgiform Attacks (SUNA and SUNCT)

These rare TACs are attacks of pain around one orbit, temple or face. They last from a second to 10 minutes. Frequency varies immensely – from once a day or less to more than 60 times per hour. Pain is accompanied by prominent autonomic features. Trigger zones: touching the face or scalp, washing, shaving, eating, chewing, brushing teeth, talking and coughing. SUNCT adds both conjunctival injection and tearing, adding the C and T.

SUNCT and SUNA are so rare that most neurologists will never see a case. Secondary SUNCT and SUNA have also been described, even more rarely, with posterior fossa and pituitary tumours.

Lamotrigine is one effective treatment. IV lidocaine can be tried, though the pain usually recurs. Carbamazepine, topiramate and gabapentin are used. Trigeminal microvascular decompression, occipital nerve stimulation and posterior hypothalamic deep brain stimulation are sometimes tried.

## Other Primary Headaches with Secondary Variants

### Primary and Secondary Cough Headache

Pain arises moments after coughing, sneezing, straining, laughing or stooping and subsides rapidly. Headache is usually bilateral and posterior. Vertigo and nausea can occur. All are rare.

Secondary cough headache occurs with Chiari malformation type 1 (Chapter 16). CSF hypotension, carotid/vertebrobasilar disease, middle cranial fossa or posterior fossa tumours, midbrain cysts, basilar impression, platybasia, subdural haematoma, cerebral aneurysm and reversible cerebral vasoconstriction syndrome are known causes. Any pulmonary disease should be identified.

For primary cough headache, the most effective treatment is indometacin. Other treatments include acetazolamide, topiramate, naproxen, propranolol, methysergide and intravenous dihydroergotamine. LP and CSF removal can be carried out – the response can be dramatic.

**Primary and Secondary Exercise Headache**

Headaches are triggered by physical exercise, with bilateral, throbbing pain for 5 minutes to 48 hours. If exertion can be predicted, then pre-emptive therapy with indomethacin 30 minutes before exercise can be tried. Propranolol is also used.

Structural intracranial lesions occur in about one-third – an intracranial mass, aneurysm or AV malformation, intracranial haemorrhage, intermittent obstruction of CSF (third ventricle colloid cyst), Chiari type 1 malformation or previous traumatic brain injury. Extracranial causes include phaeochromocytoma and cardiac cephalgia – exertional headache secondary to cardiac ischaemia.

**Primary (Benign) and Secondary Sex Headache**

Pre-orgasmic headache is a bilateral occipital or generalised headache that intensifies with sexual arousal. Orgasmic headache has an explosive onset around the moment of orgasm, followed by throbbing head pain. These last between 10 minutes and 6 hours. Most settle within 6 months. When these headaches occur frequently, propranolol, diltiazem, indomethacin or a triptan may help. Migraine, exercise headache and sex headache are associated.

Secondary sex headache is a rare presentation of an intracranial aneurysm, stroke, phaeochromocytoma and low CSF pressure.

**Primary and Secondary Thunderclap Headache**

Thunderclap means an abrupt headache that reaches its zenith within a minute. Primary thunderclap means that no underlying cause is found. Secondary thunderclap covers the headache of SAH and other intracranial catastrophes. All thunderclap headaches should be investigated with CT and usually MRI and CSF examination. Primary thunderclap is self-limiting but can recur. Nimodipine may help such cases.

**Other Primary Headaches**

Primary stabbing headache: transient, sharp jabbing pains occur in volleys within a localised frontal scalp area – may respond to indometacin or melatonin.

Nummular (coin) headache: pain focussed on an unchanging area of 1–6 cm, with local hyperaesthesia, paresthesiae or allodynia. Gabapentin can be tried.

Hypnic headache: a.k.a. alarm clock headache, also a rarity is pain that awakens the patient from sleep for 15 minutes to 3 hours, usually after the age of 50. Pain is usually featureless. Lithium, caffeine, melatonin, indometacin and flunarizine can be tried.

**New Daily Persistent Headache and Chronic Daily Headache**

NDPH is daily, unremitting and lasts more than 3 months. Most can pinpoint the date it started. In many, pain resembles either migraine or TTH. Chronic daily headache (CDH) is a term in widespread use, though no longer within formal headache classification.

## Secondary Headaches

### Medication Overuse Headache (MOH) and Withdrawal Headache

The most common cause of secondary headache follows a combination of escalating headache frequency and analgesic use, for example:

- paracetamol, aspirin or NSAIDs on 15+ days/month for >3 months.
- triptans or opiates (including codeine) on 10+ days/month for >3 months.

Frequency, not dosage, is the determinant of overuse. Where migraine ends and MOH begins may be impossible to ascertain. About half with MOH who withdraw from analgesia for two months will improve. 10% will worsen.

Caffeine withdrawal: withdrawal of daily caffeine 200 mg/day (about three espressos) can cause headaches. They resolve typically within a week.

Other drugs that may provoke headaches include nitroglycerin, atropine, digitalis, disulfiram, hydralazine, imipramine, nicotine, nifedipine, nimodipine and cocaine.

## Headache and Vascular Disorders

Thunderclap headache is a dramatic secondary headache – the typical cause is SAH. Thunderclap can also follow arterial dissection, venous thrombosis, ischaemic stroke, intracranial haemorrhage, pituitary apoplexy, reversible cerebral vasoconstriction syndrome and intracranial hypotension.

### Subarachnoid Haemorrhage
The patient with an acute 'worst headache of my life' with an entirely normal initial examination may have suffered SAH. A high index of suspicion is essential. Non-contrast CT has a pick-up rate approaching 100% within 6 hours. CSF examination may be necessary. Over three-quarters are aneurysmal: all require specialist neurovascular assessment.

### Carotid and Vertebral Artery Dissection
Dissection (Chapter 6) is spontaneous in most but can follow even minor trauma. There is pain in the neck and/or head and ischaemia distal to the dissection. 15% have headache alone. Neck pain with features of posterior circulation ischaemia should make one suspect vertebral dissection. An ipsilateral Horner's can follow carotid dissection.

### Giant Cell Arteritis
GCA occurs exclusively in those over 50 and is 10 times more common in the over 80s than in the 50–60 age group and is 2–3 times commoner in women than men. Scalp tenderness and ischaemic pain in muscles of mastication (jaw claudication) or the tongue (tongue angina) point to the diagnosis and/or visual loss. ESR and/or CRP is elevated in almost all. Diagnosis: biopsy and temporal artery histology. Prompt high-dose steroids rapidly alleviate symptoms and reduce the risk of anterior ischaemic optic neuropathy (AION, Chapter 14).

## Intracranial Mass Lesion

It is unusual for someone with an intracranial mass lesion to present with a headache alone, though this may be the patient's fear. An isolated headache is a presenting feature of a brain tumour, or even a cerebral abscess in less than 50% of such lesions, and headaches when they occur are usually of an unremarkable type. An enlarging mass lesion can, however, raise the intracranial pressure, or cause stretching of the meninges or less commonly by blockage of CSF pathways. The traditional description of a headache with raised intrac-ranial pressure causing morning headache and vomiting is rare, though this can occur with a posterior fossa mass. The diagnosis rests more on the additional complaints and/or focal signs. The fear of an intracranial lesion leads to brain imaging, now so readily available, in almost everybody who has a headache.

## Headache with High or Low Intracranial Pressure

### Idiopathic (Benign) Intracranial Hypertension
Idiopathic intracranial hypertension (IIH, Chapter 14) is most commonly seen in young women with a high body mass index (BMI). Papilloedema is usual. Treatment is directed at lowering CSF pressure – essential to prevent visual loss. Ultimately, reduction of BMI is usually curative, but because this is slow, pressure-lowering strategies include drugs (e.g. acetazolamide and bendroflumethiazide), repeated LPs and CSF shunting or optic nerve fenestration may be necessary.

### Secondary Intracranial Hypertension Resembling IIH
Intracranial hypertension with features identical to IIH can have other causes, such as a sagittal sinus thrombosis. Cerebral venous and venous sinus thrombosis are discussed in Chapter 6. Other aetiologies for high pressure are possible, though evidence is often lacking. Hypoparathyroidism, Addison's and Cushing's diseases have been implicated and also pregnancy, nalidixic acid, ciprofloxacin, tetracyclines, nitrofurantoin, growth hormone, oral contraceptives, anabolic steroids, amiodarone and lithium. Hypervita-minosis A or retinoid excess is a cause of papilloedema: stopping the vitamin relieves the symptoms. Other causes of raised CSF pressure include malignant meningeal infiltration.

### Low-pressure Headaches (Intracranial Hypotension)
Intracranial hypotension is commonly iatrogenic, following LP or epidural anaesthesia. Low CSF pressure (less than 60 mm CSF) causes headache that is usually worse on stand-ing and relieved by lying. There may be neck pain, photophobia, tinnitus or even hearing loss and nausea. Some relief may be obtained from caffeine.

CSF leakage may also occur following a tear in a spinal nerve root sheath. Spontaneous CSF leakage can occur in those with a collagen disorder such as hypermobility/Marfan's syndrome. In post-dural leak (post-LP) headache, resolution is usually spontaneous within 2 weeks.

Cranial MRI can show cerebellar tonsillar descent, sagging of the brainstem, post-contrast enhancement of the meninges and occasionally subdural fluid collections. In spontaneous intracranial hypotension, the site of CSF leakage is usually spinal. Careful imaging may be required to identify the site of leakage.

With persistent post-dural puncture headache, one treatment is an epidural blood patch with autologous blood. In refractory cases, repeated blood patching or rarely operative repair may be required.

## Headaches and Head Trauma

It will be common personal knowledge that a headache can follow a minor blow to the head, and that this can persist for longer than one might expect. There is no doubt that such post-traumatic headaches do sometimes last for days or weeks, when there has been no suggestion of a brain injury. Mechanisms are conjectural. In some cases, migraine or TTH occurs, whilst in others local scalp tenderness at the site of the blow would appear to be the cause.

Whether prolonged post-traumatic headaches or post-traumatic migraine are realities is debated in medicolegal cases, and there is a range of opinion. For the majority of neurologists, the view is that psychological causes or the effect of litigation itself prolongs the complaints when such headaches persist for more than 12 weeks.

It is of interest that the brain trauma – a defined traumatic brain injury – is not typically followed by headache at all. Neck pain and headache, often labelled by the dramatic term whiplash, are mentioned in Chapter 16.

## Infection and Other Disorders

A headache can accompany many viral respiratory infections and is self-limiting. However, the headache of incipient meningitis, viral or bacterial can be similar, and thus, it is vital to examine for neck stiffness and other meningitic features, such as a rash in anyone with a fever and headache. Chronic meningitis such as TB can also cause indolent headaches.

Headaches can follow scalp injuries and infection, paranasal sinus disease, glaucoma, facial and dental infection. The source of the problem is usually apparent.

# Acknowledgements

I am most grateful to Manjit Matharu, Paul Shanahan and Tim Young for their contribution to *Neurology A Queen Square Textbook* Second Edition and to Peter Goadsby who wrote the chapter in the First Edition.

Figure 12.1 is from Ashina A, Hansen JM, Phu Do T, Melo-Carrillo A, Burnstein R, Moskowitz MA. Migraine and the trigeminal system – 40 years and counting. *Lancet Neurol* 2019; 18: 795–804. This article summarises views about headache pathogenesis.

Table 12.1 is adapted from *Neurology A Queen Square Textbook* Second Edition.

# Further Reading, References and Websites

Ashina A, Hansen JM, Phu Do T, Melo-Carrillo A, Burnstein R, Moskowitz MA. Migraine and the trigeminal system – 40 years and counting. *Lancet Neurol* 2019; **18**: 795–804.https:// www.thelancet.com/journals/laneur/article/PIIS1474-4422(19)30185-1/fulltext

International Headache Society. International Classification of Headache Disorders (ICHD-3), 2018. http://www.ichd-3.org (accessed 26 August 2021).

Johnson SRD, Hammond A, Griffiths L, Greenwood R, Clarke CRA. Subarachnoid haemorrhage – can we do better? *J R Soc Med* 1989; **82**: 721–772.

Matharu M, Shanahan P, Young T. Headache. In *Neurology: A Queen Square Textbook*, 2nd edn. Clarke C, Howard R, Rossor M, Shorvon S, eds. Chichester: John Wiley & Sons, 2016. There are numerous references.

National Institute for Health and Clinical Excellence. Diagnosis and management of headaches in young people and adults, 2021. http://www.nice.org.uk (accessed 26 August 2021).

https://www.nhs.uk/conditions/headaches/

https://www.migrainetrust.org/

Free updated notes, potential links and references as these become available:
https://www.drcharlesclarke.com
You will be asked to log in, in a secure fashion, with your name and institution.

# 13

# Cranial Nerve Disorders

I summarise here cranial nerves I, V, VII and IX–XII. The optic nerve (II) and ocular motor nerves III, IV and VI are discussed in Chapter 14, and neuro-otology in Chapter 15.

## I. Olfactory Nerve

### Functional Anatomy

Olfaction detects odours; the anatomy is summarised in Figures 13.1 and 13.2. Olfactory bipolar neurones, unique among mammalian neurones are replaced every 4–8 weeks. A second system – trigeminal afferents – responds to irritants, pungent smells and sensations such as the coolness of menthol.

Anosmia means complete loss of olfaction; partial anosmia is the inability to detect certain smells; hyposmia is generally diminished olfaction; dysosmia is distorted olfaction – pleasant odours seem unpleasant – and phantosmia is a sensation of a constant smell.

Patients with impaired olfaction usually also complain of loss of taste, because most of our perception of flavour derives from olfaction. The basic tastes remain intact with anosmia. Many are unaware of gradual loss of olfaction. Dysosmia and phantosmia occur during olfactory epithelium degeneration and regeneration – following respiratory or paranasal sinus infection, head trauma and after chemotherapy and cranial radiotherapy.

### Examination

Ask the patient to sniff vials containing specific odours using each nostril with the other occluded – or use whatever is around, such as soap, hand cream or an orange. The crux of the matter is to distinguish odours. Kits such as the University of Pennsylvania Smell Identification Test are available. Distinguish between bilateral and unilateral anosmia. Test taste. Examine mouth and nose.

*Neurology: A Clinical Handbook*, First Edition. Charles Clarke.
© 2022 John Wiley & Sons Ltd. Published 2022 by John Wiley & Sons Ltd.

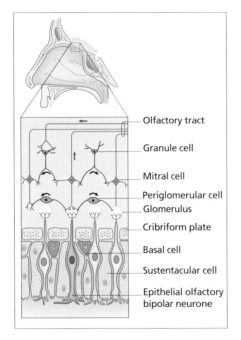

Figure 13.1  Cells of the olfactory system.

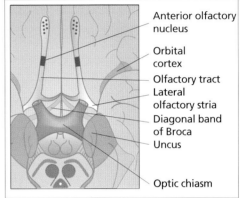

Figure 13.2   Olfactory tract region, from below.

**Olfactory Disorders**

Olfactory disorders are caused either by local obstruction in the nose or damage to the olfactory neuroepithelium, olfactory nerves or their central connections.

Ageing: about half between 65 and 80 years have some impairment, and three-quarters after 80. Olfactory receptors and neurones decrease with age. Most will be aware that anosmia can herald Covid-19 infection – but this has long been well known for many viruses. Allergic and infective nasal disorders and sinusitis can cause anosmia.

Acceleration–deceleration injuries shear the olfactory fila traversing the ethmoid cribriform plate. A fall can cause this, without loss of consciousness, via frontal *contrecoup*. Generally, from any cause, recovery  is unlikely if anosmia or hyposmia persist for longer than a year. Anosmia, unilateral or bilateral, can also follow neurosurgery.

Impaired olfaction occurs in:

- Parkinson's disease and dementia with Lewy bodies
- Alzheimer's, Huntington's disease and motor neurone disease
- Korsakoff's syndrome and multiple sclerosis.

In Parkinson's, the olfactory bulb and anterior olfactory nucleus degenerate, with early Lewy body formation. In Alzheimer's, neuronal loss develops in both olfactory bulb and limbic regions, which become laden with neurofibrillary tangles and plaques. In Parkinson's, hyposmia can predate motor symptoms by some years.

An olfactory groove meningioma is a rare cause of isolated unilateral anosmia. Other lesions such as a pituitary tumour or an aneurysm may also compress the olfactory tract.

Acids, acetone, solvents and benzene impair olfaction, usually briefly. Receptor cells are also vulnerable to drugs – antibiotics, anti-inflammatory and antithyroid drugs, chemotherapy and radiotherapy. Tobacco impairs olfaction.

Cirrhosis, renal failure, hypothyroidism and vitamin deficiency (vitamins A, $B_6$ and $B_{12}$) can cause impaired olfaction. Olfactory receptor cells may be congenitally absent in Kallmann's syndrome, Turner's syndrome and albinism.

Damage to cortical structures can lead to impaired odour identification and/or impairment of recognition memory but rarely to anosmia. Olfactory hallucinations can be the aura preceding a temporal lobe seizure but rarely are the sole manifestations (Chapter 8) – an unpleasant, stereotyped smell is typical but rarely identifiable. Hallucinations occur in depression, schizophrenia and alcohol withdrawal. A constant foul odour is often of psychotic origin.

## V. Trigeminal Nerve

The sensory territory includes the face and scalp anterior to the vertex, mucous membranes of oral and nasal cavities, paranasal sinuses, teeth, intracranial vessels and dura of the anterior and middle cranial fossae. The motor root supplies muscles of mastication. The three cutaneous sensory divisions are shown in Figure 13.3, the spinal nucleus in Figure 13.4 and the V brainstem nuclei in Figure 13.5.

Sensory examination: study all three divisions; compare with the opposite side. Include light touch, pain and temperature with a cold tuning fork. The angle of the jaw is usually outside the V nerve territory – this area and the back of the scalp are supplied by C2/3. Non-organic patterns of sensory loss tend to include the angle of the jaw or stop at the hairline, though syringobulbia, for example can cause confluent non-dermatomal loss.

Test the corneal reflex (Chapters 4 and 20) with cotton wool. The afferent arc is $V_1$ for the upper cornea and $V_2$ for the lower fifth. The efferent arc is via VII (blink) and nervus intermedius (lacrimation). In the normal corneal response, there is discomfort, with tears and conjunctival injection. In traditional neurology, an acoustic neuroma could be silent until

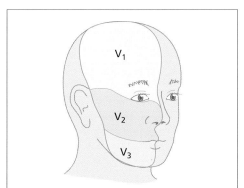

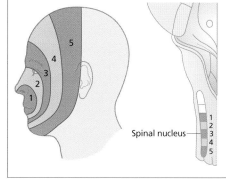

**Figure 13.3**   Cutaneous distribution of $V_1$, $V_2$ and $V_3$.   **Figure 13.4**   Spinal V nucleus: distribution.

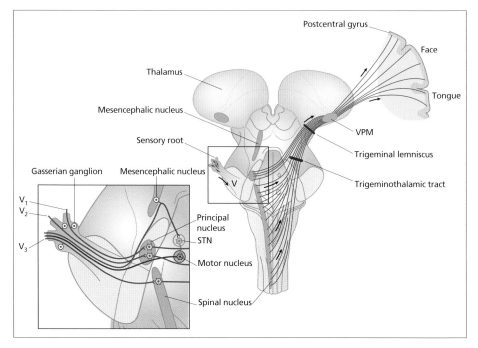

**Figure 13.5** Trigeminal pathways within the brainstem.

depressed corneal sensation was found – imaging has changed that. Widespread facial sensory loss in the absence of a reduced corneal should raise the question of a non-organic cause. Parietal lesions can rarely cause depression of contralateral corneal sensation.

## Peripheral V Nerve Lesions

Lesions of divisions and branches produce well-demarcated facial sensory loss and pain that can be severe: toothache is familiar to all. The ophthalmic, maxillary and mandibular divisions may be compressed individually or together as they exit the skull base – through the superior orbital fissure (SOF), foramen rotundum and foramen ovale – by malignant infiltration, infection or granulomas. The Gasserian ganglion at the petrous tip causes ipsilateral sensory facial symptoms, and with the VI nerve Gradenigo's syndrome. A schwannoma can arise from the trigeminal ganglion, and V involved in a cerebropontine angle (CPA) syndrome.

Unilateral numbness of the chin and lower lip is distinctive and typically indicates a metastasis involving the mental nerve – breast or prostate cancer, lymphoma, myeloma and granulomas. A numb cheek can be caused by $V_2$ compression in the infraorbital foramen. Trauma can damage supra- and infraorbital branches of $V_1$.

### Superior Orbital Fissure Syndrome

The ophthalmic division ($V_1$) within the SOF can become involved with the III, IV and VI nerves (Chapter 14). The typical presentation is with ophthalmoplegia, sensory loss and $V_1$

pain, sometimes with proptosis. Horner's syndrome and visual loss can develop. Tumours, such as nasopharyngeal cancer, trauma, infection – an epidural abscess, mucormycosis and granulomas such as sarcoid and granulomatosis with polyangiitis (GPA) are causes (Chapter 26).

### Cavernous Sinus Syndrome

This is similar to the SOF syndrome except that $V_2$ is also involved. Proptosis is unusual, except with a carotid-cavernous fistula (Chapter 14). Involvement of both oculomotor nerve and the sympathetic can cause a mid-position, non-reactive pupil.

Causes:

- Vascular – carotid aneurysm, caroticocavernous fistula and thrombosis
- Neoplasms – metastases, nasopharyngeal carcinoma, pituitary, lymphoma and meningioma
- Infection and Inflammatory – sarcoid, GPA, polyarteritis nodosa and Tolosa–Hunt syndrome.

Cavernous sinus thrombosis is a potentially fatal condition that can follow rapidly infection in the face, paranasal sinuses (particularly sphenoid) or teeth (see also Chapters 6 and 14).

### Nuclear V lesions

A trigeminal nuclear lesion from intrinsic brainstem pathology, such as a tumour, inflammatory or vascular lesion, frequently involves the lateral spinothalamic tract. A common pattern is ipsilateral facial dissociated sensory loss (pain and temperature) with contralateral dissociated sensory loss in the limbs and trunk. Infarction of the lateral medulla (Wallenberg's lateral medullary syndrome; Chapter 6) is the typical cause.

The spinal trigeminal nucleus can be disrupted anywhere between caudal pons and upper cord. The somatotopic arrangement of the nucleus maps to an onion skin type distribution, the nose and mouth being the centre of the onion (Figure 13.4). A pontine nuclear lesion can cause circum-oral or intra-oral sensory loss, while a lesion of the lower part of nucleus (e.g. in syringobulbia) can be like a balaclava, sparing the snout. Extension of the lower trigeminal spinal nucleus into the upper spinal cord means that a cord lesion can occasionally cause facial pain.

A dorsal mid-pontine lesion involving the principal sensory nucleus and motor nucleus can cause ipsilateral facial hemianaesthesia, with paresis of muscles of mastication. There may be contralateral hemiplegia and spinothalamic sensory loss in the limbs. Ipsilateral tremor, internuclear ophthalmoplegia and Horner's syndrome can also occur.

### Trigeminal Neuralgia

Trigeminal neuralgia (TN) is a common and distressing disorder. Incidence: 4/100 000/ year, prevalence much higher. Women are more frequently affected. TN, frequently caused by neurovascular compression, starts typically after the age of 60. Young patients are likely to have symptomatic TN (e.g. MS) or occasionally a mass lesion.

The pain is excruciating – shooting, stabbing and electric shock-like paroxysms from a few seconds to a minute. A refractory period of several minutes tends to follow. Pains tend to occur in bouts, sometimes with great frequency. The face may contort during an attack, hence the name *tic douloureux*. Patients are usually pain free between bouts. Pain is triggered by touching a specific area, often no larger than a few millimetres, or by talking, chewing or a cold wind. Patients stop eating, drinking or brushing teeth; men leave an area of the face unshaven. The mandibular and maxillary territories are most commonly affected initially. Pain commencing in $V_1$ should lead to consideration of an underlying cause. Bilateral TN is exceptional and can occur with MS.

Spontaneous remissions occur, for months or years, but pain almost invariably recurs. Successive bouts tend to be worse, with shorter remissions. Examination is typically normal. Subtle areas of sensory loss are seen in a minority. Some patients consult a dentist initially. Atypical facial pain is sometimes labelled as TN initially, but this pain is constant rather than paroxysmal.

### Aetiology, Pathogenesis and Management

In many cases TN is caused by compression of the V nerve root at or near the dorsal root entry zone by an ectatic vessel, often the superior cerebellar artery. Ephaptic non-synaptic transmission between trigeminal axons, within areas of demyelination caused by compression of the nerve, is proposed as the mechanism. High-resolution MRI demonstrates a vascular loop in contact with the nerve in some cases. A CPA mass – a vestibular schwannoma, meningioma, epidermoid or aneurysm – can occasionally cause TN.

Brainstem pathology: particularly MS plaques in the pons can cause TN, occasionally bilateral or, rarely, a small infarct in the pons dorsal root entry zone, amyloid infiltration or tumour.

Carbamazepine is effective in 70%. Oxcarbazepine is also used. Other drugs include lamotrigine, baclofen and gabapentin. For patients with drug-resistant TN, surgical approaches are considered. The trend is towards early surgery. Most severe TN cases will require microvascular decompression. The V nerve is exposed at the brainstem. In some, a vascular loop is seen and the vessel dissected away. Surgery has a high success rate, even when no evident compression is seen. Ablation techniques and radiosurgery are also used.

### Trigeminal Idiopathic Sensory Neuropathy and Somatisation

The patient develops gradual facial numbness, often preceded by positive sensory symptoms but usually without much pain. A few have an acute onset. The motor root is rarely affected. Some cases have a connective tissue disease. Neuroimaging is normal. Few are severely disturbed by the persistent symptoms. Odd facial sensory symptoms are a feature of somatisation (Chapter 22): non-organic patterns of sensory loss are typical.

### Herpes Zoster Ophthalmicus (HZO)

The lifetime risk of ophthalmic ($V_1$) zoster is about 1%. The elderly and immunocompromised are at risk. Preventable ocular complications are common. Pain often precedes the vesicles. Vesicles on one side of the nose and medial to the eye indicate nasociliary nerve involvement and that of the eye itself (Hutchinson's sign). Most have conjunctivitis. Without antiviral therapy, 50% develop ocular complications – keratopathy, episcleritis, corneal perforation and iritis. Retinal necrosis occurs occasionally in immunocompromised patients.

Give an oral antiviral – aciclovir, valaciclovir or famciclovir – as early as possible. Assess by an ophthalmologist. Topical steroids are indicated for anterior chamber inflammation. Taping of the lids is helpful at night.

A fifth of herpes zoster ophthalmicus (HZO) cases over 60 develop post-herpetic neuralgia (PHN), with a few persisting at 2 years. PHN can have a major impact on the quality of life. Treatment: tricyclic antidepressants and/or gabapentin and capsaicin cream.

Rare late complications of HZO include optic neuropathy and III, IV and VI lesions and/or stroke, sequelae of a granulomatous arteritis, usually some weeks after the rash. Immunisation against shingles is important.

### Atypical Facial Pain

Atypical facial pain describes pain without an apparent structural cause. Chronic pain for months or permanently, is usually unilateral and within trigeminal distribution but without sensory loss. Pain is deep and burning, without paroxysms. Patients are typically over 50, mainly female. Depressive features are prominent, but atypical facial pain cases have little in the way of other unexplained pain. Antidepressants are usually unhelpful. Invasive treatments tend to increase pain.

## VII. Facial Nerve

The facial nerve has motor, sensory and autonomic components and runs a tortuous course from pons to facial muscles, lacrimal and salivary glands. The essential anatomy is summarised in Figures 13.6–13.8.

The majority of corticobulbar fibres decussate in the pons, but the upper third of the face receives little direct cortical innervation – separate supranuclear pathways subserve voluntary and emotional facial movements. Thus, emotional movements can be preserved when voluntary movements fail following a stroke. The right hemisphere tends to be dominant for expression of facial emotion.

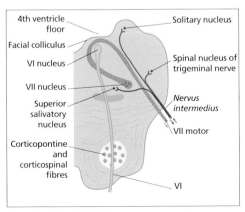

**Figure 13.6** Facial nucleus, facial and abducens (VI) nerves (pons cross-section).

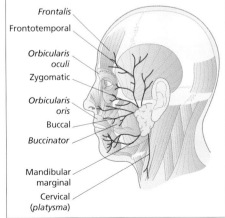

**Figure 13.7** Principal branches of VII.

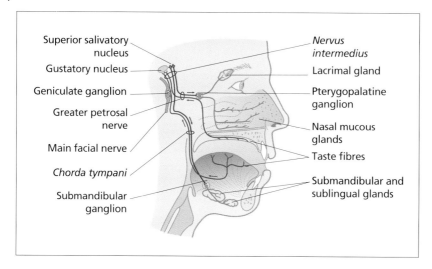

Superior salivatory nucleus
Gustatory nucleus
Geniculate ganglion
Greater petrosal nerve
Main facial nerve
*Chorda tympani*
Submandibular ganglion

*Nervus intermedius*
Lacrimal gland
Pterygopalatine ganglion
Nasal mucous glands
Taste fibres
Submandibular and sublingual glands

**Figure 13.8**  *Nervus intermedius*, greater petrosal nerve and *chorda tympani*.

The VII motor nucleus lies in the lower pons. The motor fibres sweep around the VI nucleus, to emerge anteriorly. The *nervus intermedius* is the sensory and autonomic component that joins the motor fibres just after the *genu*. After leaving the pons, the nerve traverses the CPA before entering the internal auditory meatus with the *nervus intermedius* and the VIII nerve. The nerve emerges from the skull via the stylomastoid foramen, traverses the parotid and divides to innervate facial muscles, except *levator palpebrae superioris* (III nerve) – a facial palsy does not cause ptosis.

## Examination

Look for facial symmetry – forehead creases and nasolabial folds. Slight facial asymmetry is not pathological.

Test:

- *frontalis* (eyebrow elevation)
- eye and lip closure, 'smile'
- *platysma*: 'bare your teeth and open your mouth'.

UMN lesions: relative sparing of *frontalis* and *orbicularis oculi* – voluntary and emotional movements affected differentially.

The four primary tastes – sweet, salt, sour and bitter – can be tested using sugar, salt, vinegar and quinine dabbed separately onto the tongue.

Inspect mouth, tongue and external auditory meatus (otoscopy); palpate parotid.

Facial weakness has many causes: Bell's palsy, herpes zoster (Ramsay Hunt), otitis media/cholesteatoma, *Borrelia,* HIV, TB, polio, Guillain–Barré, sarcoidosis, GPA, Sjögren's, IgG4 related, Melkersson–Rosenthal, stroke, MS, tumour, e.g. schwannoma and parotid mass.

A nuclear VII produces an LMN palsy but seldom in isolation: the VI nucleus is often involved. A contralateral hemiplegia (Millard–Gubler syndrome) can occur with a pontine vascular lesion.

## Cerebellopontine Angle (CPA) Syndrome

The petrous temporal bone completes this triangular recess (CPA) between cerebellum and lower pons. The V nerve lies at its upper corner, the IX and X nerves at the lower and the VII and VIII between them. A CPA mass lesion causes combinations of VIII, V and VII nerve lesions. Additional features: cerebellar signs, IX nerve lesion, limb UMN signs and exceptionally hydrocephalus. VIII nerve schwannoma (acoustic neuroma; Chapters 15 and 21) is one typical cause. Meningioma, cholesteatoma, metastasis and occasionally an aneurysm are others.

### A Canal Lesion or Distal to Stylomastoid Foramen

At the internal auditory meatus the VII nerve lies close to the VIII. The facial canal is where the VII nerve is affected in Bell's. The first (labyrinthine) portion of the canal is the narrowest and lacks anastomosing arterial arcades, making it vulnerable. Features depend on where damage occurs:

Damage proximal to the first branch of the VII nerve (the greater superficial petrosal nerve to the lacrimal gland) causes facial palsy with loss of lacrimation, hyperacusis (nerve to *stapedius*) and loss of taste in the anterior two-thirds of the tongue (*chorda tympani*). A lesion distal to the supply to stapedius does not cause hyperacusis. A lesion distal to the *chorda tympani* spares taste.

A temporal fracture can damage the nerve within the canal. Otitis externa in diabetics, usually from pseudomonas, and suppurative middle ear infection can spread to the skull base. Bone metastases, nasopharyngeal carcinoma, osteopetrosis and cholesteatoma sometimes compress the nerve. At or distal to its exit from the skull, a parotid tumour or parotitis can cause facial weakness. Individual branches can be damaged by surgery and trauma. A misplaced botox injection can cause temporary paralysis.

## Bell's Palsy

Bell's is an acute unilateral LMN facial palsy. Incidence: about 20/100 000/year. There is no association with season, geography or personal contact. Herpes simplex virus type 1 (HSV-1) DNA can be found in endoneurial fluid in most. Both primary HSV-1 infection and reactivation have been implicated. Microvascular ischaemic facial mononeuropathy may be causal in older patients.

Rapid facial weakness develops over 48 hours, occasionally up to 5 days with retroauricular pain. This mastoid pain can be severe, for a week or longer. Facial asymmetry with drooling often lead the patient to suspect a stroke. All facial muscles are usually equally affected. The palpebral fissure is widened, and eye closure and blinking are reduced. Ectropion may lead to overflow of tears. The extent of weakness varies but is severe in most. Mild, painless, progressive or patchy facial weakness is distinctly unusual in Bell's.

A vague alteration of sensation is common, but the corneal reflex is preserved. Loss or change in taste, often muddy/metallic, indicates *chorda tympani* involvement. Hyperacusis occurs when *stapedius* is paralysed.

Other causes of facial paralysis should be considered:

- Ramsay-Hunt syndrome: geniculate ganglion varicella-zoster reactivation. Vesicles appear in the external auditory meatus. Tinnitus, hearing loss and nystagmus are common – VIII nerve involvement and occasionally IX and X. Vesicles may be absent.
- Cholesteatoma, malignant otitis externa and parotid tumours.
- Lyme disease.
- A VII nerve lesion can occur at HIV seroconversion.
- A skull base tumour, such as a breast metastasis, can cause an isolated VII.

Investigations are generally unnecessary. MRI may show contrast enhancement of the intracanalicular and labyrinthine portions of the nerve.

Complications: inability to blink may lead to exposure keratitis. Lubricating eye drops are often required and taping the eye at night. Complete inability to close the eye requires a lateral tarsorrhaphy and/or temporary insertion of a weight into the lid.

Complete recovery over 8 weeks is the norm without treatment. Steroids and antivirals are contentious, but many use prednisolone. Antivirals may help patients with severe weakness, and an antiviral/prednisolone combination is justified also because of possible HSV reactivation. Most patients are managed in primary care.

After recovery, aberrant reinnervation of facial muscles and glands can lead to synkinesis and jaw winking – involuntary eye closure with lip or mouth movement, known as the inverse Marcus Gunn phenomenon (Marin–Amat). Lip movement may occur on blinking. Aberrant parasympathetic reinnervation can cause eye watering when eating, a.k.a. crocodile tears (Chapter 24). Hemifacial spasm can follow. For the minority with severe weakness after a year, reconstructive surgery can help. Bell's is rarely recurrent.

### Melkersson–Rosenthal Syndrome

This rare triad is intermittent VII nerve palsy, recurrent lip or facial swelling and a fissured tongue (*lingua plicata*). Non-caseating granulomas are found on lip biopsy and can sometimes be helped by steroid injections. Aetiology: possibly related to IgG4 disease (Chapter 19).

### Bilateral Facial Weakness

Bilateral LMN palsies are typically a feature of a disease – HIV seroconversion, sarcoidosis, EBV infection or Lyme disease (Bannwarth's syndrome). Other causes include a skull base fracture, pontine glioma, bone metastases, leukaemic skull base deposits and malignant meningitis and in the past bilateral mastoiditis and diphtheria. Bilateral weakness also occurs in Guillain–Barré and the Miller-Fisher variant, in myotonic dystrophy, facioscapulohumeral dystrophy, myasthenia, botulism, congenital myopathies and motor neurone disease. Möbius syndrome is a disorder with bilateral facial weakness and abducens palsy. Familial amyloid polyneuropathy can cause bilateral facial palsy with corneal lattice dystrophy.

## Hemifacial Spasm

This is benign, painless unilateral, irregular tonic and/or clonic contractions of facial muscles. Onset is usually in the fifth and sixth decades. In some, twitches start in *orbicularis oculi* and gradually spread. In others, twitching begins around the mouth or cheek. Movements are either spontaneous or triggered by chewing, speaking and stress. They persist during sleep. Hemifacial spasm can follow nerve injury or Bell's. Bilateral spasm is rare. Slight facial weakness is sometimes present. Hemifacial spasm is usually caused by compression of the nerve root entry zone by a branch artery. A CPA mass lesions is rarely the cause. MRI demonstrates a vessel in contact with the nerve in some.

Botox into affected muscles is used for those who need treatment. Drugs are rarely effective. Microvascular decompression of the nerve gives resolution in over 50%. Hemifacial spasm occasionally occurs with ipsilateral TN, a combination called *tic convulsif*. Paroxysms of pain and spasm occur independently.

## Other Involuntary Facial Movements

Myokymia of orbicularis oculi (lower eyelid twitching) is normal but causes anxiety in neurology trainees. Extensive facial myokymia with persistent worm-like wriggling of the chin is sinister and follows brainstem MS or a pontine glioma. Myokymia occurs in ataxias, e.g. spinocerebellar atrophy type 3 (SCA3).

Tics and tardive dyskinesias frequently involve the face; blepharospasm is a focal dystonia (Chapter 7). Fasciculation can develop in MND and in Kennedy's disease (Chapter 10).

Focal motor seizures can affect facial muscles. *Epilepsia partialis continua* (Chapter 8) is a rare cause of persistent facial movements. Orofacial dystonia can occur in the rare neuroacanthocytosis.

### Progressive Hemifacial Atrophy

This rarity, a.k.a. Parry–Romberg syndrome, is progressive hemifacial atrophy – of skin, soft tissue and bone, sometimes with changes within the brain. This begins in childhood, with wasting in one or more trigeminal nerve dermatomes, though sensation remains normal. The condition is related to linear scleroderma – a vertical forehead fissure, the *coup de sabre*, sometimes delineates atrophic areas. Brain imaging can show ipsilateral grey and white matter lesions in some. Epilepsy can occur.

# Lower Four Cranial Nerves: IX, X, XI and XII

## IX. Glossopharyngeal Nerve

The IX nerve is predominantly sensory but has motor and parasympathetic components. It arises from the lateral medulla as rootlets rostral to those of nerves X and XI. All three nerves then traverse the jugular foramen. The motor root supplies pharyngeal constrictors and elevators. The sensory root carries taste and touch from the posterior one-third of the tongue, posterior pharyngeal wall, Eustachian tube, tympanic membrane and chemo- and baroreceptors. Parasympathetic fibres from the inferior salivatory nucleus leave the nerve at the petrous ganglion to pass into the tympanic and petrosal nerves to terminate in the parotid. Anatomy of nerves IX, X, XI and XII is shown in Figures 13.9–13.12.

Examination of the IX nerve is near impossible in isolation. In a IX nerve lesion, there is altered sensation of the soft palate and pharynx, but neighbouring nerves are also usually affected. Testing taste over the tongue posterior third is impractical. Weakness of *stylo-pharyngeus* that elevates the palate is also difficult to detect. With corticobulbar disease, as part of a pseudobulbar palsy, IX is affected. Peripheral lesions usually occur in jugular foramen and CPA syndromes. The nerve can be damaged in the retropharyngeal space, for example by a nasopharyngeal carcinoma.

Glossopharyngeal neuralgia is rare, unilateral intense and paroxysmal – sharp and stabbing in the throat, usually for seconds. Similar to TN, actions such as yawning and swallowing trigger pain. Bradycardia and syncope can occur. The cause usually remains obscure, although a CPA lesion, demyelination or a vascular loop has been found. Carbamazepine and gabapentin are effective. Microvascular decompression or nerve section is sometimes needed.

## X. Vagus Nerve

The connections of the vagus and its relations to IX, XI and XII are outlined in Figure 13.9. The vagus exits at the jugular foramen with the spinal accessory nerve XI and with IX. Two ganglia are formed (jugular and nodose), and from this region a number of rami – auricular (external ear), meningeal (posterior fossa dura) and pharyngeal (soft palate and pharynx). There are two principal laryngeal nerves, superior and recurrent

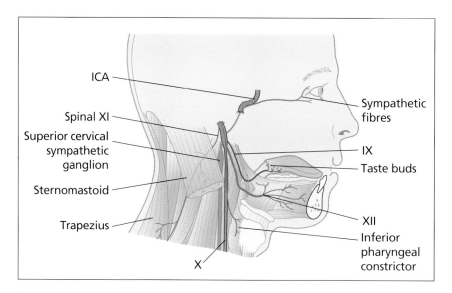

**Figure 13.9** Nerves IX, X, XI and XII: distribution. ICA, internal carotid artery.

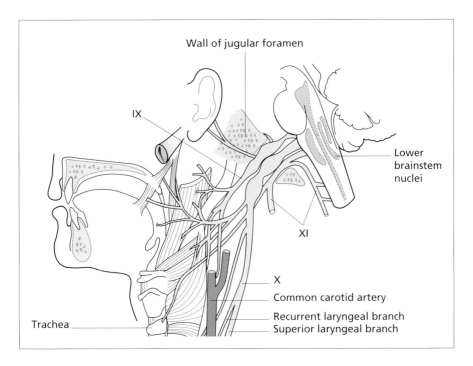

**Figure 13.10**   Nerves IX, X and XI: skull base and brainstem.

(Figure 13.10). The vagus carries the parasympathetic supply to thoracoabdominal organs, with fibres from the *nucleus ambiguus* innervating the striated muscles of larynx, pharynx and palate, with the exception of *stylopharyngeus* (IX) and *tensor veli palatini* (V). Sensory input from viscera and taste from the palate/epiglottis travel to the *nucleus solitarius*.

A X lesion interferes with speaking/articulation, cough, swallowing and palatal movement. Bilateral lesions cause complete palatal, pharyngeal and laryngeal paralysis – severe dysphagia, dysphonia, stridor, inability to cough, regurgitation and aspiration. A unilateral X causes hoarseness and dysphagia. The vocal cords cannot be opposed, making coughing dependent on forceful expiration, described as bovine. With difficulty clearing the throat of secretions, the voice sounds wet. The soft palate droops to the weak side while the uvula is pulled towards the intact side on phonation, with unilateral depression of the gag reflex. Autonomic dysfunction is discussed in Chapter 24.

### Investigation and Causes

Investigation: imaging, general medical and ENT evaluation.
   Causes are summarised here:

- An acute hemisphere stroke often causes transient swallowing difficulty, but with bilateral innervation compensation occurs rapidly. Bilateral supranuclear lesions cause pseudobulbar palsy (see below).

- Syringobulbia and MND can cause bilateral nuclear X lesions, producing a bulbar palsy. Multiple system atrophy can also affect the nuclei to cause stridor.
- As X exits the skull, IX, X, XI and XII are often involved together. Cancer, inflammatory disorders and infection (TB) may all be responsible (see jugular foramen syndrome). In the neck, where X runs in the carotid sheath, damage can follow carotid dissection or surgery.
- Distally, an isolated vagal palsy causes unilateral vocal cord palsy and laryngeal anaesthesia but spares pharyngeal and palatal muscles. The superior laryngeal nerve, arising distal to the pharyngeal nerve, is primarily sensory – lesions tend to be symptomless. Precise localisation may be impossible.
- Recurrent laryngeal nerve lesions cause dysphonia, transient if unilateral, and severe if bilateral. The left recurrent laryngeal nerve is the more frequently involved. Thyroid masses, lymph nodes and cancer can affect the nerves in the neck, and they can be damaged during surgery.

## XI. Accessory Nerve

The spinal accessory nerve is the motor nerve to the upper portion of trapezius and sternocleidomastoid. Unusually, XI has twin origins: the caudal portion of the *nucleus ambiguus* forms the internal ramus (minority). The accessory nuclei of the upper cervical cord (C1–4) form the spinal root and external ramus (majority). The pathway begins through the foramen magnum, with ascent of the spinal root. The nerve exits from the skull via the jugular foramen (Figure 13.11). Thence, the internal ramus supplies the larynx and pharynx with X; the external ramus supplies the sternocleidomastoid and trapezius muscles. Fibres of the cranial root of the nerve destined to form the internal ramus are part of X, and thus, XI is primarily a spinal nerve with an intracranial course rather than a true cranial nerve. Afferent twigs from cervical and thoracic nerves combine with spinal XI as it pierces trapezius – an anomalous arrangement. The spinal XI has an intimate relationship with the internal jugular vein.

### Examination and Localisation

Test the right sternomastoid: ask the patient to turn the head to the left against resistance. Contraction of both sternomastoids produces head flexion. Trapezius raises the abducted arm above the horizontal and moves the scapula.

With an accessory nerve lesion the shoulder droops on the affected side, with wasting of the upper trapezius and weakness of shoulder elevation and arm abduction above 90°. Winging of the scapula occurs when the arm is moved laterally – in contrast to serratus anterior weakness (long thoracic nerve) when winging follows forward pressure with the palm against a flat surface. With a hemisphere stroke, trapezius is weak on the side of the hemiparesis, while the opposite sternomastoid is weak – the head turning towards the side of the hemiparesis is weak.

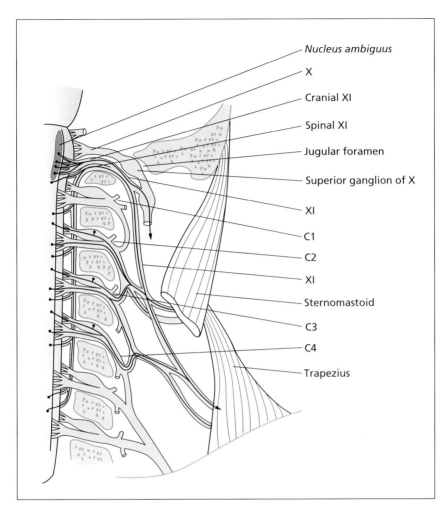

**Figure 13.11** Nerve XI, jugular foramen, *nucleus ambiguus* (AP view, upper cord and skull base).

## XI Nerve Damage

The leading culprit is trauma during lymph node biopsy in the posterior cervical triangle. Carotid endarterectomy, internal jugular vein cannulation and neck TB are also causes. Weakness is often associated with pain around the shoulder or deep in trapezius. The cause of this pain is unclear but probably relates to the way trapezius is (or was, pre-injury) innervated. Surgery: grafting, end-to-end repair and other procedures are often unhelpful.

A rare spontaneous painful XI neuropathy also occurs, allied to neuralgic amyotrophy. Pain subsides over weeks, but full recovery is unusual. The spinal nucleus of XI can be damaged in the cord, and the intracranial portion of the nerve, often with IX and X in the posterior fossa (see jugular foramen syndrome). Generalised neuromuscular processes such as myotonic dystrophy and myasthenia gravis can also affect muscles.

## XII. Hypoglossal Nerve

XII supplies tongue muscles (Figure 13.12). *Genioglossus* protrudes the tongue, *styloglossus* draws it back and up and *hypoglossus* depresses it. The nucleus is in the floor of the fourth ventricle, and the nerve emerges in the ventrolateral sulcus. XII leaves the skull through the hypoglossal foramen, nearby the jugular foramen, close to both the internal carotid artery and the internal jugular vein.

### XII: Examination and Pathology

Observe the tongue both resting and moving – forward–backward and side–side. Unilateral (or bilateral) wasting can be seen: furrowing, atrophy, discolouration and fibrillation. Tongue fibrillation, seen typically in MND, should only be diagnosed with the tongue at rest within the mouth; some flickering movements when protruded are normal. A XII nerve lesion causes tongue deviation to that side when protruded. Subtle weakness: ask the patient to press the tongue against each cheek and feel its strength. Palpate mouth and tongue.

Bilateral LMN lesions produce a small weak tongue, dysphagia and severe dysarthria (see Bulbar palsy). The tongue can also be spastic, with small, slow clumsy movements (see Pseudobulbar palsy). A tumour such as nasopharyngeal carcinoma, lymphoma and a metastasis are typical causes, often with other cranial nerve palsies and also trauma and sepsis. An isolated XII is sometimes seen with carotid artery dissection (Chapter 6) and

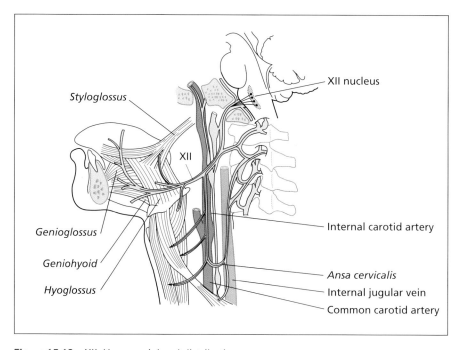

**Figure 13.12** XII: Nerve peripheral distribution.

following endarterectomy. Numbness of half of the tongue with occipital and upper neck pain on head turning is known as the neck–tongue syndrome, caused by compression of the ventral ramus of C2 that carries sensory fibres from the tongue via XII.

### Jugular Foramen Syndrome

Lesions of IX, X and XI are also known as Vernet's syndrome. Vernet with a XII lesion is known as Collet-Sicard, and with the addition of a Horner's, Villaret's syndrome. Causes are a tumour, infection such as malignant otitis externa, zoster, trauma and thrombosis of the jugular bulb.

## Bulbar and Pseudobulbar Palsy

These describe the weakness and/or poor movement of muscles supplied by lower cranial nerves (largely IX, X and XII), whose nuclei lie in the medullary bulb. UMN lesions cause pseudobulbar palsy. Lesions of the nuclei, fasciculi, cranial nerves and muscles – including myasthenia – produce bulbar palsy: weakness can be unilateral. Pseudobulbar palsy is bilateral. There is choking, dysphagia and dysarthria and sometimes emotional lability with pseudobulbar palsy. Patients with severe Parkinson's also have poverty of movement of bulbar muscles.

## Multiple Cranial Neuropathies

These are relative rarities. Some causes are summarised here:

- Meninges/skull: infection, carcinoma, lymphoma, epidural abscess, clivus/skull base tumour, osteopetrosis, Paget's, fibrous dysplasia, trauma and radiotherapy
- Infection: *Borrelia*, TB, syphilis, fungi, *cysticercus,* HZV, HSV, EBV, CMV, HIV and HTLV-1
- Neuropathy: Guillain–Barré, Miller–Fisher, idiopathic and diabetes mellitus
- Inflammatory: sarcoidosis, Behçet's, amyloid, GPA, PAN, Churg–Strauss, giant cell arteritis, SLE, Sjögren's, scleroderma and mixed connective tissue disease
- Pituitary: apoplexy and lymphocytic hypophysitis
- Vascular: aneurysm, dissection and endarterectomy

A recurrent idiopathic multiple cranial neuropathy occurs in South-East Asia. Clusters of nerve lesions, such as a III, V and VII arise, remit and recur over several years.

### Cranial Epidural Abscess

Pyogenic cranial epidural abscess (also Chapter 9) is a rare cause of sequential unilateral cranial nerve lesions, typically in the elderly with diabetes. For example, hearing loss with a discharge from the external auditory meatus can be followed by a VII palsy and progressively by lower cranial nerve palsies, even to include the XII. The abscess, a sheet of pus several millimetres thick, can also track upwards to V, the three ocular motor nerves and even to the optic nerve. An epidural abscess can be hard to see on imaging. Surgery and antibiotics are required. Mortality is high.

## Acknowledgements

I am most grateful to Jeremy Chataway, Robin Howard and Paul Jarman for their contribution to *Neurology A Queen Square Textbook*. 2nd edn. I was also a contributor.

Neuroanatomy Figures: the late Professor MJ Turlough Fitzgerald, Emeritus Professor of Anatomy, National University of Ireland, Galway most generously provided illustrations for Neurology *A Queen Square Textbook* 2nd & 1st edns from his own *Clinical Neuroanatomy and Neuroscience*.

Figures 13.4 and 13.5 are from Patten J. *Neurological Differential Diagnosis*. 2nd edn. Springer 1996.

## Further Reading and Information

Chataway J, Clarke C, Howard R, Jarman P. Cranial nerve disorders. In *Neurology: A Queen Square Textbook*, 2nd edn. Clarke C, Howard R, Rossor M, Shorvon S, eds. Chichester: John Wiley & Sons, 2016. There are numerous references.

Mtui E, Gruener G, Dockery P. *Fitzgerald's Clinical Neuroananatomy & Neuroscience*, 8th edn. Mtui E, Gruener G, Dockerty P. New York: Elsevier, 2020.

Patten J. *Neurological Differential Diagnosis*, 2nd edn. London: Springer, 1996.

For free updated notes, potential links and references as these become available:
https://www.drcharlesclarke.com
You will be asked to log in, in a secure fashion, with your name and institution.

# 14

## Neuro-Ophthalmology

This chapter outlines conditions that affect the visual pathways, eye movements and pupils. I separate clinical problems broadly into:

- Visual loss: unilateral, bilateral, acute and subacute (progressive), transient and permanent
- Optic disc swelling
- Eye movement and pupil disorders.

## Visual Pathways

These are summarised in Figure 14.1, and typical field defects in Figure 14.2.

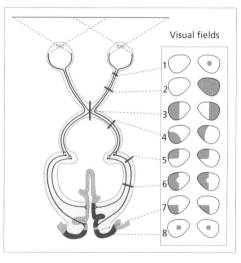

Figure 14.2   Typical visual field defects.
1. Central scotoma (intrinsic optic nerve lesion)
2. Blind R eye (complete optic nerve lesion)
3. Bitemporal hemianopia (optic chiasm)
4. Incongruous hemianopic defect (optic tract)
5. Upper quadrantic homonymous defect (temporal optic radiation)
6. Lower quadrantic homonymous defect (parietal optic radiation)
7. Homonymous hemianopia with macular sparing (visual cortex)
8. Bilateral occipital polar defects (rare)

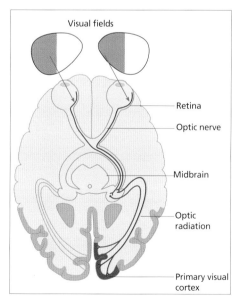

Figure 14.1   Visual pathway: essential anatomy.

*Neurology: A Clinical Handbook*, First Edition. Charles Clarke.
© 2022 John Wiley & Sons Ltd. Published 2022 by John Wiley & Sons Ltd.

## Retina and Optic Nerve

The eight cell and fibre layers are shown in Figure 14.3.

- Photoreceptors (2) – rods and cones – are applied to the pigment epithelium (1)
- Ganglion cells (7) are the source of action potentials conducted by axons that form both retinal nerve fibre layer (8) and optic nerve.
- Two sets of retinal neurones – horizontal cells and amacrine cells – are arranged transversely.

The essential circuitry is shown in Figure 14.4.

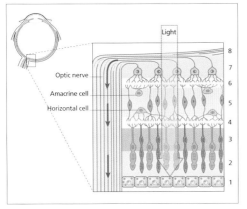

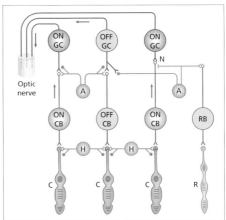

**Figure 14.3** The eight retinal layers.
8. Nerve fibre layer
7. Ganglion cell layer (OFF and ON cells)
6. Inner plexiform layer (with amacrine cells)
5. Inner nuclear layer (OFF and ON bipolars)
4. Outer plexiform layer (with horizontal cells)
3. Outer nuclear layer (of rods and cones)
2. Photoreceptor layer
1. Pigment epithelium layer

**Figure 14.4** Circuit diagram of retina. A, amacrine cell; C, cone; CB, cone bipolar; GC, ganglion cell; H, horizontal cell; N, nexus (gap junction); R, rod; RB, rod bipolar.

### Photoreceptors, Bipolars, Amacrine and Ganglion Cells

Cone photoreceptors sensitive to bright light, colour and shape are clustered around the fovea. Photoreceptor end feet synapse with bipolar and horizontal cell processes. Cone bipolar cells are either:

- ON bipolars switched ON by light or inhibited when light levels fall. They synapse on ON cone ganglion cells.
- OFF bipolars have an opposite response: they synapse on OFF ganglion cells.

Horizontal cells extend dendrites between photoreceptors and bipolars to inhibit them, restricting activity to the area stimulated.

Rod photoreceptors are active in low illumination and insensitive to colour.

Rod bipolars activate ON and OFF rod ganglion cells via amacrine cells. There are more than 10 amacrine cell types. Their function is to turn ON or OFF ganglion cells, enhance contrast and detect subtle movement.

Ganglion cells, of either ON or OFF variety, are activated by bipolar neurones. An ON ganglion cell is activated by a point light source and inhibited via horizontal cells and appropriate bipolars by a surrounding ring of light, known as annular inhibition. An OFF ganglion cell reacts in reverse – inhibited by a point source but excited by a ring of light.

Retinal colour recognition, for red, green and blue, is achieved via ganglion cells. These are either: ON-line for green + OFF-line for red, ON-line for red + OFF-line for green and ON-line for blue + OFF-line for yellow. Colour recognition is achieved by cones sensitive to specific wavelengths.

### Rods, Cones, Ganglion Cell Axons, Fovea and Foveola

Most rod and cone ganglion cells are parvocellular (small, P cells) – small receptive fields receptive to shape and colour. A minority are magnocellular ganglion cells (large, M cells) – large fields, receptive to moving objects.

The fovea has a central section, the foveola with the highest sensitivity (Figure 14.5):

- Midget cones have one-to-one synapses with midget bipolar cells and ganglion cells.
- Cell bodies have long neurites – allowing light to strike midget cones directly.

Each optic nerve carries over one million axons, with supporting glia, blood supply and meningeal sheath.

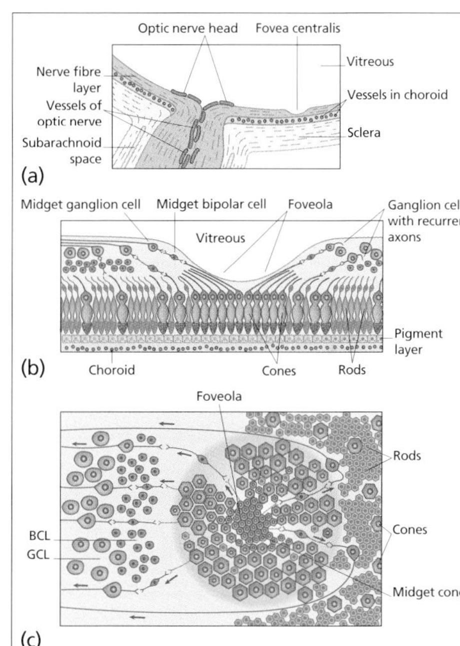

### Optic Chiasm, Optic Tract and Radiation

The chiasm, optic tract and optic radiation are shown above in Figures 14.1 and 14.2.

Each optic tract (the uncrossed temporal-half and crossed nasal-half retinal axons) divides into a medial and a lateral root. The medial root enters the midbrain. This carries:

- Fibres serving the pupillary light reflex – to the pretectal nucleus
- Fibres from retinal M cells – scanning movements – to the superior colliculus
- Fibres to the reticular formation (parvocellular) – arousal function
- Fibres from superior colliculus to pulvinar and visual association cortex – the extrageniculate visual pathway.

**Figure 14.5** (a) Fovea and optic nerve. (b, c) Fovea and foveola: section and surface diagram. BCL, bipolar cell layer; GCL, ganglion cell layer.

The axons of lateral root of the optic tract synapse in the lateral geniculate body (LGB). The LGB is six layered:

Three laminae receive crossed fibres and three uncrossed. The deepest laminae (magnocellular) receive axons from retinal M ganglion cells (movement detection). The outer laminae (parvocellular) receive axons from P ganglion cells (detail and colour).

The optic radiation (*syn.* geniculocalcarine tract) is a prominent white matter bundle.

- The radiation enters the posterior part of the internal capsule, runs beneath the temporal cortex and alongside the lateral ventricle.
- Meyer's loop contains forward-sweeping fibres in the anterior temporal lobe, from the upper part of the visual fields that run to the lower occipital cortex.

## Occipital Cortex

Within the visual a.k.a. striate cortex, the optic radiation synapses with spiny stellate cells of cortical layer IV. The striate cortex (striae of Gennari) bears the name of an eighteenth century Parma student anatomist. Ganglion cells are arranged in alternating columns (alternating inputs between left and right eyes). Thus, impulses from identical points on each retina arrive side by side in the cortex. Differentiation is achieved by a cell hierarchy:

- Spiny stellate cells produce simple responses – to fine slits of light in one orientation.
- Some pyramidal cells produce complex responses – to broad slits (bars), orientated at a particular angle and either stationary or moving in one direction.
- Other pyramidal cells are hypercomplex, responding to L-shaped configurations.
- Simple cell axons converge on to complex cells; complex cell axons converge on to hyper-complex cells.

The primary visual cortex can be thought of as a pixellated screen, detecting position, shape and movement. Area 17 (V1) does not interpret what we see. Recognition is achieved by connections with the visual association cortex, temporal lobes and with memory.

### Visual Association Cortex and V1–V5

Brodmann areas 18 and 19, also known as peristriate or extrastriate (*syn.* visual association) cortex, contain cortical cell columns concerned with feature extraction. Some cell groups respond to shape, some to perception of height/depth and others to colours. The regions contain cell groups that recognise these particular attributes of objects. Afferents arrive primarily from area 17.

The V1–V5 nomenclature is widely used. The lateral and medial parts of area 19 (V4, V5) contain specialised connections – 'where' and 'what' visual pathways:

- 'What' is the ventrally placed, medial stream for object recognition (V4).
- 'Where' is the lateral, dorsally situated stream concerned with location (V5).

### 'What'

Three types of recognition take place here (Figure 14.6):

- For forms, shapes and categories of objects: in the lateral zone.
- For faces: in the mid zone.
- Colours: medially.

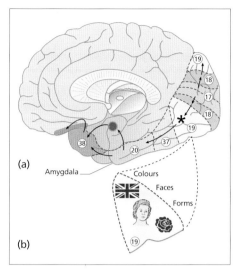

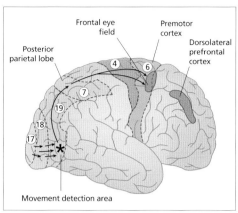

**Figure 14.7** 'Where' visual pathway – right hemisphere, lateral surface. Asterisk: movement detection area in Area 19. Right frontal cortical eye field activates conjugate saccades towards left field.

**Figure 14.6** 'What' visual pathway – right hemisphere medial surface. (a) Asterisk: visual identification area, left visual field. (b) Detail of Area 19 – colours, faces and forms.

Sophisticated recognition of objects and faces involves area 20 (inferotemporal cortex) and area 38 (temporal pole). Threatening objects generate activity via these areas and within the amygdala.

### 'Where'

The lateral part of area 19 is responsive to movement in the contralateral hemifield (Figure 14.7). The main projection is to area 7 (posterior parietal cortex), long known as the area affected in disorders such as astereognosis (Chapter 4). Area 7 is involved in:

- Movement perception
- Stereopsis (three-dimensional vision)
- Spatial sense (relative position of objects to each other).

Area 7 also receives fibres from the pulvinar known as blindsight fibres.

### Cortical Eye Fields

Conjugate eye movement is controlled by discrete regions within the grey matter (Figure 14.8).

Three mechanisms are involved in driving conjugate gaze. (The word conjugate means joined together: *jugum* is the yoke between two oxen in Latin):

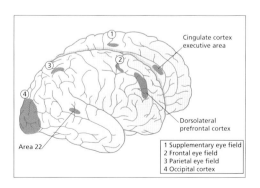

**Figure 14.8** Cortical eye fields.

- *Scanning*: saccades (i.e. rapid movement from one target to another).
- *Tracking*: smooth pursuit of a target across the visual field.
- *Compensation*: maintenance of gaze during head movement via vestibulo-ocular fixation reflex.

Voluntary saccades are initiated in the frontal eye fields. Smooth pursuit movements originate in the occipital and parietal cortices. Velocity detectors in the upper pons receive information via the optic tract. Fixation is achieved by visual pursuit modulated by vestibular and cerebellar input.

Automatic scanning movements are generated in the medial portion of the optic tract via the pulvinar area and influenced by the cerebellum and vestibular system. This explains movements such as hands being in position to catch a ball before it becomes visible.

Eye and pupil movement below the level of the cortical eye fields consists of:

- Conjugate gaze mechanisms within the brainstem
- Pupillary light reflexes
- Individual cranial nerves III, IV and VI and the muscles supplied
- Near and far responses.

## Gaze Centres in the Brainstem

Horizontal (lateral) gaze centres lie in the right and left PPRF adjacent to each VI nucleus (Figure 14.9). Upward gaze is controlled by the rostral interstitial nucleus (RiN) close to the pretectal nucleus (III nucleus level). The medial longitudinal fasciculus (MLF) connects each PPRF and the VI nucleus with the portion of the III nucleus that supplies the medial rectus – thus yoking together ABDuction in one eye with ADDuction in the other.

## The Light Reflex: Pupil Constriction

The pathway from retinal ganglion cell to postganglionic parasympathetic fibres and onwards to the iris (*sphincter pupillae*) is shown in Figure 14.10. The sympathetic pathway (pupil dilatation) and the near reflex are mentioned below.

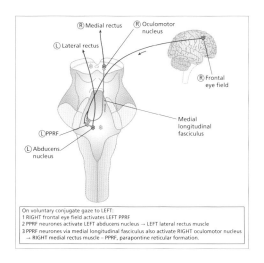

On voluntary conjugate gaze to LEFT:
1 RIGHT frontal eye field activates LEFT PPRF
2 PPRF neurones activate LEFT abducens nucleus → LEFT lateral rectus muscle
3 PPRF neurones via medial longitudinal fasciculus also activate RIGHT oculomotor nucleus → RIGHT medial rectus muscle – PPRF, parapontine reticular formation.

**Figure 14.9** Voluntary conjugate eye movement (midbrain, posterior view).

## III, IV and VI Nerves and Nuclei

The essential anatomy is summarised in Figure 14.11.

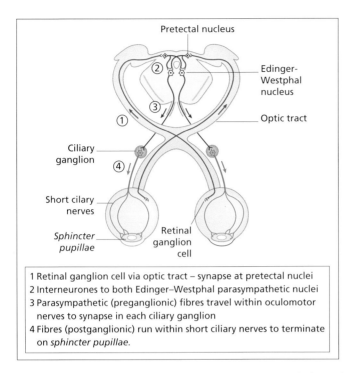

1 Retinal ganglion cell via optic tract – synapse at pretectal nuclei
2 Interneurones to both Edinger–Westphal parasympathetic nuclei
3 Parasympathetic (preganglionic) fibres travel within oculomotor
   nerves to synapse in each ciliary ganglion
4 Fibres (postganglionic) run within short ciliary nerves to terminate
   on *sphincter pupillae.*

**Figure 14.10**   Pupillary constriction to light (midbrain, level of superior colliculus).

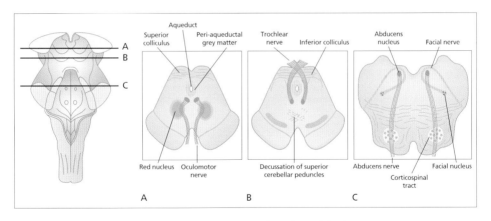

**Figure 14.11**   Origins of III, IV and VI: transverse sections through brainstem.

### Oculomotor Nucleus and the III Nerve

This nucleus, adjacent to the periaqueductal grey matter at superior colliculus level, consists of neurones that supply:

- Five striated muscles: medial, superior, inferior recti, inferior oblique and *levator palpbe-
  brae superioris.*
- Muscles supplied by the parasympathetic system: *ciliaris* (ciliary muscle) and *sphincter
  pupillae* via the Edinger–Westphal nucleus.

Each III nerve passes through the midbrain tegmentum, emerges into the interpeduncular fossa, crosses the apex of the petrous temporal bone, enters the cavernous sinus and leaves in two divisions within the superior orbital fissure. Parasympathetic fibres travel in the lower division and leave in the branch to the inferior oblique muscle. They synapse in the ciliary ganglion, pierce the sclera and, via the short ciliary nerves reach *ciliaris* and *sphincter pupillae*.

### Trochlear Nucleus and the IV Nerve

The nucleus is at the level of the inferior colliculus. Each IV nerve then decussates, emerges from the back of the brainstem and enters the cavernous sinus (just below III), to reach the superior oblique muscle via the superior orbital fissure.

### Abducens Nucleus and the VI Nerve

Each VI nucleus, lower in the brainstem than III and IV, lies in the mid pons at the level of the facial nucleus. The nerve runs a long intracranial course, initially beside the basilar artery and thence over the petrous temporal bone. Within the cavernous sinus it lies beside the internal carotid artery (Figure 14.12). Like III and IV, VI passes through the superior orbital fissure. VI innervates the lateral rectus muscle.

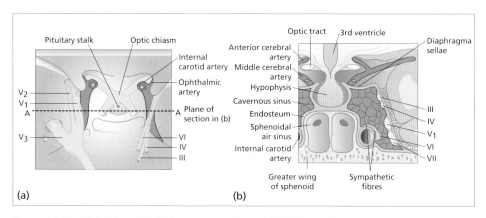

**Figure 14.12** III, IV, VI and V within cavernous sinus. (a) Middle cranial fossa from above (cavernous sinus removed). Left: relations of V. Right: relations of III, IV and VI. (b) Coronal section through pituitary (AA).

### *Ocular Muscle Motor Units and Sensory Connections*

These motor units contain 5–10 muscle fibres (cf. 500 or more in large limb muscles) and comprise A, B and C muscle fibres:

- A fibres (fast twitch): involved in saccades
- B fibres (slow twitch): smooth pursuit
- C fibres: maintain the visual axes.

Proprioceptive pathways from the extraocular muscles extend widely – to the mesencephalic nucleus of V and to the cuneate nucleus in the medulla. Afferent projections from neck muscles and vestibulocerebellum to these nuclei assist head movements in response to changes in gaze.

### The Near Response

Three responses combine to enable gaze to focus on a near object:

- Convergence is brought about by contraction of the medial recti.
- The ciliary muscle contracts – the lens bulges passively, the thicker lens shortening its focal length (Figure 14.13).
- *Sphincter pupillae* contracts – concentrating light through the central lens.

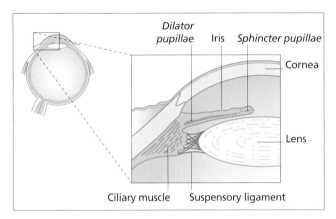

**Figure 14.13** *Dilator* and *sphincter pupillae*, lens and ciliary muscle.

Retinal impulses pass via the lateral geniculate body to the occipital cortex and thence to the visual association cortex that analyses the object in view. Thence, the efferent pathway reaches the Edinger–Westphal nucleus and vergence cells within the reticular formation.

### The Far Response

To bring a distant object into focus, the ciliary muscle must be inhibited – allowing the suspensory ligament to become tight and flatten the lens. Sympathetic impulses cause this relaxation of the ciliary muscle. *Dilator pupillae* contracts.

### Sympathetic Pathway to the Eye and Face

The sympathetic system originates in the hypothalamus. Central efferents decussate in the midbrain and are joined by ipsilateral fibres running within and from the reticular formation. The pathway descends in the cord, emerges in the first ventral thoracic root and reaches the sympathetic chain. These preganglionic fibres synapse in the superior cervical ganglion. Post-ganglionic fibres run within the adventitia of branches of the internal and external carotid arteries. The internal carotid system is accompanied by two sets of fibres. One joins $V_1$ in the cavernous sinus but leaves this nerve in the short and long ciliary nerves to the smooth muscles of the eye (*dilator pupillae, ciliaris* and *levator palpebrae superioris*). The second forms a plexus around the internal carotid artery. Branches reach the skin of the forehead and scalp. Horner's syndrome is discussed below. External carotid sympathetic fibres are intimately related to all branches of the external carotid artery: superficial and middle temporal, facial, maxillary, middle meningeal, posterior auricular and lingual arteries.

## Examination

Visual acuity, colour vision and visual fields: see Chapter 4. Fundus examination requires practice, patience and a good ophthalmoscope.

Consider:

- Disc and cup morphology: size, crowded nerve fibres, hypermetropia
- Disc colour: pallor – atrophy; large/pale in myopia (normal)
- Disc swelling: true disc swelling or, for example drusen?
- Nerve fibre layer: ? thinning with optic nerve disease
- Retinal haemorrhages: form and position
- Retinal arteries and veins: qualities – a-v nipping, cotton wool spots, venous pulsation, emboli?
- Macula: normality, macular star.

## Visual Loss: Uni- and Bilateral Visual Failure

The many causes are drawn together in Table 14.1.

**Table 14.1**  Visual failure.

| |
| --- |
| *Ocular and retinal* |
| Refractive errors, cataracts, glaucoma, macular degeneration, uveitis, retinal disease – diabetes, vascular disease, dystrophies, paraneoplastic degeneration |
| *Unilateral and bilateral optic nerve* |
| e.g. bilateral optic nerve lesions – anterior pathway inflammation and compression, vascular events, papilloedema, toxins, nutrition, drugs and radiation, hereditary optic neuropathies |
| *Chiasm* |
| e.g. chiasmal compression (pituitary), chiasmal (optic nerve) glioma and meningioma |
| *Post-chiasmal* |
| Optic tract, optic radiation, visual association area, cortical visual loss |
| *Non-organic (functional)* |

Was the onset acute, subacute or gradual? Has vision deteriorated, improved or remained static?

Abrupt loss – complete or partial: if abrupt, painless and permanent, a vascular cause such as central retinal artery (CRA) occlusion is likely or a retinal/vitreous detachment.

Subacute (progressive) visual loss over days with pain is in keeping with inflammation – generally in MS optic neuritis, pain precedes vision loss. Persistent pain raises questions of a compressive or infective cause.

Sudden permanent monocular or bilateral visual loss typically follows a vascular event – arteritic and non-arteritic, systemic inflammation such as sarcoid, retinal or vitreous detachment and haemorrhage and traumatic optic neuropathy. Other causes include occipital lobe infarction, sagittal sinus thrombosis, pituitary apoplexy, posterior reversible encephalopathy and toxins. Visual loss can also be non-organic.

Gradual loss is usually a complaint, but it can be an incidental finding when the acuity is checked:

- Acuity less than 6/9 requires investigation when acuity was previously normal.
- Progression of any visual loss requires investigation.
- Post-chiasmal lesions (optic tracts) are relatively unusual.
- Optic radiation lesions and occipital lobe infarction tend to present acutely.
- Functional visual loss occurs.

Transient visual loss with recovery and frequently unilateral is summarised below:

- Vascular – emboli and/or ischaemia, giant cell arteritis, vasculitis
- Hypoperfusion – hypotension, anaemia, hyperviscosity, carotid artery disease
- Ocular – intermittent angle closure glaucoma, retinal/vitreous detachment
- Demyelination – Uhthoff's phenomenon with MS-ON
- Obscurations – papilloedema
- Non-organic or no cause found.

## Optic Nerve Disease

Various terms are used – optic neuropathy, optic neuritis, retrobulbar neuritis, perineuritis, neuroretinitis, papilloedema, papillophlebitis, periphlebitis, papillopathy and neuromyelitis. All optic nerve diseases cause visual impairment. Six inflammatory optic neuropathies are mentioned here before the wider classification.

- Optic neuritis with MS and the clinically isolated syndrome (CIS)
- Optic neuritis with neuromyelitis optica (NMO-ON, a.k.a. Devic's disease)
- Optic neuritis: chronic relapsing inflammatory optic neuropathy (CRION)
- Infections and other causes – optic neuritis/perineuritis
- Sarcoid-related optic neuropathy
- Neuroretinitis – the macular star.

Optic neuropathies are either typical or atypical. Typical means the common optic neuritis (ON) associated with MS – with characteristic recovery. Demyelinating ON can occur alone – the CIS – or as atypical ON with neuromyelitis optica (NMO-ON). All are immune mediated and confined to the nervous system (MS, CIS, NMO-ON: Chapter 11). Atypical ON can also be part of a systemic disorder, such as sarcoid.

### Optic Neuritis with MS

This is the commonest cause of subacute unilateral visual loss in a young Caucasian adult. Most experience some pain on eye movement before loss of vision. Visual loss progresses over days and can be either minimal or progress, even to no light perception. Colour vision and the pupil light reflex are impaired, with a central field defect. Disc swelling is seen in one-third, when the term optic neuritis is used. When disc appears normal, the neuropathy is termed retrobulbar neuritis. Most recover to VA 6/9 or better. After recovery, disc pallor may be seen. The clinical context often points to MS. Routine bloods are normal. Brain MRI usually shows high signal in the optic nerve and may show MS white matter lesions. Steroids reduce recovery time (Chapter 11).

### Optic Neuritis with Neuromyelitis Optica (NMO-ON, a.k.a. Devic's Disease)

NMO-ON is rarer and tends to cause severe periocular pain with visual loss. Spontaneous recovery is less likely than with MS-ON (Chapter 11). Imaging: no absolute features – a plaque in the optic nerve is likely to be posterior and/or in the chiasm.

### Optic Neuritis: Chronic Relapsing Inflammatory Optic Neuropathy

CRION refers to unusual cases with painful prolonged and isolated subacute visual loss of unknown cause. In most, the second eye becomes involved. There is a response to steroids but relapse when these are withdrawn, in contrast to MS-ON. Investigations are normal. There is no other evidence of MS or NMO nor any systemic condition.

### Infections and Other Causes – Optic Neuritis/Perineuritis

Rarer causes of optic neuritis include infection such as pneumococcal meningitis that can cause devastating visual loss as can TB or fungal invasion. Optic neuritis is one of many complications of neurosyphilis, Lyme disease and zoster. Optic neuritis with orbital signs or prolonged severe pain should flag up these possibilities. The nerve sheath can be involved, a.k.a. optic perineuritis. Viral infections can also cause an optic neuropathy as a post-infectious syndrome (Chapter 9). Infiltration with lymphoma, malignant meningitis or sarcoid can cause perineuritis.

Sarcoid-related optic neuropathy: usually the optic nerve is infiltrated with granulomata visible at the disc or compressed by a granulomatous mass. Sarcoid chiasmitis also occurs (Chapter 26). Sarcoid ON can also be indistinguishable from MS-ON with spontaneous recovery.

### Neuroretinitis – the Macular Star

In neuroretinitis the disc becomes swollen, and exudates develop radially around the macula, a.k.a. the macular star. *Bartonella* – cat scratch disease – has been implicated. Neuroretinitis is not associated with MS.

### Optic Neuropathy – the Wider Classification

The extent of optic neuropathy is covered within Table 14.2. Selected conditions are reviewed briefly here.

**Table 14.2** Optic neuritis/optic neuropathy.

| |
| --- |
| Central retinal artery and vein occlusion |
| Immune mediated, with or without systemic inflammation, a.k.a. demyelination |
| Infection, infiltration and compression |
| Anterior optic neuropathy with disc swelling (often monocular) |
| Anterior optic neuropathy without disc swelling (ganglion cell failure – typically bilateral, symmetrical) |
| Hereditary optic neuropathies |
| Posterior (retrobulbar) optic neuropathy without disc swelling |
| Chronic ocular ischaemia |
| Toxic, nutritional and radiation-induced optic neuropathies and trauma |

## Retina and Optic Nerve Vascular Anatomy

The retinal ganglion cell layer is supplied entirely by the central retinal artery (CRA), an end-artery branch of the ophthalmic. CRA occlusion, usually embolic, causes total visual loss. In 15%, the cilioretinal artery from the choroidal circulation supplies the macula. Occlusion of the cilioretinal artery produces a scotoma from the blind spot to the macula – a rare event in isolation.

The prelaminar portion of the optic disc – its most anterior portion – is supplied by the short posterior ciliary arteries. These are also branches of the ophthalmic artery, but they are not end arteries. Zinn–Haller anastomoses surround each optic nerve, immediately behind the globe – arterioles pierce the sclera to supply the optic nerve head and the choroid. Ischaemic events in posterior ciliary artery territory tend not to be related to embolic events, cf. the CRA, but to low perfusion. The optic disc is vulnerable because it is at a watershed between branches of the short posterior ciliary vessels.

Internal and external carotid artery anastomoses within the orbit are extensive. The retrolaminar portion of the optic nerve and the remainder of the intraorbital nerve are supplied by pial vessels and by penetrating branches of the ophthalmic artery. The intracanalicular portion of the nerve is supplied by branches of the ophthalmic artery. The intracranial portion of the nerve is supplied by pial vessels.

## Central and Branch Retinal Artery Occlusion

In central retinal artery occlusion (CRAO), abrupt painless total loss of vision is typical. In branch occlusion, field defects do not cross the retinal horizontal raphe: altitudinal defects, or portions thereof, are the rule. Any portion of the retina supplied by a cilioretinal artery – typically the macula – is spared. Acutely, there is retinal oedema, a hallmark of infarction of inner retinal layers that include the ganglion cell layer. The macular cherry red spot – a feature of CRAO – is normal in colour – the red spot is simply the product of an intact choroidal supply, thrown into contrast by pale, infarcted retina (Figure 14.14).

If CRA flow is restored within minutes, then monocular blindness will be transient.

Various types of embolus – calcific (Figure 14.15), cholesterol or platelet/fibrin – can give some clue to the source.

Retinal artery occlusion can also occur in giant cell arteritis and other vasculitides (Chapter 26 and below).

Treatment: acetazolamide IV and ocular massage, with or without paracentesis to lower intraocular pressure and thus improve perfusion, is an established practice but has no evidence base. There is sometimes partial recovery. Thrombolysis is not helpful.

## Central and Branch Retinal Vein Occlusion

There is usually abrupt painless blurred vision. A central retinal vein occlusion (CRVO) is easily recognised – there is disc swelling, retinal vein congestion and extensive haemorrhages. Partial occlusion, a.k.a. venous papillopathy or papillophlebitis, can cause

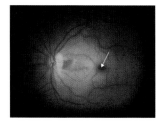

**Figure 14.14** Central retinal artery occlusion; cherry-red spot (white arrow) Afro-Caribbean case.

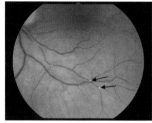

**Figure 14.15** Cholesterol emboli (black arrows).

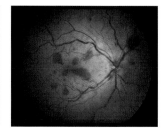

**Figure 14.16** Central retinal vein occlusion: scattered deep haemorrhages.

difficulty – unilateral disc swelling, but with minimal haemorrhages, that can be misdiagnosed as raised intracranial pressure (Figure 14.16).

CRVO tends to occur in later life, but it can occur in young fit people – dehydration may play a part. There is no acute treatment.

## Arteritic Anterior Ischaemic Optic Neuropathy: Giant Cell Arteritis (GCA)

Everyone should be familiar with this potential cause of visual loss. In GCA, some loss of vision, and even blindness in a matter of hours, is common. Premonitory transient visual loss can precede this for seconds when the patient stands up. Preceding systemic symptoms should be sought in anyone with sudden visual loss. Headache and tenderness of the extracranial arteries are typical. Polymyalgia rheumatica may coincide with GCA, precede or follow it. GCA is rare below the age of 50 (Chapter 26). In GCA, many arteries and arterioles are involved – their lumens occluded by intimal hypertrophy. The CRA, choroidal vessels, the entire globe or the orbit can be involved, because both internal and external carotid branch arteries are inflamed. Typically a swollen disc develops when vision becomes impaired.

A high ESR, greater than 50 mm, and greatly raised CRP are typical, but a normal ESR and CRP do not completely exclude GCA. A temporal artery biopsy should be carried out (Figure 14.17). It may be necessary to disregard blood tests and commence steroids. Oral high-dose prednisolone or methylprednisolone IV should be commenced immediately. A rapid response of the headache is typical. Recovery in an eye with established damage is minimal. Steroids can usually be stopped within two years.

AION can occur with polyarteritis, Churg–Strauss, rheumatoid, ANCA-positive vasculitis and SLE. Visual recovery is usual if treatment is immediate.

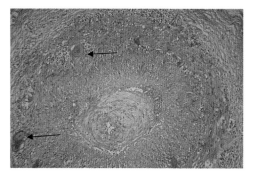

**Figure 14.17** Giant cell arteritis histology: granulomatous inflammation, fragmentation of internal elastic lamina and occlusion of arterial lumens (arrows).

## Non-Arteritic Anterior Ischaemic Optic Neuropathy

The patient complains of sudden or suba-cute visual loss over hours to days. Ischaemia of the posterior short ciliary arteries that supply the prelaminar optic nerve head causes this ischaemic neuropathy. The optic disc becomes swollen acutely and atrophic after 4–6 weeks – typically in the upper pole. A few weeks later, sectoral optic atrophy develops with loss of nerve fibres from the disc upper pole (Figure 14.18).

Most cases have small crowded discs with hypermetropia. Associations include sys-temic hypotension, obstructive sleep apnoea and glaucoma. AION follows a drop in the perfusion pressure at the optic nerve head. There is a risk of AION in the other eye in about a quarter. Most cases are relatively young and do not have vascular disease. No treatment is effective. This is also caused exceptionally by an embolus from an atrial myxoma.

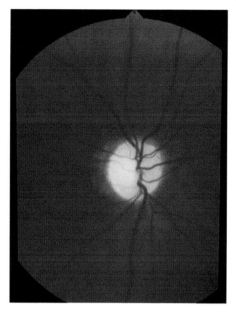

**Figure 14.18**  Right-sided optic atrophy.

## Posterior Ischaemic Optic Neuropathy

Posterior ischaemic optic neuropathy (PION) occurs in GCA, in vasculitis and following severe hypotension. There is acute or subacute painless vision loss and at first a normal fundus. Optic atrophy follows. When PION follows blood loss, vision impairment can be bilateral.

## Chronic Ischaemia and Slow Flow Retinopathy

Chronic ischaemia can lead to disc swelling with variable visual loss. One example is dia-betic papillopathy – a chronically swollen disc develops in poorly controlled diabetes. In accelerated hypertension, disc swelling also follows disc ischaemia. In both, optic nerve infarction can lead to permanent vision loss.

Slow flow retinopathy develops when there is severe impairment of both internal and external carotid supply to the orbit. Patients complain of transient loss of vision on stand-ing. Vision may be only mildly impaired, but there is congestion of retinal veins, haemor-rhages and macular oedema. When severe, the entire globe can become ischaemic, with vessel formation at the iris – *rubeosis iridis* – that can lead to glaucoma. A slow flow retin-opathy can also develop with a carotid-cavernous fistula (Chapter 6) and in GCA.

## Tumours, Compressive and Infiltrative Optic Neuropathy

Visual loss can be unilateral or bilateral. When unilateral, there is a relative afferent pupillary defect. The disc may be normal, swollen or infiltrated. Collaterals sometimes form to bypass the retinal circulation.

- Compressive optic neuropathy: intraorbital tumour, meningioma – nerve sheath, sphenoid wing, a pituitary tumour, craniopharyngioma, thyroid eye disease, sphenoid mucocoele, orbital pseudotumour and orbital haemorrhage, Paget's disease of bone, fibrous dysplasia.
- Infiltrative optic neuropathy: optic nerve glioma and glioblastoma, metastatic and nasopharyngeal carcinoma, lymphoma and leukaemia, carcinomatosis, malignant meningitis, sarcoid, TB.

### Meningioma

A meningioma can arise from arachnoid cells of the nerve sheath, generally in the orbital portion. Optic nerve sheath meningiomas tend to occur in middle-aged women and may be a feature of neurofibromatosis type 2. Stereotactic radiotherapy may slow progression. A meningioma can also arise from the sphenoid wing, tuberculum sellae or olfactory groove. A large olfactory groove or sphenoid wing meningioma can produce optic atrophy in one eye from compression with papilloedema in the other from raised intracranial pressure (Foster–Kennedy syndrome).

### Optic and Opto-Chiasmal Glioma

These anterior visual pathway tumours are the so-called benign gliomas of childhood and glioblastomas in adults. Childhood gliomas usually arise in the chiasm. The child presents with proptosis and visual loss. There may be nystagmus with head nodding. Discs: swollen or atrophic. Hypothalamic involvement, hydrocephalus and raised intracranial pressure can develop and/or meningeal spread. NF1 may be present. Surgery is solely palliative, and radiotherapy rarely helpful. A glioblastoma tends to arise in males of 40–60 years and cause rapid monocular visual loss, retrobulbar pain and disc oedema. Prognosis is poor.

### Hereditary – AD Optic Atrophy and Leber's

AD optic atrophy typically commences by the teenage years with gradual binocular visual loss. It commonly causes loss of central vision with a bilateral symmetrical central or centrocaecal scotomata. Gene: *OPA1* – chromosome 3.

Leber's (LHON) typically presents in a young adult with subacute painless visual loss over 3 months. There is marked impairment of acuity. The disc may be normal initially, but hyperaemia develops with swelling around the disc (pseudopapilloedema) and telangiectatic vessels nearby. Optic atrophy follows. Disc abnormalities may be present for years prior to the visual loss and may be seen in unaffected carriers. LHON is a mitochondrial disorder, maternally inherited (Chapter 10).

### Toxic, Nutritional, Radiation-Induced Optic Neuropathies and Trauma

All can present with bilateral visual loss, centrocaecal scotomata and impaired colour vision. Disc(s): hyperaemic initially – pallor follows.

- Tobacco–alcohol amblyopia occurs with excessive tobacco, alcohol or poor nutrition. Blindness can follow methanol toxicity and vitamin $B_{12}$ deficiency. Nutritional optic neuropathy occurs in starvation and malabsorption.
- Toxic amblyopia (Chapter 19) is associated with amiodarone, ciclosporin and digoxin. In a curious epidemic of optic neuropathy in Cuba in the 1990s, there were also peripheral neuropathy, myelopathy and sensorineural hearing loss, possibly toxic or nutritional.
- Radiation: visual loss can follow, from 4 months to some years after radiotherapy (Chapters 19 and 21).
- Trauma can damage the nerve directly, its blood supply or follow a blow to the orbital rim. Avulsion can occur.

## Swollen Disc(s) – Papilloedema

Disc swelling has many causes. Definitions vary: one view is that papilloedema should be reserved for swelling with raised intracranial pressure (Figure 14.19). However, papilloedema means oedema of the optic nerve head. Optic neuritis can produce an identical appearance. Disc anomalies can also cause difficulty.

- Raised intracranial pressure: intracranial mass lesion, hydrocephalus, idiopathic intracranial hypertension, venous obstruction, e.g. sagittal sinus thrombosis, respiratory failure, high-altitude cerebral oedema, excess CSF production, e.g. choroid plexus papilloma, arachnoid obstruction by blood/protein, A-V fistula.
- Local optic nerve disease: anterior optic neuropathies and nerve tumours, uveitis, low intraocular pressure, central retinal vein occlusion – all usually with visual loss.
- Disc anomalies, a.k.a. pseudopapilloedema: drusen, tilted disc, myelinated nerve fibres, hypermetropia, disc hamartomas.

As intracranial pressure rises, disc swelling develops (Figure 14.20) and then hyperaemia. Spontaneous venous pulsations disappear. Peripapillary flame-shaped haemorrhages develop.

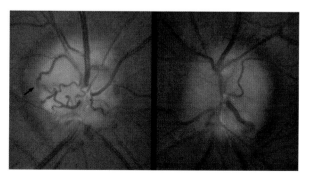

Figure 14.19  Chronic bilateral papilloedema and dilated veins with raised intracranial pressure.

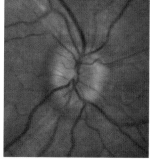

Figure 14.20  Early papilloedema.

Retinal and/or macular folds may form. Even when papilloedema is prominent, acuity and colour vision can remain normal, but the blind spots enlarge, with field constriction. Visual obscurations can occur, sometimes frequently; these herald optic nerve infarction and should be addressed urgently. With chronic papilloedema, discs become pale and their margins clearer. Haemorrhages resolve.

Atrophic papilloedema follows – disc pallor, poor acuity reduced and constricted fields.

**Idiopathic Intracranial Hypertension**

Idiopathic intracranial hypertension (IIH) is a likely diagnosis when papilloedema occurs without other evident neurology in an obese young woman. Headache is common; vomiting unusual. Visual obscurations, lasting seconds or minutes following postural changes, are common. A VI nerve palsy develops in many. Other features are occasionally seen – hyposmia, III and VII nerve palsies, tinnitus, eye pain and neck pain.

Papilloedema is typically dramatic but may be asymmetrical or even unilateral. Optic atrophy can develop. IIH is usually self-limiting, over months, but may cause severe vision loss before it subsides. Management and secondary causes are covered in Chapter 12.

## Uveo-Meningitic Syndromes

These disorders affect the iris, ciliary body and choroid – *i.e.* the uveal tract and/or the retina and/or the meninges. They are:

- Inflammatory: sarcoid, Behçet's, Vogt–Koyanagi–Harada, MS, SLE, GPA
- Infections: borrelia, syphilis, TB, leprosy, meningococcus, candida, coccidioidomycosis, CMV, HSV, HZV, HIV, hepatitis B, SSPE
- Cancer: lymphomas, leukaemia, metastases, paraneoplastic
- Ophthalmological: *retinitis pigmentosa*, posterior placoid pigment epitheliopathy, evanescent white dot syndrome, posterior scleritis.

## Phakomatoses

In these diseases – mainly inherited – tumours arise in ectodermal tissues such as the eye, CNS and skin.

- Neurofibromatosis types 1 and 2 (Chapter 26):
  NF1 is the commonest; some are new mutations.
  Ocular features:
  – optic nerve glioma in childhood
  – iris hamartoma, a.k.a. Lisch nodules, melanocytic naevi
  – pulsating exophthalmos due to sphenoid dysplasia – rare
  – retinal and choroidal hamartoma, congenital glaucoma, subcapsular cataract.

In NF2, one hallmark is a vestibular nerve schwannoma. Many have posterior subcapsular cataracts and occasionally an optic nerve sheath meningioma. Other ocular findings:

pigment epithelial changes, disc glioma, medullated nerve fibres, choroidal naevus and hamartoma and occasionally Lisch nodules.

- Von Hippel–Lindau disease: an AD predisposition to develop CNS and retinal hae-mangioblastomas, renal cell carcinoma, phaeochromocytoma, renal, pancreatic and epididymal cysts.
- Tuberous sclerosis: a.k.a. Bourneville's disease, a triad of epilepsy, retinal tumours and *adenoma sebaceum.*
- Sturge–Weber – facial and meningeal (encephalotrigeminal) angiomatosis: ocular features – glaucoma and choroidal, conjunctival and episcleral haemangiomas – no genetic basis.

## Diplopia and Eye Movement Abnormalities

Double vision is caused by:

- Extraocular muscle and neuromuscular junction dysfunction.
- Orbital and cranial nerve lesions.
- Nuclear and supranuclear lesions.

Monocular diplopia is generally caused by refractive error, a lens problem or is non-organic. Diplopia may be absent if there is impaired acuity in one eye, and/or when the false image can be suppressed, for example when misalignment is long-standing. Eye movements examination: see Chapter 4.

### Orbital Conditions and Ophthalmoplegia

Some orbital diseases are summarised here.

- Inflammatory – pseudotumour, Tolosa–Hunt, orbital myositis, dysthyroid eye disease
- Primary orbital tumours, metastates, lymphoma, sphenoid wing meningioma
- Orbital/muscle infiltration and infection – e.g. sarcoid, amyloid, acromegaly, vasculitis, TB, mucor, cellulitis, paranasal sinus mucocoele
- Trauma and extraocular muscle entrapment
- Caroticocavernous fistula, cavernous sinus thrombosis.

### Orbital Inflammatory Syndromes

Orbital inflammation causes pain, conjunctival injection, lid oedema, proptosis and oph-thalmoplegia. Inflammatory disorders of unknown cause include:

- Orbital pseudotumour – inflammation involves the orbit, sclera, ocular muscles and lids.
- Tolosa–Hunt syndrome – inflammation involves the superior orbital fissure and cavern-ous sinus.
- Orbital myositis – any extraocular muscle can be involved; usually unilateral. There is restriction of movement, pain on eye movement and conjunctival injection.

**Orbital Infection, Mass Lesions and Infiltration**

Infection within the orbit is an emergency. In orbital cellulitis, there is fever, ophthalmo-plegia and lid swelling. Proptosis may develop. TB and mucor can involve the orbit and also granulomas such as sarcoid and rarities such as granulomatous polyangiitis. A lymphoid tumour or a metastasis is a typical mass lesion.

### Cavernous Sinus Thrombosis

This tends to follow paranasal sinus infection, with headache, fever and pain and total external ophthalmoplegia. Disc swelling follows, with optic neuropathy and/or retinal ischaemia. Meningitis or cerebral abscess can develop. Diabetes, malignancy and collagen vascular disease can predispose to cavernous sinus thrombosis.

### Caroticocavernous Fistulae

Caroticocavernous fistulae (CCF) are A-V shunts between the intracavernous carotid artery and cavernous sinus.

- Direct CCF: arterial supply comes from the internal carotid and
- Indirect (low flow) CCF: supply via carotid extradural, meningeal branches.

The commonest is a direct CCF following a TBI. Other causes are rupture of an intracav-ernous aneurysm, rarely vasculitis, Ehlers–Danlos or fibromuscular dysplasia. With a direct CCF there can be dramatic pulsatile proptosis, chemosis, arterialisation of conjunc-tival vessels and an orbital bruit. Ophthalmoplegia and visual loss follow. Indirect CCFs are typically non-traumatic, with milder features.

## Ocular Myopathies

Slowly progressive external ophthalmoplegia has many causes. See also Chapter 10.

- Mitochondrial disorders
- Congenital myopathies – e.g. central core, centronuclear, nemaline
- Oculopharyngeal muscular dystrophy
- Myotonic dystrophy, myasthenia gravis, LEMS, botulism
- Rarities: abetalipoproteinaemia, spinocerebellar ataxias.

## Palsies of III, IV and VI Nerves

### Oculomotor Nerve (III Nerve Palsy)

The commonest cause of an isolated, complete III nerve palsy is a posterior communicat-ing artery aneurysm. Diabetes is the commonest cause of a pupil-sparing III nerve palsy. Other causes are listed in Table 14.3.

**Table 14.3** III nerve palsy: causes.

| Location | Aetiology | Features |
|---|---|---|
| Nucleus | Infarction, haemorrhage<br>Trauma, tumour<br>Infection | Ipsilateral but weak contralateral superior rectus; ptosis: bilateral, or absent |
| Nerve fascicles | Infarction, haemorrhage<br>Trauma, tumour<br>MS, syphilis | Ataxia, tremor, hemiparesis, chorea |
| Subarachnoid space | Aneurysms (posterior communicating, ICA, basilar, posterior cerebral)<br>Ischaemia, trauma<br>Tumour, infection | Usually isolated, with pain |
| Tentorial edge | Raised intracranial pressure<br>Trauma | Uncal herniation |
| Cavernous sinus, superior orbital fissure | | IV, V, VI, VII, Horner's |
| Orbital | Trauma, tumour<br>Inflammatory<br>Infection<br>Dural AVM<br>Sphenoid sinus mucocoele | Optic neuropathy, chemosis, conjunctival injection, proptosis |

## Abducens (VI) and Trochlear (IV) Nerve Palsies

The VI nerve, with its lengthy course, can be damaged in many situations (Table 14.4). With a trochlear (IV) nerve palsy, a relative rarity, the commonest cause is trauma – but many conditions that cause a VI nerve palsy can also cause a IV nerve palsy.

**Table 14.4** Abducens (VI) nerve palsy.

| Location | Aetiology | Additional features |
|---|---|---|
| Nuclear | Möbius, Duane, infection, tumour, MS<br>Wernicke, trauma | Contralateral internuclear ophthalmoplegia |
| Nerve fascicles | Infection, MS, tumour<br>Inflammation, Wernicke | +/− Horner's |
| Subarachnoid | Aneurysm – ICA<br>SAH<br>Trauma, infection<br>Inflammatory<br>Tumour<br>Raised intracranial pressure | Contralateral hemiparesis |

*(Continued)*

**Table 14.4**   (Continued)

| Location | Aetiology | Additional features |
|---|---|---|
| Petrous apex | Infection, otitis media | VI, VII, deafness |
| | Gradenigo's | Facial pain |
| | Thrombosis – inferior petrous sinus, transverse/sigmoid sinus, trauma | |
| | Tumour | |
| Cavernous sinus and superior orbital fissure | ICA aneurysm/dissection | III, IV, $V_1$, Horner's |
| | Cavernous sinus thrombosis | |
| | Caroticocavernous fistula | |
| | Sphenoid mucocoele | |
| | Tolosa–Hunt, tumours | |
| Orbital | Tumour, inflammation, infection | Ophthalmoplegia, proptosis, chemosis |
| | Trauma | |

Multiple unilateral ocular motor palsies are caused typically by cavernous sinus and superior orbital fissure disease. Muscle diseases, myasthenia, Miller Fisher syndrome, infiltrative brainstem lesions, infection, vasculitis and cancer are other causes.

## Gaze and Central Eye Movements

We need to be able to shift gaze rapidly:

- to bring an object into foveal vision – via the saccadic system and
- to stabilise that new image – even if the object moves – with pursuit and vergence movements.

Vestibulo-ocular and optokinetic reflexes help deal with head and body movement.

### Saccades, Gaze Palsies and Oculogyric Crises

Assessment: Chapter 4. Horizontal gaze palsy – restriction of conjugate lateral movements usually implies either an ipsilateral pons or a contralateral frontal lesion. Vertical gaze palsy can be caused by many lesions from the cortex to the midbrain vertical gaze centre.

Oculogyric crises are episodes of fixed conjugate upwards, and occasionally lateral eye deviation, first described in *encephalitis lethargica*. They occur with metoclopramide, neuroleptics and with brainstem encephalitis, parkinsonian syndromes or as a paraneoplastic phenomenon. Obsessive thoughts and dystonic movements also occur.

### Internuclear Ophthalmoplegia (INO)

A typical INO is caused by a lesion of the medial longitudinal fasciculus (MLF) that connects the VI nucleus to the contralateral medial rectus (oculomotor) nucleus. There is incomplete and slow ADDuction of the eye ipsilateral to the MLF lesion, with ataxic nystagmus in the other eye.

When INO is bilateral, vertical nystagmus on upgaze is usual. INO occurs in MS, brainstem vascular disease, Wernicke's and as a rare paraneoplastic sign. Varieties of INO are also described.

### Skew Deviation, Ocular Tilt Reaction and Nystagmus

Skew means a vertical misalignment – one eye up, one eye down, either the same in all positions of gaze or varying or even alternating between left and right gaze. Skew deviations occur following damage to the vestibular nuclei, MLF and with cerebellar disorders. A head tilt may try to compensate. Nystagmus is dealt with in Chapter 4 and within Neuro-Otology (Chapter 15).

## Chiasmal and Retrochiasmal Visual Pathways

Features of chiasmal disease are mentioned in Chapter 4, and pituitary lesions in Chapter 21. Bitemporal hemianopia is the characteristic sign. There are several finer points in relation to the chiasm, rarely of major importance:

- Post- and pre-fixed chiasm
- Diplopia, difficulty with depth perception, post-fixation blindness
- Band or bow-tie atrophy of the optic disc.

### Homonymous Hemianopia

Homonymous hemianopia is caused by a unilateral lesion posterior to the optic chiasm – optic tract, lateral geniculate body (LGB), optic radiation and visual cortex. These field defects cause difficulty reading and scanning. Patients fail to notice obstacles on the affected side. Driving, shopping, shaving, applying make-up and food preparation are affected. Transient homonymous hemianopia occurs in migraine, TIAs and seizures. The commonest cause of a fixed homonymous hemianopia is vascular. A tumour, trauma and surgery are also causes.

### Visual Cortex and Visual Association Areas

Conditions mentioned below are dealt with elsewhere.

- Cortical blindness
- Anton–Babinski syndrome
- Blindsight
- Charles Bonnet syndrome – pseudo-hallucinations with impaired vision
- Visual hallucinations
- Balint's syndrome
- Visual agnosia, prosopagnosia, alexia and neglect.

Many other sensations are described, sometimes with partial visual loss. Among these are:

- oscillopsia – movement of the environment
- achromatopsia – poor colour recognition and the reverse hyperchromatopsia
- macropsia and micropsia – an object appears large or small
- polyopia – a single object seen as multiple.

**Functional (Non-Organic) Visual Disorders**

Functional disorders are discussed in Chapter 21. Of note:

- Functional visual loss is common. Typical field defects are concentric constriction or spiralling.
- Within ophthalmology there is a view that most functional disorders are within voluntary control – not in keeping with the current attitudes.
- Organically based visual disturbances follow migraine, minor head injuries and syncope. Though minor, they can cause disproportionate alarm.

## Pupil Abnormalities

Pupillary changes can indicate the presence of a disease. Afferent limbs are via the optic nerves to the Edinger–Westphal nuclei, where parasympathetic efferent outflow originates. Preganglionic fibres in the III nerves synapse in the ciliary ganglia. Post-ganglionic fibres reach the iris sphincter, via the short posterior ciliary nerves.

### Complete and Relative Afferent Pupillary Defect

With blindness in one eye following retina or optic nerve pathology, light shone into the blind eye produces no reaction in either pupil: a complete afferent defect. Light shone in the normal eye constricts both pupils. This is the situation in any complete optic nerve lesion. A preserved light reflex with unilateral blindness is often functional.

A relative afferent pupillary defect (RAPD, a.k.a. Marcus Gunn pupil) indicates typically asymmetrical optic nerve disease – identified by the swinging light test.

- When the torch is shone into the weaker eye, for example in a patient with MS-ON, with acuity down to 6/18, there is slight constriction of both pupils. The afferent defect reduces the amount of light reaching the Edinger–Westphal nucleus.
- When the torch is shone into the unaffected eye, there is some slightly greater constriction of both pupils.
- When the light is swung *back*, into the weaker eye, its pupil will dilate. This dilatation is the hallmark of a relative afferent pupillary defect.

### *Argyll Robertson Pupil and Parinaud's*

An Argyll Robertson pupil, the venerable sign of neurosyphilis, is now rare. The pupil, typically small and irregular, does not react to light but does so to accommodation, a.k.a. light-near dissociation. There is damage ventral to the aqueduct. Occasionally also seen in diabetes, MS or myotonic dystrophy.

Parinaud's dorsal midbrain syndrome describes five signs:

- Dilated (or mid-dilated) pupils that do not react to light but do so to accommodation.
- Voluntary up-gaze paralysis.

- Convergence-retraction nystagmus on attempted up-gaze.
- Eyelid retraction, a.k.a. Collier's sign.
- Convergence paralysis.

Parinaud's is a sign of a pineal gland tumour. MS, angioma and stroke are less-common causes.

## Efferent Light Reflex Defects

These can be divided into pre- and post-ganglionic parasympathetic lesions. In acute preganglionic block, there is a large unreactive pupil, with light and accommodation reflexes absent. A preganglionic lesion can be associated with a compressive III nerve lesion, such as a posterior communicating artery aneurysm. Mydriatic eye drops can also cause a dilated pupil.

### Holmes–Adie Syndrome

HAS has two features: an abnormal, dilated pupil and tendon areflexia. The pupil shows little or no reaction to light, but some sectors of its margin constrict causing the pupil to be misshapen. The pupil has an exaggerated near response, but this constriction is slow, a.k.a. tonic. Deep tendon reflexes, especially knee jerks, become absent – unassociated with symptoms. HAS is more common in females and tends to develop in one pupil initially. Once present, it persists. A few develop sweating abnormalities, a.k.a. Ross's syndrome. HAS is often noticed by chance. It is due to damage to the ciliary ganglion and/or dorsal root ganglia of unknown cause. Such pupils can occur in dysautonomias and neuropathies.

### Horner's – A Pupillary Sympathetic Defect

Horner's is caused by dysfunction of the sympathetic supply to the iris. There can be damage anywhere along the sympathetic pathway:

- central lesions – first order
- preganglionic – second order, and
- post-ganglionic – third order.

Horner's is important: many of its causes require attention.
Cardinal signs are:

- miosis – constricted pupil
- ptosis – loss of sympathetic tone in Müller's muscle
- conjunctival injection and facial anhidrosis.

Other features: slight lower lid elevation, a.k.a. upside-down ptosis – a narrow palpebral fissure with apparent enophthalmos.

Causes are listed in Table 14.5. Horner's itself is so characteristic that pharmacological tests are rarely needed.

Traumatic birth injury can cause a congenital Horner's, with a Klumpke upper limb paralysis. Heterochromia iridis may develop. Bilateral Horner's occur in autonomic neuropathies. Raeder's syndrome comprises Horner's and facial pain, often with trigeminal and oculomotor nerve lesions. Cluster headaches cause a transient Horner's.

**Table 14.5** Causes of unilateral Horner's.

| Type | Anatomy | Typical pathologies |
| --- | --- | --- |
| First-order neurone | Brainstem, cervical cord | MS, tumour, Wallenberg's, syrinx |
| Second-order neurone | T1, superior cervical ganglion | Cord lesion, trauma, cervical rib |
| | | Arterial dissection/aneurysm |
| | | Central venous catheterisation |
| | | Abscess, infection, lymphadenopathy |
| | | Lung apex: TB, cancer |
| Third-order neurone | ICA, skull base, cavernous sinus, superior orbital fissure, orbit | Aneurysm/ICA dissection |
| | | Cavernous sinus thrombosis, fistula |
| | | Skull base tumour, Raeder's |
| | | Arnold–Chiari |
| | | Infection, meningioma, trauma |
| | | Nasopharyngeal carcinoma |
| | | Orbit – trauma, tumour, granuloma, infection |
| | | Neuroblastoma (in children), HZV |

# Acknowledgements

I am most grateful to James Acheson, Fion Bremner, Elizabeth Graham, Robin Howard, Alexander Leff, Gordon Plant, Simon Shorvon and Ahmed Toosy for their contributions of text and retinal photographs in Neurology A Queen Square Textbook Second Edition upon which this chapter is based.

The late Professor MJ Turlough Fitzgerald, Emeritus Professor of Anatomy, National University of Ireland, Galway most generously provided all the neuroanatomy illustrations for *Neurology A Queen Square Textbook* Second & First Editions from his book *Clinical Neuroanatomy and Neuroscience*.

# Further Reading and Information

Acheson J, Bremner F, Graham E, Howard R, Leff A, Plant G, *et al.* Neuro-ophthalmology. In *Neurology: A Queen Square Textbook*, 2nd edn. Clarke C, Howard R, Rossor M, Shorvon S, eds. Chichester: John Wiley & Sons, 2016. There are numerous references.

Free updated notes, potential links and references as these become available:
https://www.drcharlesclarke.com
You will be asked to log in, in a secure fashion, with your name and institution.

# 15

# Neuro-Otology: Disorders of Balance and Hearing

## Essential Anatomy

The vestibular sense organs and labyrinth are outlined in Figure 15.1, and their brainstem connections in Figure 15.2.

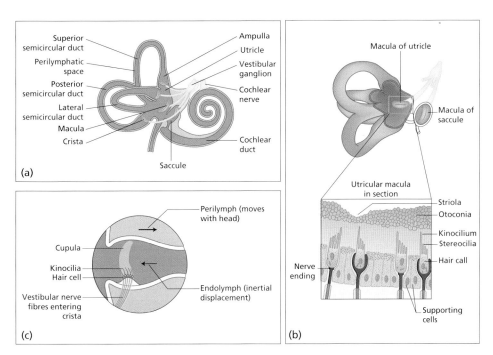

**Figure 15.1** Vestibular apparatus: (a) Five vestibular sense organs. (b) Cells of static labyrinth. (c) Cupula and kinocilia hair cells.

*Neurology: A Clinical Handbook*, First Edition. Charles Clarke.
© 2022 John Wiley & Sons Ltd. Published 2022 by John Wiley & Sons Ltd.

## Afferents and Efferents

Information comes from three systems:

- vestibular labyrinths
- vision
- joint and muscle position sense.

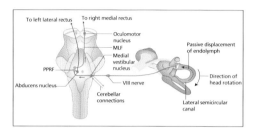

**Figure 15.2** Semicircular canals and brainstem: head rotation and conjugate lateral gaze. MLF: medial longitudinal fasciculus. PPRF, parapontine reticular formation.

This afferent data converges on the vestibular nuclei, with input from the reticular formation, cortex, cerebellum and basal ganglia. Efferents from vestibular nuclei project to oculomotor nuclei, neck, trunk, limbs and cortex.

The vestibular system has three functions:

- Perception of orientation, motion and acceleration/deceleration
- Control of posture when static or moving
- Gaze stabilisation during movement.

The three sets of semicircular canals are aligned such that when one labyrinth is either excited or damaged, both eyes move conjugately in response. For example, the horizontal semicircular canals gauge head rotational acceleration: they drive the eye muscles of that plane – lateral and medial recti. There is compensation for head movement and gaze stabilisation – a vestibulo-ocular reflex. Planes of movement:

- Yaw: head rotation
- Pitch: head flexion/extension, and
- Roll: lateral head tilt.

Maculae, located in the utricle and cristae in each ampulla, contain sensory hair cells with projecting kinocilia. Linear acceleration and gravitational forces are transduced by the otolith organs of the utricle and saccule. Angular acceleration is transduced by the cristae. Normally visual, proprioceptive and vestibular inputs are matched.

Vertigo occurs when a mismatch between sensory information and reality leads to the illusion of movement. Vestibular symptoms occur either in response to movement of the environment, such as with motion sickness, or from pathology within the stabilising systems, such as in benign paroxysmal positional vertigo (BPPV), with impaired proprioception, or anxiety. Severe vertigo is highly unpleasant: the accompanying nausea, vomiting and malaise are mediated via vestibulo-autonomic pathways.

## Dizziness and Vertigo Assessment

Dizziness encompasses many unpleasant feelings: lightheadedness, imbalance and/or vertigo. Vertigo is the illusion of movement of the body or surroundings – rotating, tilting or rocking to and fro. Nystagmus is involuntary oscillatory movement in one or both eyes and has either a peripheral or central origin. Eye movement, gait and balance examination: Chapters 4 and 13. The history is all important, and basic outpatient tests are also useful.

In the Doll's head eye manoeuvre, the patient sits in front of the examiner and fixates on their face. You turn the patient's head from side to side. In the complete absence of a vestibulo-ocular reflex, eye movements will be jerky, interrupted by catch-up saccades towards the fixation target.

In the Head Impulse test (Halmagyi and Curthoys), the examiner turns the patient's head briskly in steps. A fast right head turn will make a patient with a right-sided vestibular loss introduce visible catch-up saccades towards the target, *i.e.* towards the left, in order to re-fixate. The test helps confirm an acute, unilateral and peripheral lesion. Canal paresis of >75% produces a positive result, but with a less severe unilateral lesion, it is often inconclusive.

The Dix–Hallpike and roll manoeuvres can help distinguish peripheral nystagmus, for example of BPPV from a central nystagmus.

- Seat the patient on a couch so that when moved laterally, their head can extend over the end of the couch.
- Warn about dizziness/vertigo, remove their spectacles and ask the patient to maintain gaze on your forehead.
- Hold their head firmly and turn it 30–45° to their left and move the patient rapidly into the lying position to the right, their head hanging over the end of the couch. The posterior semicircular canal of the lower ear is thus moved through its plane of orientation. Look for nystagmus.
- Repeat for the other side.

The simpler supine roll is carried out by laying the patient on the couch and rolling the head from side to side.

In BPPV, vertigo and nystagmus develop after a latent interval and then fatigue. With central positional nystagmus, typically there is no latency, little vertigo and no fatiguing – occasionally, this is the only sign of central pathology.

## Nystagmus Varieties

### Jerk, Normal, Deliberate and Pendular Nystagmus

Jerk nystagmus consists of a slow drift and a corrective fast jerk saccade. The fast component defines its direction. Amplitude is usually increased on gaze in the direction of the fast component (Alexander's law). Nystagmus is also defined by its trajectory – horizontal, torsional/rotary, vertical/upbeat, downbeat or mixed. Jerk nystagmus can be caused by either peripheral or central abnormalities. Peripheral disorders such as BPPV cause a unidirectional jerk nystagmus with the fast phase directed away from the affected side. Amplitude increases as the eyes are turned in the direction of the fast phase. Nystagmus is reduced by visual fixation and intensified by loss of fixation – darkness or Frenzel goggles. Associated features may include tinnitus, vertigo, hearing loss and falling, towards the lesion.

Normal endpoint nystagmus occurs on extreme lateral gaze. Optokinetic nystagmus (OKN) is induced by visual stimuli such as a rotating drum or when gazing from a moving vehicle. OKN is retained with non-organic visual loss. Some people can produce horizontal, vertical or rotary eye movements deliberately. Eyelid twitches can occur with nystagmus. Rarely, lid nystagmus occurs with MS. Some lid flutter can occur in Parkinson's.

Pendular nystagmus is typically congenital with similar velocity in each phase. Movements are usually vertical, with a torsional component in the primary position and constant with gaze direction. Movements may differ between each eye. Acquired pendular nystgamus causes oscillopsia, seen occasionally in MS, following a brainstem stroke or encephalitis. Forms of pendular nystagmus include *spasmus nutans*, oculopalatal myoclonus, see-saw nystagmus and oculomasticatory myorhythmia (Whipple's disease). Ocular movements in coma: Chapter 20.

### Gaze-Evoked, Gaze-Paretic Jerk and Caloric Nystagmus

Gaze-evoked nystagmus is induced by holding gaze off-centre – the eyes drift back into the primary position, followed by a corrective saccadic movement. If paresis of gaze is present, either because of a peripheral or central lesion, the nystagmus is termed gaze-paretic. Similar fatigue nystagmus can occur in myasthenia. Gaze-evoked nystagmus is also caused by alcohol, anti-epileptics, sedatives and by a cerebellar or brainstem lesion. Caloric nystagmus: cold/warm water in the external auditory meatus causes a jerk nystagmus (see Caloric testing).

Alexander's law:

- First-degree nystagmus: visible on gaze deviation in the direction of the fast phase
- Second-degree nystagmus: present in primary gaze as well as the direction of the fast phase
- Third-degree nystagmus: also visible when the eyes are deviated in the opposite direction.

## Nystagmus with Central Lesions

### Torsional Central Nystagmus and Central Vestibular Horizontal Nystagmus

Torsional central nystagmus beats away from a unilateral brainstem lesion. There is generally skew deviation (Chapter 14) and oscillopsia. Central vestibular horizontal nystagmus is a low-amplitude nystagmus, with fast phase towards the side of the lesion. Such nystagmus can follow brainstem infarction, MS, a tumour or encephalitis. Vestibular nuclei and cerebellar flocculus lesions cause many forms of nystagmus.

### Downbeat, Upbeat, See-Saw Nystagmus and Oculopalatal Tremor

Downbeat jerk nystagmus causes oscillopsia and gait imbalance and is associated with a cervicomedullary junction lesion, spinocerebellar degeneration, anti-epileptics, lithium and alcohol. Upbeat nystagmus has a slow downward drift and a fast upward phase; this occurs in cerebellar degeneration, brainstem and cerebellar stroke, MS, with drugs and Wernicke's encephalopathy. See-saw is a rarity with alternating elevation and intorsion of one eye while the opposite eye falls and extorts – seen typically with bitemporal hemianopia from a large suprasellar mass such as a craniopharyngioma.

Oculopalatal tremor, another rarity, is a slow vertical regular pendular movement, synchronous with the palatal movement can follow brainstem infarction or cerebellar degeneration.

### Oculomasticatory Myorhythmia, Alternating and Convergence-Retraction Nystagmus

Oculomasticatory myorhythmia is a rarity associated with Whipple's disease – a continuous slow rhythmic convergent–divergent nystagmus, with synchronous contractions of the jaw, face and palate. Periodic alternating nystagmus is also rare: nystagmus occurs in one direction for a minute or two, stops and then beats in the opposite direction – seen with Arnold–Chiari malformation, cerebellar degeneration, MS and a brainstem tumour.

Convergence-retraction nystagmus in Parinaud's syndrome is rapid convergence of both eyes that retract into the orbits. There is co-contraction of the horizontal recti on attempted convergence and upgaze, pupillary light-near dissociation and bilateral lid retraction. Typical cause: a pineal tumour.

### Nystagmus in Childhood

Latent nystagmus is a congenital jerk nystagmus that appears when one eye is covered. Congenital nystagmus – generally horizontal and either pendular or mixed. Nystagmus block syndrome is a horizontal congenital nystagmus, minimal in ADDuction and marked in ABDuction. Pendular nystagmus from visual loss: vertical pendular nystagmus such as with an optic nerve glioma. *Spasmus nutans*, another rarity – nystagmus with head nodding – usually resolves by 3 years.

### General Medical Problems

Dizziness and even vertigo can be caused by general medical problems:

- Orthostatic hypotension (sustained BP fall >20 mmHg on standing)
- Vasovagal episodes, low output, e.g. aortic stenosis, dysrhythmia
- Breathlessness, hyperventilation, anxiety
- Hypoglycaemia, anaemia, acute infections, chronic fatigue.

## Vestibular Investigations

Specialist tests consist of eye movement recordings, postural and rotational change measurements, evoked potentials and caloric response assessments.

## Caloric Testing

The Hallpike–Fitzgerald bithermal caloric test demonstrates a peripheral vestibular deficit. With the head at 30° to the horizontal, the horizontal semicircular canals are in the vertical plane. Following irrigation of the external ear with water at 7 °C below body temperature, and then at 7 °C above it, a gradient is set up between the external ear and the two limbs of the horizontal canal. With warmth, there is ampullopetal flow, with cupular deflection towards the utricle, causing activation of the vestibulo-ocular-reflex, vertigo and horizontal nystagmus towards the stimulated ear. The endpoint of the nystagmus is recorded.

Normally, nystagmus ceases 90–140 seconds after irrigation. There are two abnormal patterns.

- Directional preponderance: thermal irrigation produces an excess of nystagmus in one direction. This indicates imbalance of vestibular tone from either a peripheral vestibular lesion (labyrinth, VIII nerve or nuclei) or a central lesion.
- Total canal paresis: absence of nystagmus following both 30° and 44° irrigations.

The duration of nystagmus can be entered into the 'Jongkees Formula' to estimate the degree of paresis. Bilateral decreased responses indicate either bilateral vestibular damage or the habituation seen in acrobats, ice skaters and ballet dancers.

Whilst calorics are valuable, test results do not correlate with the degree of dizziness. Also, if a patient has some directional preponderance or canal paresis, this can simply reflect a past problem. A unilateral decreased response cannot take into account any distant previous vestibular damage that has recovered clinically and may have passed unnoticed. Caloric testing in the symptomless population can show surprising abnormalities and sometimes marked asymmetry. Results must always be correlated with the clinical picture – such matters can be of relevance in legal claims.

## Vestibular Disorders

### Benign Paroxysmal Positional Vertigo

BPPV is common: by the age of 70, about a quarter of the population have experienced BPPV, from accumulation of otolith debris. A bolus of crystals heavier than the surrounding endolymph gravitates to the most dependent part of the canal (Figure 15.3). Acting like a plunger, the bolus exerts an ampullofugal pull on the cupula, triggering vertigo. Most cases (F:M 2:1) arise without any obvious cause. Following trauma, it is hard to know whether such a common condition would have occurred anyway, but it is sometimes accepted that BPPV can follow minor trauma.

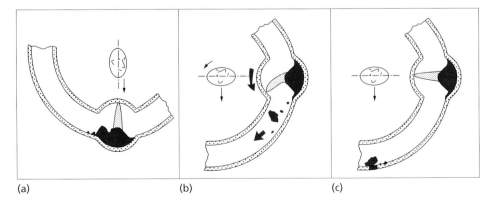

(a)  (b)  (c)

**Figure 15.3**  Canalolithiasis. Diagram of a clump of otoconial debris in the posterior semicircular canal (a). With head movement (b) in the plane of the canal, the debris acts like a plunger (c) on the cupula and endolymph.

BPPV is a distinct, dramatic condition, not to be confused with feeling mildly off-balance. Distress, as with any vertigo, is disproportionate to its seriousness. BPPV is easy to diagnose, helped greatly by positional manoeuvres and tends to resolve spontaneously within days or weeks. In some, vertigo can be recurrent.

**Posterior Semicircular Canal BPPV and Others**
This (p-BPPV) is the commonest. There is sudden vertigo with nystagmus lasting less than a minute, triggered by a head movement, such as rising from bed. Criteria for p-BPPV:

- Latency: vertigo and nystagmus commence after a change in posture within 20 seconds
- Nystagmus gradually reduces after 10–40 seconds and disappears
- Rotary-vertical nystagmus
- Reversal: on returning to the upright position, vertigo and nystagmus may return in the opposite direction
- Fatiguability: on repeating a manoeuvre, both vertigo and nystagmus lessen.

Horizontal canal, apogeotropic horizontal canal and anterior canal BPPV are rarer.

## Vestibular Neuritis

This is a common cause of an acute, persistent vertigo, a.k.a. vestibular neuronitis, vestibular neuro-labyrinthitis, acute vestibulopathy and labyrinthitis – a sudden unilateral vestibular paresis, usually of unknown cause. There is:

- Acute rotary vertigo
- Blurred vision/oscillopsia
- Postural imbalance
- Nausea and vomiting.

Pointers to a virus are:

- Preceding URTIs
- Autopsy: degeneration of vestibular nerve trunks and latent HSV1 in vestibular ganglia.

Similar vertigo can be caused by MS – a plaque in the VIII nerve root entry zone – and posterior circulation vascular disease, if rarely.

Onset is sudden and distressing. Throughout the first several days the patient feels intensely unwell. All head movement exacerbates symptoms. By 6 weeks, most have recovered. No investigation is usually needed. With acute severe isolated persistent vertigo, whilst the likelihood is VN, posterior circulation infarction should be considered, though other features are usually present (Chapter 6).

## Vestibular Migraine

Many migraine patients describe dizziness and occasionally vertigo prior to a headache. Basilar migraine cases can have distinct auras of dysarthria, vertigo, tinnitus and hyperacusis (Chapter 12). Vestibular migraine criteria are outlined in Table 15.1.

Benign recurrent vertigo describes sudden intense vertigo, postural imbalance +/− nausea and spontaneous/positional nystagmus, but without headache, sometimes regarded as a migraine equivalent.

**Table 15.1** Vestibular migraine criteria (International Headache & Bárány Societies, 2012).

Migraine, with >5 episodes of moderate/severe vestibular symptoms for 5 minutes – 72 hours:
- Rotational and/or positional vertigo
- Illusory self or object motion and/or head motion intolerance

One or more migraine features with >50% of vestibular episodes:
- Headache with >2 characteristics: one-sided, pulsating, moderate/severe pain, aggravation by physical activity
- Photophobia and phonophobia and/or visual aura
- Not better accounted for by another vestibular or headache diagnosis.

### Motion Sickness

This common problem is caused by vestibular stimulation from pitch, roll and yaw. Motion sickness occurs at sea and in cars – and with less usual conveyances such as horse-drawn carriages, camels and elephants. Motion sickness is now rare during commercial flights but a problem during space travel – and one reason why airships did not flourish.

At sea, nausea, sweating, dizziness, vertigo and profuse vomiting develop over several hours or less, with an irresistible desire to return to *terra firma*. Intense malaise should not be underestimated. Early symptoms are helped by visual contact with the horizon, eating, avoiding a stuffy cabin and engine fumes. Alcohol makes matters worse. The motion of a small vessel is less dramatic close to its centre of gravity, and many prefer to 'go below' despite losing contact with the horizon.

### Ménière's Disease

In Ménière's, a.k.a. *endolymphatic hydrops*, there are prolonged attacks of vertigo and progressive hearing loss, tinnitus and aural fullness. The mechanism is failure of endolymph resorption, of unknown cause: over-accumulation causes distortion of the membranous labyrinth.

Attacks of vertigo tend to be severe with vomiting and can prostrate the patient. Drop attacks (Tumarkin's crises) can occur and occasionally syncope. With the inevitable progression canal paresis develops and typically hearing loss. Bilateral disease is common.

Hydrops starts in the helicotrema. This leads to ruptures of Reissner's membrane that separates the perilymph from the endolymph, which accounts for the aural fullness. Temporary paresis of the VIII nerve fibres occurs. There is also initial neural excitation, causing vertigo and an irritative nystagmus. Later, there is blockade of action potentials leading to destructive nystgamus. Permanent changes develop within the membranous labyrinth, with loss of cochlear and vestibular neurones.

### Bilateral Vestibular Failure

BVF is a rare cause of disabling unsteadiness. Some cases have an underlying disease, such as a progressive cerebellar syndrome. Gentamicin ototoxicity, vasculitis and malignant meningitis are also the causes. BVF can follow bacterial meningitis. Symptoms depend on whether BVF is sudden, sequential or long-standing. With acute total bilateral BVF, there is sudden unsteadiness, oscillopsia and vertigo. BVF present from infancy, such as following meningitis, is surprisingly well tolerated.

### Vestibular Paroxysmia and Episodic Ataxia

Existence of this rarity is supported by its response to carbamazepine. There are:

- Intense attacks of rotational or to-and-fro vertigo lasting seconds to minutes
- Attacks frequently provoked by a particular head position
- Impaired hearing during an attack, or permanently.

  VP is attributed to neurovascular compression, like trigeminal neuralgia.
  Episodic ataxia type 2 (Chapter 17) – another rarity – can present with vertigo and ataxia.

### Chronic and Persistent Postural-Perceptual Dizziness (PPPD)

Most cases of long-standing dizziness have a history of vestibular symptoms, poor central vestibular compensation and/or psychological complaints. Examination is usually normal. Vestibular investigation may unearth abnormalities. PPPD describes this – a label used increasingly as an explanation for disability.

## Management: Drugs and Physical Manoeuvres

Acute unilateral vestibular dysfunction causes alarming vertigo, nausea, vomiting, sweating, pallor and even diarrhoea. Simple reassurance helps and keeping still. Vestibular sedatives can help acutely but should be used sparingly because they interfere with vestibular compensation. Anticholinergics (hyoscine), antihistamines (promethazine, prochlorperazine, cyclizine and metoclopramide) and calcium-channel antagonists (cinnarizine and flunarizine) are used. For seasickness, prophylactic cinnarizine, hyoscine, cyclizine and stem ginger are of value. Habituation usually takes place over several days, but some remain prone to seasickness. Benzodiazepines help with anxiety.

The widely available Cawthorne–Cooksey exercises stimulate visual, vestibular and proprioceptive input to enhance compensation. Simple advice often helps:

- Explanation – enhancement of natural compensation, anxiety management.
- Emphasis upon movements that actually provoke dizziness, with brief frequent repetition.

### Particle Repositioning Procedures and CBT

BPPV is the most common vestibular disorder. The Epley particle-repositioning and Semont liberatory manoeuvres are usually carried in specialist clinics. Both are highly effective. Less formal manoeuvres, such as sudden passive head movements, also help – easily and safely carried out anywhere. Vestibular symptoms can cause agoraphobia, anxiety, panic, depression and/or avoidance behaviour. CBT can be helpful.

## Ménière's, Central Vestibular Dysfunction and Migraine

For Ménière's, treatment is either symptomatic, e.g. betahistine and/or aimed at influencing the presumed underlying *endolymphatic hydrops*. Recommendations include lifestyle adaptations, a low-salt diet, bendroflumethiazide, chlorthalidone and acetazolamide. Intra-tympanic gentamicin has become a treatment for intractable vertigo, when hearing is preserved. Hyperbaric oxygen has been said to help and the Meniett device delivers micropressure waves to the inner ear. Surgical management includes endolymphatic sac decompression and destructive procedures.

Central dysfunction with neurological disease is difficult to help. Clonazepam, 3,4-diaminopyridine, gabapentin and baclofen can be tried and intensive vestibular rehabilitation. The management of migrainous vertigo is that of migraine (Chapter 12).

## Hearing Disorders

In the over 50s, about one-third have some loss of hearing, with socioeconomic and psychological consequences. Tinnitus is sound perception from within the body rather than the external world. Hyperacusis is reduced tolerance to noise. Hearing loss is either conductive, following middle ear tympanic membrane disorders, or sensorineural.

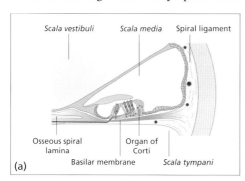

(a)

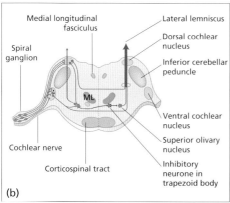

(b)

**Figure 15.4** (a) Cochlea (in section). (b) Cochlear nerve, ventral cochlear nucleus (midbrain – cross-section). ML: medial lemniscus.

### Auditory Anatomy and Investigation

The external and middle ear collect and amplify sound. Inner hair cells of the organ of Corti transduce mechanical into electrical activity. Outer cochlear hair cells act as modulators and amplifiers. Signals are transmitted along the afferent auditory pathway (VIII nerve→ipsilateral cochlear nucleus→contralateral superior olivary complex→lateral lemniscus→inferior colliculus→medial geniculate body →auditory cortex) See Figure 15.4.

Basic examination is dealt with in Chapter 4. Hearing loss is assessed in specialist clinics.

Auditory tests:

- Quantify audiometric thresholds at each frequency
- Differentiate between conductive and sensorineural hearing loss
- Differentiate between cochlear and retro-cochlear abnormalities
- Identify central auditory dysfunction and non-organic impairment.

## Conductive Loss: Middle Ear and Tympanic Membrane

Disorders include acute, serous and chronic otitis media. Other causes are:

- Cholesteatoma – an epithelial cell collection – e.g. following chronic middle ear infection. A cholesteatoma may erode bone.
- Otosclerosis, an AD disorder, apparent in early adulthood (*TGBF1* gene). Bone deposition leads to fixation of the stapes footplate with conductive hearing loss. Sclerosis can extend to the otic capsule to cause sensorineural loss.
- Glomus tumours are rare jugulotympanic paragangliomas that expand within the petrous temporal bone and into the labyrinth: pulsatile tinnitus and a vascular mass behind the tympanum are typical.

## Age Related and Genetic Hearing Loss

Progressive age-related deterioration of auditory sensitivity (presbyacusis) is the leading cause of adult hearing impairment. Specific genes predispose to environmental triggers to cause degenerative changes. Remarkably, the pathophysiology of presbyacusis remains poorly defined.

In childhood genetic forms, AR hearing loss accounts for nearly half of childhood hearing loss cases – a profound congenital impairment. Some children have a rare AR auditory neuropathy related to mutations of the otoferlin gene or *12S rRNA*.

## Environmental, Trauma, Drug Related and Syndromic Hearing Loss

### Acoustic Trauma
- Noise-induced trauma is a preventable cause of sensorineural hearing loss – occupational and/or recreational exposure.
- Acute barotrauma – diving, depressurisation and explosions cause tympanic membrane haemorrhage, rupture, conductive hearing loss and/or perilymph fistula.
- Head injury can cause middle ear, inner ear, VIII nerve and/or central auditory loss. Labyrinthine concussion and fractures of the petrous temporal bone cause sensorineural and/or conductive hearing loss.

### Drugs
Many are ototoxic – chloroquine, aminoglycosides and salicylates. Platinum-based chemotherapy damages the inner ear hair cells. Vincristine produces cochlear nerve damage. Streptomycin causes damage to cochlear receptors.

### Metabolic Disease and Autoimmune Disorders
- Diabetes mellitus: auditory and/or vestibular abnormalities – neuropathy and/or angiopathy.
- Renal failure is associated with hearing loss. Ototoxicity from disease, drugs and axonal uraemic neuropathy is implicated.
- Autoimmune inner ear disease (AIED) causes progressive typically bilateral hearing loss without other systemic abnormalities caused by presumed autoimmune attack on inner ear proteins. Steroids and immunosuppression help.

- Cogan's syndrome is a rare, presumed autoimmune disorder, affecting the eye and ear in children and young adults following a URTI with rapid progression to total deafness. Lymphadenopathy, night sweats, aortic valve disease, pleuro-pericarditis and myocardial infarction can occur.
- Vogt–Koyanagi–Harada syndrome (VKH) is a rare disorder of melanocyte-containing organs: bilateral uveitis with cutaneous lesions (vitiligo, alopecia and poliosis), CSF pleocytosis and hearing loss.
- Behçet's commonly presents with orogenital ulceration, arthritis and headache. One-third have high-frequency cochlear hearing loss and vestibular involvement.
- Susac's syndrome is a rare micro-angiopathy – encephalopathy, retinopathy and hearing loss – assumed to have an autoimmune basis (Chapter 26), mainly in young women. Low-frequency, unilateral or bilateral sensorineural hearing loss is often the presenting feature, with tinnitus and vestibular disturbance. Encephalopathy causes cognitive impairment.
- Other autoimmune conditions: SLE, rheumatoid, ulcerative colitis, scleroderma, polyarteritis nodosa, Sjögren's, giant cell arteritis and GPA.

### Retro-Cochlear Hearing Disorders

Retro-cochlear hearing loss accounts for some genetic and acquired cases:

- Charcot–Marie–Tooth disease and HNPP (Chapter 10)
- Neurofibromatosis type 2
- Friedreich's ataxia (Chapter 17): hearing impairment is an unusual feature
- Refsum's: (Chapter 19) defective phytanic acid oxidation – *retinitis pigmentosa*, polyneuropathy, anosmia and hearing loss
- Mitochondrial disorders: sensorineural hearing loss occurs in Kearns–Sayre syndrome, MELAS and MERRF (Chapter 10)
- Muscle disorders: facioscapulohumeral dystrophy and myotonic dystrophy.

### Infections

Viruses: sudden sensorineural hearing loss in adults is often presumed to be viral. The Ramsay-Hunt syndrome is characterised by facial palsy, hearing loss and herpetic vesicles around the pinna and external auditory meatus. Sensorineural hearing loss occurs in over half – the result of cochlear or retro-cochlear involvement.

HIV/AIDS and syphilis: in HIV, auditory abnormalities range from conductive to sensorineural hearing loss, with mild audiometric changes, to abnormalities in central auditory dysfunction. In otosyphilis, a rarity, there can be sudden sensorineural hearing loss and/or a Ménière's-like condition.

Bacterial meningitis: sensorineural hearing loss in children and adults with pyogenic or TB meningitis is common. A fever with sudden loss of hearing is meningitis until proved otherwise. Once hearing loss is established, it is usually irreversible. Lyme disease can cause sensorineural hearing loss.

### Extrinsic and Intrinsic Tumours

CPA tumours, cerebellar medulloblastoma, vestibular schwannoma, meningioma, cholesteatoma, ependymoma, *glomus jugulare* tumour, metastasis, malignant meningitis and paraneoplastic syndromes can present with retro-cochlear hearing loss.

Vestibular schwannomas account more than 75% of CPA lesions. Most are unilateral, arising from the vestibular portion of the VIII nerve. Common presenting features are deafness and tinnitus. In all with unilateral sensorineural hearing impairment, asymmetric bilateral sensorineural loss or unilateral tinnitus, it is essential to exclude a vestibular schwannoma by detailed imaging.

### MS, Sarcoid and Superficial Siderosis

About 10% of MS cases have some hearing loss. Plaques develop in the VIII nerve root entry zone, cochlear nucleus and in the pons. In sarcoidosis, bilateral deafness can occur (Chapter 26). Deafness is usually of VIII nerve origin. Granulomas can also cause necrosis of the incus and encase the *chorda tympani*. In the rare superficial siderosis (Chapter 17), symptoms include sensorineural deafness, cerebellar ataxia and pyramidal signs, dementia, anosmia and anisocoria.

### Vascular Disease

Stroke, both haemorrhagic and ischaemic, can cause hearing disorders at many levels. Brainstem cavernomas can cause deafness. Aneurysm of the anterior inferior cerebellar artery can occasionally mimic a vestibular schwannoma. Sudden deafness can occur following inferior collicular, inferior pontine and lateral pontine infarction, vertebral artery dissection, anterior inferior cerebellar artery occlusion and, rarely, migraine.

### Temporal Lobe Disease

Cortical hearing loss is rare but is typically caused by vascular disease or trauma affecting both temporal lobes. The primary auditory cortex lies in the anterior–posterior transverse temporal gyrus of Heschl. Each ear has bilateral representation. In true cortical deafness, a patient can have no subjective experience of hearing and demonstrates profound hearing loss on pure-tone audiometry. This can be misdiagnosed as peripheral if detailed tests are not conducted, but there is usually other evidence of brain damage.

### Auditory Agnosia and Corpus Callosum Surgery

Auditory agnosia is a rare selective disorder of sound recognition that typically follows a stroke: 'I can hear you talking, but I cannot understand it'. The agnosia is subdivided into those unable to recognise one type of sound, such as speech, music and a dog barking, and those who cannot discriminate at all between verbal and non-verbal sounds. Verbal auditory agnosia, a.k.a. word deafness, describes severely impaired speech perception but intact recognition of non-verbal material such as music.

Another rarity can follow surgical section of the posterior corpus callosum. This produces a pattern termed Auditory Disconnection Profile. These cases tend to have normal performance on some monaural speech tests but some bilateral hearing loss.

### Auditory Processing Disorder (APD)

An APD case has a normal audiogram but difficulty with background noise, often excessive, and may have degraded or rapid speech. In an adult a structural (organic) cause is rarely found. In children, APD can accompany language, learning and behavioural difficulties.

## Hearing Loss: Management

This includes:

- Prevention: protection from noise hazards; avoidance of ototoxic drugs
- Treatment of systemic conditions
- Auditory rehabilitation, hearing aids and implants.

### Conductive Hearing Loss

Any obstruction within the external and middle ear by a foreign body, wax, polyp, tumour or infection must be corrected. Residual hearing loss, otosclerosis, hereditary osseous dysplasias and some congenital malformations are managed using hearing aids and/or surgically.

### Sudden and Chronic Progressive Sensorineural Hearing Loss

In many, no firm diagnosis is made. In sudden hearing loss, there is no evidence-based treatment: partial spontaneous recovery is usual. Therapies include inhalation of $CO_2$–oxygen mixtures, hyperbaric oxygen, antivirals, immunosuppression, calcium-channel blockers and steroids.

With progressive impairment, management obviously depends on the aetiology. Chronic sensorineural impairment is managed by treatment of any relevant medical condition, rehabilitation of residual hearing and environmental modifications. Hearing aid selection is the key element for many. Implantable devices have revolutionised auditory rehabilitation. Various implants are helpful in profound hearing impairment.

### Auditory Training and Strategies

Auditory training modifies cortical neural representation. Computer-based programmes include:

- Earobics (www.earobics.com)
- FastForWord (www.scilearn.com)
- Phonomena (www.mindweavers.co.uk)
- Brain Fitness for older adults (www.positscience.com).

## Acknowledgements

I am most grateful to Rosalyn Davies, Linda M. Luxon, Doris-Eva Bamiou and Adolfo Bronstein for their contribution to *Neurology A Queen Square Textbook* Second Edition on which this chapter is based.

Neuroanatomy Figures: the late Professor MJ Turlough Fitzgerald, Emeritus Professor of Anatomy, National University of Ireland, Galway most generously provided illustrations for *Neurology A Queen Square Textbook* 2nd & 1st editions from his own *Clinical Neuroanatomy and Neuroscience*.

Figure 15.3 is from Brandt T, Steddin S, Daroff RB. Therapy for benign paroxysmal positioning vertigo (BPPV). *J Vestib Res* 1993; 3: 373–382.

## Further Reading and Information

Brandt T, Steddin S, Daroff RB. Therapy for benign paroxysmal positioning vertigo (BPPV). *J Vestib Res* 1993; 3: 373–382.

Davies R, Luxon LM, Bamiou D-E & Bronstein A. *Neuro-otology*: problems of dizziness, balance & hearing. In *Neurology: A Queen Square Textbook*, 2nd edn. Clarke C, Howard R, Rossor M, Shorvon S, eds. Chichester: John Wiley & Sons, 2016. There are numerous references.

Mtui E, Gruener G, Dockery P. *Fitzgerald's Clinical Neuroanatomy & Neuroscience*, 8th edn. New York, Elsevier, 2020.

Vestibular migraine: Bárány Society & International Headache Society. Lempert, T *et al.* (2012). *J. Vestibular Research*, 22 (4),167–172.

Free updated notes, potential links and references as these become available:
https://www.drcharlesclarke.com
You will be asked to log in, in a secure fashion, with your name and institution.

# 16

# Spinal Cord and Spinal Column Disorders

It is useful to consider the spine in several ways:

- Emergencies: spinal cord compression, infection and an acute cauda equina syndrome – all can be subtle.
- Degenerative disease in the neck and lumbar region: common–in an interface between neurology, neuroradiology, neurosurgery and orthopaedics.
- Less-common conditions: from $B_{12}$ deficiency (subacute combined degeneration), syringomyelia and arteriovenous malformations to spinal tumours, skull base problems and many more.

Terminology is outlined in Chapter 4.

## Emergencies

Spinal cord compression: a spastic paraparesis developing over hours or days, thoracic spinal pain and a sensory level with lower limb weakness are easily recognisable. The more gradual emergence of scuffing of the toes and numbness, without pain, is less obvious and also a potential medical/neurosurgical emergency. Infection is also vital to recognise.

*Cauda equina* compression from a large acute central L4/L5 disc or multiple discs with a narrow lumbar canal affects all lumbosacral roots. Typically, there is severe low back pain, loss of bladder and bowel control and numbness of the buttocks and saddle, with weakness of ankle dorsiflexion (L4), toes (L4, L5), eversion and plantar flexion (S1). Ankle jerks are lost. This may also be easy to recognise, but a central disc can sometimes generate little pain, weakness that may not obvious and a vaguely numb saddle area with urinary retention, and develop over an hour or less.

Urgent imaging and neurosurgical assessment are required for all. Delay even for a few hours can lead to irreversible deficits.

## Cervical Spine Degeneration and Pathology

Cervical spine degeneration, a.k.a. cervical spondylosis, is almost universal above 40. MR imaging bears little relation to symptoms: major changes can be symptomless. Assess whether there is root pain, or myelopathy.

*Neurology: A Clinical Handbook*, First Edition. Charles Clarke.

Age-related degeneration typically affects mid-cervical levels. In younger people, movement/degeneration occurs first at C5–6 and C6–7. As the years go by, C4–5 and C3–4 become affected. Disc degeneration occurs with osteophytes around annular attachments to end plates with degenerative hypertrophy of facet joints. Disc dehydration/degeneration can cause either kyphosis or reversal of the normal curve – a straight neck. Vertebral subluxation also contributes.

## Lateral and Central Cervical Disc Protrusion

With a lateral cervical protrusion (Figure 16.1) root pain is frequent, typically a dull lateral neck ache worse on movement, radiating down one arm – a pain that waxes and wanes. However, such pain is sometimes acute and excruciating. Most acute severe cases settle within days or weeks. Weakness and numbness may point to a root level. Cough impulse pain can accompany a lateral disc prolapse.

Central cervical disc protrusion (Figure 16.2) and/or osteophytic cord compression, with or without canal stenosis, causes myelopathy. Cord compression can be dramatic or subtle. Most with cervical cord compression require surgery. Anterior horn cells can be damaged; arterial insufficiency, venous congestion and repetitive minor trauma can contribute.

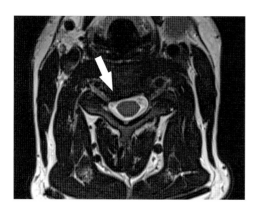

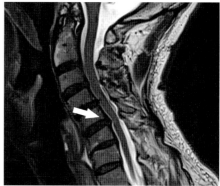

**Figure 16.1**  Axial T2W MR: right lateral disc protrusion at C3–C4.

**Figure 16.2**  Sagittal T2W MR: central disc protrusion at C5–C6.

## Management of a Painful Cervical Root Lesion

- A severely painful acute lateral cervical prolapse requires immobilisation and plentiful analgesia.
- Less severe pain – avoid lifting and improve posture: keep active.
- Paracetamol and NSAIDs, occasionally opiates.
- Physio, acupuncture, TENS, ultrasound, heat and cold, massage, hydrotherapy, chiropractic or osteopathic treatment can all help neck pain. Physical manoeuvres should be avoided if there are any physical signs of cord origin.

## Cervical and Thoracic Spinal Surgery

Surgery for root compression is either via anterior cervical discectomy or posterior foraminotomy. Cord compression requires surgery the aim is to prevent deterioration, but improvement can sometimes follow. Surgery is either via anterior cervical discectomy and/or corpectomy or posterior laminectomy and/or laminoplasty.

Fusion with discectomy is a common procedure, but there are then added stresses on adjacent discs. Disc implants can be used. There is wide variation in surgical practice.

Degenerative thoracic spine disease presents with radicular pain but little else until cord compression develops from a thoracic disc protrusion – a paraparesis with a sensory level. Surgery is usually via thoracotomy.

# Lumbar and Sacrococcygeal Spine

Low back pain is exceedingly common – typically a dull ache, often movement sensitive, and sometimes acute and severe. By 50, most of us will have had pain, sufficient to prevent normal activities and/or seek advice. The gelatinous *nucleus pulposus* surrounded by the *annulus fibrosus* forms the disc. With ageing and day-to-day movement, there are changes in the collagen matrix. Protective measures fail – weakening of the annulus and rupture of the nucleus follows – typically during a spinal load. The nucleus is an immunologically privileged site: disc extrusion sets up intense inflammation. Ultimately, resorption of disc material follows.

It may be impossible on clinical and/or radiological grounds to sort out the origin of lumbar pain – be it from the disc/vertebra, facet joints, ligaments or muscles.

Try to assess:

- Is this lumbosacral root pain?
- Is cauda equina compression possible?
- Is canal stenosis likely?
- Is this facet joint pain?
- Is something sinister afoot or is there infection?

With a lumbosacral root lesion (Figure 16.3), pain and LMN signs may point to the root compressed, but this is not entirely reliable. A dropped ankle jerk points to S1. *Extensor digitorum brevis* wasting indicates L5. Sensory change reflects the root dermatome. L4–5 and L5–S1 are the most common levels, the disc prolapse often compressing the root below.

*Cauda equina* compression is dealt with above and illustrated in Figure 16.4.

## Lumbar Canal Stenosis

Lumbar canal stenosis develops because of facet joint or *ligamentum flavum* hypertrophy, disc prolapse or spondylolisthesis and/or the canal is narrow from birth. As the cross-sectional area diminishes, root symptoms and/or neurogenic claudication follows because of root compression and/or ischaemia. Lumbar canal stenosis, commoner in males, causes low back pain, with leg pain/weakness worsened by exercise and standing upright. These spinal claudication

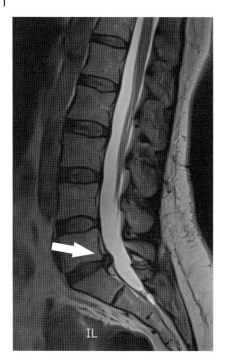

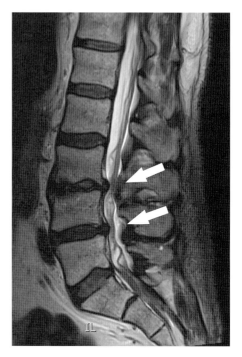

**Figure 16.3**  Sagittal T2W MR: central disc protrusion at L5–S1.

**Figure 16.4**  Sagittal T2W MR: multiple lumbar disc protrusions in a narrow canal causing *cauda equina* compression.

cases may adopt a flexed posture; they find it easier to walk leaning forward. They may squat to relieve pain and sometimes are able to cycle longer than walk. Some have variable sensory symptoms and even rarely an autonomic problem such as developing an erection on walking. The natural history is of slow progression. Neurological examination may be normal initially. Weakness and reflex loss can be exercise dependent. Vascular claudication tends to cause calf pain and does not vary with posture. Treatment: laminectomy with or without discectomy.

## Low Back Pain: Management

Pain needs prompt attention. When low back pain has become established, rather than a transient, acute problem, MR imaging and general investigation become necessary. When pain is severe, bed rest and analgesia – paracetamol, an NSAID, a benzodiazepine and/or an opiate – are needed. A common error is insufficient, regular analgaesia. Bed rest beyond 4 days should be avoided if possible. Mobilise: but discourage lifting, prolonged sitting and abnormal postures. Establish a gentle exercise programme. Posture, sleeping position and, later, lifting technique are important. Most with leg pain of root origin and/or disc pain improve over several weeks or months.

Physiotherapy, TENS, chiropractic treatment, osteopathy, acupuncture, epidural and facet injections can help. There are many long-established self-help programmes, for example Williams exercises – lying supine and flexing the knees – and also gentle stretch-ing by reaching to the top of a door and taking the weight off the spine.

When pain is paraspinal, that is along the lateral lumbar spine, a facet joint manipulation can help:

- Lay patient supine on a firm flat surface
- Flex the hip, on the painful side, gently and passively to more than 90°
- Slowly and firmly internally rotate the hip – grasp the ankle and gently force the knee towards and past the midline.

Relief can be dramatic. Manipulation should be avoided when there are neurologi-cal signs.

### Lumbar Disc Surgery and Fusion

Lumbar microdiscectomy is the standard surgical technique for removing a disc prolapse. Percutaneous techniques – laser, thermocoagulation, chymopapain and other are also used. Lumbar fusion is used for vertebral instability from trauma, infection, degenerative disease or a tumour, but for mechanical back pain alone, fusion remains controversial. Disc prostheses are also used. As with neck surgery, there is wide variation in practice.

## Paraparesis/Paraplegia, Myelitis, Transverse Myelitis and Myelopathy

One difficulty is that these terms are used in different contexts. All imply disease of the spinal cord.

- Paraparesis describes weakness of the lower limbs, spastic or flaccid. Paraplegia describes complete paralysis. Quadriparesis/tetraparesis and quadriplegia/tetraplegia refer to all four limbs.
- Myelitis is literally cord inflammation, but there is confusion with poliomyelitis – an anterior horn cell cord disease. Acute transverse myelitis refers to cord inflammation without a compressive cause – for example from a viral infection.

The term myelopathy avoids any causal implication. Table 16.1 draws together condi-tions that cause cord disease.

### Metabolic Conditions

Subacute combined degeneration of the cord (SACD) from vitamin $B_{12}$ deficiency causes a treatable myelopathy with prominent dorsal column features. Characteristic findings are paresthesiae, unsteadiness, mild UMN leg weakness, depressed reflexes, extensor plantars and impaired toe joint position and vibration sense. Megaloblastic anaemia is not invaria-ble. SACD was fatal before the discovery of vitamin $B_{12}$. Folic acid deficiency should

**Table 16.1**  Some causes of myelopathy.

| | |
|---|---|
| Neurological conditions | MS, Devic's, syringomyelia, MND, cortical/brain lesion(s) |
| Cord compression | Its many causes |
| Metabolic conditions | B$_{12}$ deficiency, also rarities – copper deficiency, hepatic failure, organophosphate poisoning, fluorosis, lathyrism, cassava poisoning, subacute myelo-optico neuropathy, tropical myeloneuropathy |
| Cord vascular disease | Cord infarction, haemorrhage, AVM, vascular neoplasm |
| Hereditary spastic paraplegia | X-linked, AR, AD |
| Inflammatory | SLE, Sjögren's, scleroderma, rheumatoid, antiphospholipid syndrome, sarcoid, Behçet's, vasculitides, ulcerative colitis, HIV |
| Neoplasm | Glioma, ependymoma, meningioma, neurofibroma, lymphoma, myeloma, metastasis, malignant meningitis |
| Paraneoplastic | Small cell lung cancer and lymphoma |
| Spinal infection: bacteria, viruses, parasites and fungi | Staphylococci, mycoplasma, TB, borrelia, rickettsia, syphilis, tetanus, enterovirus – coxsackie, poliovirus, enterovirus 71, flavivirus – West Nile, HZV, HSV 1, 2, HIV, HTLV-1 & 2 (Tropical Spastic Paraparesis), CMV, EBV, influenza, Covid-19, schistosoma, toxoplasma, malaria, cysticercus, aspergillus |
| Post-infectious/ immunisation | ADEM, rabies immunisation |
| Toxins and drugs | Snake and spider bite, arsenic, diethylene glycol, nitrous oxide, cyanide, chemotherapy, heroin |
| Spine and spinal cord major trauma | See below and whiplash |
| Miscellaneous | Decompression sickness, electrical injury, necrotising myelitis, radiation |

produce similar problems, but there is no evidence that it does. Acquired copper deficiency, an absolute rarity, causes a syndrome similar to SACD – with malabsorption, dialysis or parenteral nutrition.

## Cord Vascular Disease

### Cord Infarction and Spinal Haemorrhage

Cord infarction usually presents acutely (see also Chapters 6 and 26), with spinal pain followed by paraplegia, sensory loss and urinary retention (Figure 16.5). The anterior spinal artery is the commonest vessel involved. Spinal haemorrhage can be intramedullary, subarachnoid, epidural and subdural. Again, presentation is typically acute with spinal pain, +/− myelopathy and sphincter loss. Spinal subarachnoid haemorrhage causes severe back pain, +/− root pain followed by features of subarachnoid bleeding.

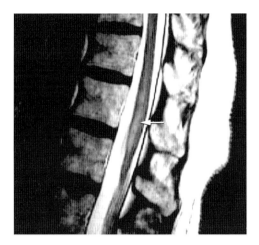

**Figure 16.5** Sagittal T2W MR: thoracic cord infarction.

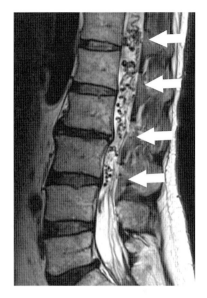

**Figure 16.6** Sagittal T2W MR: spinal AVM – multiple tortuous vessels with signal voids in the thoracolumbar region.

## Cord Arteriovenous Malformations

An AVM (Figure 16.6) usually presents progressively though there can be sudden haemorrhage. There are four types:

- dural arteriovenous fistula (AVF) – commonest
- glomus AVM – a nidus of vessels with multiple feeders
- juvenile, a.k.a. metameric, AVM – intradural and/or extradural
- cord surface AVM – intradural, extramedullary.

## Cord Vascular Neoplasms

A cavernous haemangioma, a.k.a. cavernoma, is a mass of blood-filled sinusoidal spaces surrounded by haemosiderin-stained parenchyma. A spinal cavernoma is typically symptomless but can bleed and/or cause cord compression. Surgery is considered for a cavernoma that has caused symptoms.

Haemangioblastoma occurs sporadically or with von Hippel–Lindau syndrome (Chapters 14, 17, 21 and 26).

## Hereditary Spastic Paraparesis

HSP causes spasticity and lower limb weakness. Transmission can be X-linked, AD or AR. In some, there is cord disease alone (pure HSP). Mutations in many SPG genes have been described, for example SPG1–48. In pure HSP, a young adult presents with progressive gait disturbance, little weakness and severe spasticity. Many remain ambulant. Older-onset forms of HSP tend to progress. In childhood, HSP can present with delayed motor milestones. In complicated HSP – there are many varieties – spastic paraparesis/tetraparesis is associated with features such as optic atrophy, retinopathy, movement disorder, cognitive impairment, deafness, epilepsy, polyneuropathy, amyotrophy and cardiac disease.

## Spinal Infection

All spinal components can be infected by bacteria, fungi, viruses and parasites (see also Chapter 9). The intervertebral disc(s), a.k.a. discitis, and vertebra (osteomyelitis) are most frequently infected. Infection can also develop in the extradural and/or intradural space with abscess formation and/or septicaemia. An extradural abscess can present acutely, but an abscess can develop slowly over months with few of the systemic symptoms that one might expect. Intramedullary infection is unusual.

## Spine and Spinal Cord Major Trauma

Common causes are road accidents and sporting injuries. The Frankel A–E grades for cord trauma are:

(A) No motor or sensory function below lesion.
(B) Incomplete: no motor function below lesion but preservation of sensation.
(C) Incomplete: power preserved below lesion, but MRC Grade <3.
(D) Incomplete: power preserved below lesion – 50% muscles >MRC Grade 3.
(E) Normal motor and sensory function (usually with spinal fracture).

### Acute Spinal Injury Management and Rehabilitation

Resuscitation/treatment of life-threatening injuries are immediate priorities, but assume that in any major trauma there may be a cord injury. The spine must be immobilised until neurological and mechanical integrity is established. Management of spinal fractures and cord injury is outside the scope of this chapter. The trend is towards early intervention. All need specialist assessment.

Spinal injury rehabilitation, pioneered in the Second World War, was the forerunner of neurological rehabilitation (Chapter 18). The goal is to increase functional capability. Challenges include chest and urinary infection, pressure sores, autonomic problems, spasticity, syringomyelia, DVTs and profound practical, sexual and psychological issues. Experimental therapies have led to many claims for the repair of cord injuries, but nothing yet has produced real benefit.

### Whiplash

This emotive word – the crack of whip is at the speed of sound – implies that the head and hence the neck has been moved with some violence. Whiplash describes sequelae of neck pain and other complaints largely in people following rear-end shunt traffic accidents – that is, the patient was seated in the vehicle in front and struck by another from behind. There has sometimes been neck extension and/or flexion but neither neck fractures, bone instability, disc protrusions nor cord damage. Neck pain, broadly of soft tissue origin, tends to start several hours after such an event. Headache and poor concentration are also common complaints with vague vestibular symptoms. There are no neurological abnormalities other than on occasion, non-organic upper limb weakness and non-dermatomal sensory findings. There is neither clinical, radiological nor electrophysiological evidence of nerve or root damage. Pain typically settles within a few weeks. Mobilisation is usually helpful.

Complaints of an enduring nature tend to be made by medicolegal claimants and one view, shared by many, but by no means all is that:

> '. . .the extent to which the symptoms have an organic basis is controversial and medico-legal practice is swamped with claims of disabling symptoms caused by whiplash many of which probably have no justification. It is interesting to note the findings of a Lithuanian study, where few drivers have insurance and disability compensation is unlikely. In this survey there was no significant difference in the incidence of chronic neck pain in people who were involved in a road traffic accident and the general population'.

Hyperextension/hyperflexion neck injury, soft tissue trauma to ligaments and muscles and root tension/traction injuries are also terms used. Attendance at A&E is frequently followed by the recommendation of a collar to which many become attached. Despite this somewhat negative overview, there is no doubt that persistent neck pain does sometimes follow these events, and occasionally, a previous symptomless cervical disc can cause complaints.

## Craniocervical Junction – Basilar Invagination and Atlantoaxial Disease

These relative rarities are summarised here. Basilar invagination, a.k.a. basilar impression – though some differentiate between the two – describes skull base deformity with or without upward displacement of vertebral elements and, hence, distortion of neural tissue. Recognition: clinical features, plain X-rays and MRI.

- Acquired basilar invagination is caused by bone softening, such as in Paget's and *osteogenesis imperfecta*.
- In congenital forms, the clivus and anterior skull base are abnormally flattened, or there are anomalies such as a Chiari malformation and/or a syrinx.
- In achondroplasia, a narrow foramen magnum may also be present.

Atlantoaxial dislocation follows incompetence of either transverse ligaments or abnormalities of the dens itself. Instability – an atlantodens interval greater than 4 mm – occurs following inflammation, trauma and in developmental anomalies, such as Klippel–Feil. Ligamentous laxity also carries a risk of dislocation, such as in Down's. Instability can develop around a degenerate odontoid, a.k.a. pseudotumour.

## Chiari Malformations and *Os Odontoideum*

These anomalies are:

Chiari I: dorsal extension of cerebellar tonsils below the foramen magnum, found on imaging in around 0.5% of symptomless people. Occasionally disease develops, such as syringomyelia.

Chiari II: an anomaly generally evident after birth – myelomeningocoele and hydrocephalus. Management: usually surgical.

Chiari III: similar to Chiari II with downward cerebellar displacement into a posterior encephalocele, typically life-threatening.

A symptomless Chiari I malformation is usually left alone. Pregnancy should be monitored – pushing during labour can cause further tonsillar descent; epidural anaesthesia can exceptionally produce coning.

An *os odontoideum* is an ossicle above the centre of the axis, in the position of the odontoid with a hypoplastic or absent dens. This occurs in Down's, in various dysplasias and in Morquio syndrome. C1/C2 fusion is sometimes recommended.

## Craniocervical Junction Disorders

These developmental and acquired conditions may not cause problems at all or do so only when decompensation occurs, gradually or rapidly. Lower brainstem, cranial nerves, cervical roots and upper cervical cord can be compressed, with changes in blood supply. Possible consequences:

- Dysphagia, dysarthria, nystagmus
- Headache/neck pain: typically suboccipital→vertex
- Head tilt
- Hearing loss – occasionally in children
- Trigeminal pain: Vth nerve and/or V nuclei compression
- Cranial nerve lesions: IX, X, XI and XII
- Cord compression
- Dissociated sensory loss
- Sleep apnoea, drop attacks, syncope.

Occasionally, myelopathy is confined to the upper limbs. Sequential, a.k.a. clock-face limb involvement, can occur with foramen magnum compression: spastic weakness begins in one upper limb, followed by the contralateral lower limb and then the contralateral upper limb. Cruciate paralysis (bilateral upper limb weakness with relative sparing of the lower limbs) occasionally occurs – pressure on the upper pyramidal tracts.

If brainstem or cord compression occurs, surgery is considered – a highly specialised field.

## Syringomyelia and Syringobulbia

A syrinx is a cystic cavity within either cord (syringomyelia, Figure 16.7) or brainstem (syringobulbia) lined typically by cord parenchyma – distinct from a cavity in continuity with the central canal lined by ependymal cells (hydromyelia). The cavity forms gradually following transmission of CSF pressure during coughing and/or raised intra-abdominal or thoracic pressure.

Syringomyelia may occur without an evident cause or can follow:

- Trauma, usually following a cord injury: nearly 10% of cord injury cases develop a syrinx, typically some years post-injury. The cavity can remain symptomless.
- Congenital conditions: Chiari malformations, basilar invagination and Dandy–Walker.
- Tumours – e.g. intramedullary astrocytoma and ependymoma.
- Following infections – pyogenic meningitis and TB.

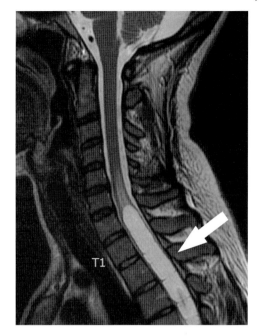

**Figure 16.7** Sagittal T2W MR: syringomyelia – large fluid-filled cavity in the cervicothoracic cord.

Features reflect pathology that starts centrally. The enlarging cavity damages crossing spinothalamic fibres to produce a half-cape or cape loss of pain and temperature sensation, with posterior columns relatively preserved. Painless hand and upper limb injuries, wasting and weakness follow. There is amyotrophy (muscle atrophy) at the level of the cavity and reflex loss. Below, UMN features emerge, with spastic lower limbs with sphincter problems. In advanced stages, neuropathic Charcot joints develop. Syringobulbia can cause onion-skin facial sensory loss from damage to the spinal nuclei or tract(s) of V and also tongue wasting, face pain and palatal/bulbar weakness. Central apnoea can develop.

Non-progressive post-traumatic syringomyelia or hydromyelia is often best left alone. Progressive symptoms may need surgery – a shunt can be inserted between the syrinx and subarachnoid space, pleural or peritoneal cavities. Procedures carry high rates of syrinx recurrence.

## Rheumatological and Bone Disorders

### Rheumatoid Disease

Rheumatoid has predilection for distal joints rather than the spine (Chapter 26). However, cord and disc problems can follow ligament/bone destruction and osteoporosis. Rarely, a rheumatoid dural pachymeningitis occurs. Atlantoaxial subluxation, basilar impression, sub-axial subluxation and cervical cord lesions occasionally develop, with inflammatory tissue, a.k.a. *pannus*. Surgery may be needed.

### Spondyloarthropathies

These include ankylosing spondylitis, psoriatic arthritis and arthritis + inflammatory bowel disease. Ankylosing spondylitis is the commonest – gradual low back pain and stiffness of large joints. One hallmark is inflammation around tendon insertion sites on vertebral bodies – a.k.a. syndesmophytes – to produce a straight rigid spine. Complications: atlantoaxial subluxation, disc destruction, lumbar canal stenosis and *cauda equina* syndrome.

### Paget's Disease of Bone

Rare below 40, Paget's becomes increasingly common – to about 10% at 90. Paget's is often symptomless, but it can cause bone pain, local deformity, pathological fracture and occasionally sarcomatous change. Paget's in the skull or spine can lead to numerous rare sequelae – headache, cranial neuropathies, myelopathy, cauda equina syndrome and root lesions. The commonest cranial neuropathy is sensorineural deafness. Optic atrophy, trigeminal neuralgia and hemifacial spasm have been described. Skull changes can lead to basilar invagination. High blood flow through pagetic bone can occasionally produce a steal syndrome. Paget's responds partially to bisphosphonates.

#### Osteopenic Disorders

These include hypoparathyroidism, Cushing's, osteomalacia, osteoporosis and *osteogenesis imperfecta*. Osteoporosis is often symptomless. The commonest problem is a compression or wedge fracture – back pain or radicular pain and occasionally cauda equina or cord compression.

*Osteogenesis imperfecta*, the rare collagen disorder, causes bone fragility. Most mutations are found in the genes (*COLIA1* and *COLIA2*) encoding the α1 and α2 collagen chains. Basilar invagination can occur.

#### Superficial Siderosis and Arachnoiditis

In siderosis, a distinct rarity, there is subarachnoid haemosiderin deposition (Chapter 26). Previous neurosurgery, root avulsion and a vascular anomaly are causes.

Arachnoiditis means adhesions in the intradural space following trauma, infection, surgery or subarachnoid bleeding. Arachnoiditis is often symptomless, but pain can follow, root symptoms and exceptionally myelopathy if the cord becomes tethered. In the lumbar region, nerve roots form adherent bundles and/or lie centrifugally, producing an apparently empty lumbar sac on MRI. Myodil myelography (not used in the United Kingdom since 1984) was once a possible cause and source of litigation – there was frequently no evidence to associate radiological findings with symptoms.

## Spinal Dysraphism, Scoliosis and Kyphosis

Spinal dysraphism describes failure of neural tube closure *in utero*. Myelomeningocoele is the commonest form – less than 1/1000 live births. Such neural tube defects are caused by many mechanisms: chromosomal abnormalities, single gene defects and teratogens such as valproate and carbamazepine. Myelomeningocoeles account for most cases of dysraphism, with exposed neural tissue a common feature. Hydrocephalus requiring surgical treatment develops in some with a Chiari II malformation and/or syringomyelia.

Scoliosis means lateral spinal deviation. This can be idiopathic. Scoliosis may be apparent at birth or become evident in adolescence. There may be failure of vertebral segmentation, e.g. Klippel–Feil and Alagille's syndrome, or a neuromuscular cause such as following polio and with Duchenne dystrophy.

Kyphosis: greater than 30° is abnormal. This may be congenital, from vertebral body abnormalities, due to Scheuermann's kyphosis, post-trauma, osteomalacia, osteoporosis or a tumour.

## Other Rare Causes of Spinal Deformity

### Osteochondrodysplasias and Dysostoses

Osteochondrodysplasias are abnormalities of cartilage and/or bone growth. Short-limbed dwarfism is typical with AD achondroplasia, with mutations in fibroblast growth factor (FGFR3) pathways in many cases. About half with achondroplasia have thoracolumbar kyphosis; some have canal stenosis. They tend to have macrocephaly and a small foramen magnum. Sleep apnoea and atlantoaxial instability can occur. Dysostoses are malformations of individual bones singly or in combination and include the craniosynostoses – Crouzon and Apert syndromes.

### Metabolic Storage Disorders

These include mucopolysaccharidoses, glycoprotein-storage disorders, gangliosidoses and mucolipidoses. Some cases have skeletal dysplasias, such as hooked vertebrae, broad ribs and flared pelvis. Kyphosis is common. Other issues include cognitive deterioration, carpal tunnel syndrome and deafness. In Morquio syndrome (mucopolysaccharidosis IV), there can be atlantoaxial instability and cord compression.

# Acknowledgements

I am grateful to Simon Farmer and David Choi for their contribution to *Neurology A Queen Square Textbook* Second Edition on which this chapter was based.

I am also most grateful to Dr Patricio Paredes, Head of The Neuroradiology Unit and Dr Pablo Soffia, Chairman of The Department of Radiology, Clínica Alemana-Universidad del Desarrollo, Santiago, Chile who were most helpful in providing the high quality images whilst I was there.

# Further Reading and Information

Clarke CR, Harrison MJ. Neurological manifestations of Paget's disease. *J Neurol Sci* 1978;
  38: 171–178.

Farmer S, Choi D. Spinal cord and spinal column disorders. In *Neurology A Queen Square Textbook,* 2nd edn. Clarke C, Howard R, Rossor M, Shorvon S, eds. Chichester: John Wiley & Sons, 2016. There are numerous references.

Hopkins A, Clarke C, Brindley G. Erections on walking as a symptom of spinal canal stenosis. *J Neurol Neurosurg Psychiatry* 1987; 50: 1371–1374.

Free updated notes, potential links and references as these become available:
https://www.drcharlesclarke.com
You will be asked to log in, in a secure fashion, with your name and institution.

# 17

# Ataxias, Cerebellar Disorders and Related Conditions

Ataxia is derived from the Greek meaning lack of order or coordination – features seen typically in diseases of the cerebellum and its connections. Anatomy is covered in Chapter 2, and examination in Chapter 4.

## Acquired Ataxia Syndromes

### The Posterior Fossa Mass Lesion

This is a potential neurosurgical emergency. Headache, vomiting and vertigo are typical, with or without emergence of cerebellar signs and papilloedema. Any suggestion of a posterior fossa mass is an emergency that requires immediate imaging. Deterioration can take place rapidly, over hours or even minutes. Brain tumours are dealt with in Chapter 21. A cerebellar abscess may cause a fever; TB can be more indolent. Neurocysticercosis occurs in endemic regions (Chapter 9). Cerebellar haemorrhage/haematoma can also be acute.

### Acute Cerebellar Ataxia

Acute cerebellar ataxia of childhood is post-infective. Viruses include echoviruses, coxsackie A and B, enteroviruses, EBV, HSV1, HHV6, parvovirus B19 and hepatitis A. This can follow immunisation for varicella, hepatitis B, rabies, meningococcal group C and human papilloma virus, but rates are far lower than following infection and rabies is fatal, in any event.

Ataxia usually presents between 1 and 8 years. The prodromal illness is sometimes unrecognised. The child develops severe ataxia, particularly midline. Additional features include myoclonus, opsoclonus and ocular flutter. Outlook is good, though it may take several months for recovery. Exceptional cases occur in adults.

Ataxia is well recognised in ADEM (Chapter 9) following varicella, measles, rubella and mumps, Bickerstaff's encephalitis and the Fisher variant of GBS.

Other microorganisms can produce ataxia – mycoplasma, borrelia, typhoid and malaria.

## Progressive Ataxia with a Chronic or Subacute Course

In childhood, SSPE is a potential cause (Chapter 9). Congenital rubella can produce a cerebellar syndrome with dementia, optic atrophy and myoclonus. HIV can cause encephalopathy with ataxia. Vanishing White Matter Disease is a rare inherited childhood leukoencephalopathy – progressive decline and cerebellar ataxia. Prions: ataxic features can develop in both iatrogenic and variant CJD and Gerstmann–Sträussler–Scheinker syndrome.

## MS, Vascular and Inflammatory Disease

An isolated cerebellar syndrome is a rare presentation of MS. Sarcoid, SLE, vasculitides, antiphospholipid syndrome and Sjögren's can all cause ataxia but rarely. A cerebellar haemangioblastoma (Chapters 14, 21 and 26) can present as a mass lesion or be found incidentally. Other vascular anomalies such as a dural fistula and an AVM are rare causes of an ataxic syndrome (Chapter 6).

## Alcohol, Solvent Abuse and Acquired Metabolic Disorders

Ethanol is the commonest (Chapter 19): acute toxicity produces staggering with slurred speech. Chronic abuse can produce progressive gait and limb ataxia with dysarthria. Neuropathy is frequently present. Imaging: cerebellar atrophy. Lifelong abstinence may help. Thiamine is essential.

Solvents: acute exposure to toluene and other solvents (Chapter 19) produces a reversible ataxia. Prolonged exposure can produce disabling persistent ataxia, seen in adolescent glue sniffers. Behavioural problems and cognitive deficits occur.

Metabolic disorders include Wernicke's and hepatic encephalopathy, pontine and extrapontine myelinolysis with hyponatraemia. Hypothyroidism can cause a cerebellar syndrome.

## Drugs, Heavy Metals and Physical Agents

- Antiepileptic drugs, especially phenytoin, carbamazepine and barbiturates, cause a cerebellar syndrome when the dose is too high – with nystagmus, dysarthria and gait ataxia. Susceptibility varies and cannot be judged by serum level alone. Long-term anti-epileptics can cause a permanent cerebellar syndrome.
- Lithium toxicity can produce a persistent deficit.
- A rare reversible ataxia occurs with piperazine, high-dose 5-fluorouracil and with cytosine arabinoside.
- Heavy metals: thallium, lead and methyl mercury (Chapter 19).
- Hypoxia, heat stroke and hypothermia (Chapter 19) can all produce cerebellar features.
- High-altitude cerebral oedema (Chapter 19) can cause a cerebellar syndrome with headache and papilloedema.

## Others

Paraneoplastic cerebellar degeneration can cause (Chapter 21) subacute midline cerebellar ataxia with chaotic eye movements and oscillopsia. There are rare cases where no cancer is found.

Superficial siderosis: chronic bleeding, usually from an unknown source, can cause slowly progressive ataxia, sensorineural deafness and +/− pyramidal signs. Dementia, incontinence, anosmia, anisocoria and sensory signs can develop. MR imaging: dark haemosiderin around posterior fossa structures and spinal cord on T2W.

### Late-Onset Cerebellar Degenerations

Multiple system atrophy (MSA) usually starts between 50 and 70 years of age, progressing to severe disability within 7 years. MSA can present with a parkinsonian syndrome (Chapter 7), with autonomic dysfunction (Chapters 24 and 25) or as a cerebellar syndrome.

Idiopathic late-onset ataxia is slowly progressive after 50 years of age. Pyramidal signs can follow.

Gluten: cases with this rarity have intestinal histology suggestive of gluten enteropathy and/or antigliadin antibodies, though the latter are common in the general population.

## Inherited Ataxia Syndromes

### Autosomal Recessive Ataxias

Friedreich's ataxia (FRDA) is the most common. The relevant AR mutations are summarised in Table 17.1 Generally, onset of ataxia is below 20 years.

Table 17.1   AR cerebellar ataxias.

| Syndrome | Gene defect | Clinical pointers |
|---|---|---|
| Friedreich's ataxia (FRDA) | GAA repeat and some point mutations | Neuropathy, pyramidal signs, skeletal abnormalities, diabetes and cardiomyopathy |
| *Ataxia telangiectasia* (AT) | *ATM* mutation | Telangiectasia (not always evident), oculomotor apraxia, movement disorder, immune deficiencies and increased cancer risk |
| AT-like disorder | *hMRE11* | |
| Cockayne's syndrome | Type A – *ERCC8* gene | Cachexia, small stature, cognitive impairment and retinopathy (pigmentary) |
| | Type B – *ERCC6* gene | |
| *Xeroderma pigmentosum* | | Increased skin cancer |
| Ataxia with oculomotor apraxia (AOA1) | Aprataxin | Oculomotor apraxia |
| Ataxia with oculomotor apraxia (AOA2) | Senataxin | Oculomotor apraxia, chorea, neuropathy, high cholesterol and hypoalbuminaemia |
| Spastic ataxia of Charlevoix-Saguenay (ARSCACS) | Sacsin | Demyelinating neuropathy and retinal layer hypertrophy |

*(Continued)*

**Table 17.1** (Continued)

| Syndrome | Gene defect | Clinical pointers |
| --- | --- | --- |
| Marinesco–Sjögren's syndrome | *SIL1* | Cataracts and cognitive impairment |
| Progressive myoclonic ataxia a.k.a. Ramsay-Hunt ataxia | Complex | Epilepsy frequent; overlaps with progressive myoclonic epilepsy |
| Behr's & related ataxias, e.g. 3-methylglutaconic aciduria type III (Costeff's) | C12*orf*65, OPA3 *et al* | Optic atrophy, spasticity and cognitive impairment |
| Deafness: congenital or childhood onset | Complex | Several syndromes; overlap with Usher's |
| AR late-onset ataxia | Heterogeneous | Variable additional features |

## Friedreich's Ataxia

FRDA is characterised by progressive gait and limb ataxia, axonal sensorimotor neuropathy, pyramidal tract involvement, hypertrophic cardiomyopathy, skeletal abnormalities, optic atrophy, deafness and diabetes, typically evident between 8 and 15 years. Exceptional cases occur later.

Frataxin was found in 1996 – a mutation is a trinucleotide repeat (GAA) in intron 1. The normal GAA repeat length varies from 7 to 22 units, whereas the disease range is 100–2000; the shorter the length of the repeat, the later the onset and milder the phenotype. The frataxin protein is involved in iron metabolism within mitochondria.

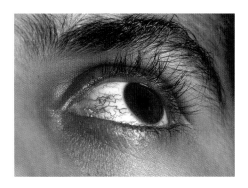

**Figure 17.1** *Ataxia telangiectasia*: typical conjunctival telangiectases.

## Ataxias with Defective DNA Repair

*Ataxia telangiectasia* (AT) is a movement disorder with progressive ataxia, dystonia and chorea. Typical conjunctival and skin lesions develop in the first decade (Figure 17.1). Growth is delayed and mild learning difficulties common. AT is associated with defective humoral and cell-mediated immunity and is caused by *ATM* gene mutations. Variants have no telangiectasia, and later, onset occur. AT-like disorder is a rarer disease caused by mutations in *hMRE11*. *Xeroderma pigmentosum* and Cockayne's syndrome are also caused by DNA repair defects.

## Ataxias with Oculomotor Apraxia

Oculomotor apraxia: Intermittent failure of voluntary saccades. AOA1 follows mutations in the aprataxin gene. Chorea, peripheral neuropathy and learning difficulties also develop. MRI: cerebellar atrophy. AOA2 is similar – mutations in senataxin. Alpha-fetoprotein is elevated.

## Ataxia: Metabolic Causes

### Ataxia and Vitamin E Deficiency

Many cases have an evident cause for vitamin E deficiency – abetalipoproteinaemia, liver disease or malabsorption following cystic fibrosis or bowel resection. Isolated vitamin E deficiency without malabsorption can cause gait ataxia, limb incoordination, areflexia and large fibre sensory loss. Abnormality in α-tocopherol transfer protein (αTTP) gene leads to impaired ability to incorporate vitamin E into liver lipoproteins. Vitamin E therapy helps stabilise the situation.

### Episodic Metabolic Ataxias

Each of these rarities has a similar phenotype – episodic ataxia, dysarthria, vomiting, confusion and involuntary movements. Seizures and learning difficulties may develop.

- *Ornithine transcarbamylase (OTC) deficiency*: The commonest urea cycle enzyme defect is X-linked. Males die in infancy. In females, features vary – from severe deficits to few symptoms, apart from mild protein intolerance. OTC deficiency can present in adults. A heavy protein meal, infection or valproate can even precipitate encephalopathy. Protein restriction and IV fluids may help during an episode.
- *Hartnup's disease*: This aminoaciduria caused by mutations in *SLC6A19* can cause an episodic ataxia, a movement disorder, psychiatric illness, cognitive decline and a pellagra-like rash. Unlike urea cycle disorders, a high-protein diet and oral nicotinamide may help.
- *Pyruvate dehydrogenase deficiency*: PDH is heterogeneous – most follow mutations in the X-linked E1 alpha enzyme subunit gene (PDHA1).
- *Biotin-dependent carboxylase deficiencies*: episodic ataxias are described.

### Progressive Metabolic Ataxias

Many metabolic diseases have ataxia as a component. Most are identified in early life. These include sphingomyelin lipidoses, metachromatic leukodystrophies, galactosylceramide lipidosis (Krabbe's), hexosaminidase deficiencies and adrenoleukomyeloneuropathy.

- *Late-onset hexosaminidase A deficiency*: this can cause progressive ataxia with proximal weakness, with cerebellar atrophy.
- *Niemann–Pick disease type C*: ataxia can occur, with supranuclear gaze palsy. Foamy storage cells are found in the marrow. Type C is caused by abnormalities in the *NPC* gene on chromosome 18.
- *Cholestanolosi*s (a.k.a. cerebrotendinous xanthomatosis): this AR disorder is caused by defective bile salt metabolism, from a deficiency of mitochondrial sterol 27 hydroxylase encoded by *CYP27A1*. This begins after puberty with ataxia, dementia, spasticity and neuropathy. It also leads to premature atherosclerosis, cataracts and tendon xanthomas.

## Autosomal Dominant Cerebellar Ataxias

There are now over 30 loci for ADCAs, numbered as each locus was found. Spinocerebellar ataxia type 1 (SCA 1) was one of the first diseases to have its gene mapped in 1977. The consequence of the most common mutation is an expanded CAG repeat.

ADCAs have two classifications, one based on the SCA mutation, and the other (Harding) clinical classification runs from I to III:

- ADCA I: progressive ataxia with variable cognitive impairment, pyramidal and extrapyramidal signs, supranuclear gaze palsy and neuropathy. Disease usually starts after 25 years of age, with occasional childhood cases.
- ADCA II has features of ADCA I, with macular dystrophy that singles out this rarity. Virtually, all are caused by *SCA7* gene mutations.
- ADCA III: generally of later onset than I and II – pure ataxias.

Signs in ADCA I and II emerge only as disease progresses. An isolated progressive ataxia for 10 years is strong evidence for ADCA III. Testing for SCA 1, 2, 3, 6 and 7 identifies the mutation in >50% of probable ADCAs. The remaining 50% are either rarer SCA5 – SCA 12, 14 and 17 – or unknown. The predominant mutations are in the gene that encodes glutamine – polyglutamine disorders are also found in Huntington's and Kennedy's syndrome (Chapters 7 and 10).

Dentatorubral-pallidoluysian atrophy (DRPLA), an AD disorder found principally in Japan, has variable combinations of ataxia, dystonia, myoclonus, seizures, dementia and parkinsonism – another expanded CAG repeat disorder.

## Episodic Ataxia: Genetic Forms

Marked variation in ataxia characterises this group. Ion channel mutations are involved.

### Episodic Ataxia Type 1

EA1 is a rare disorder with brief attacks, lasting seconds or minutes – sometimes many each day. Sudden movement or shock can bring on an attack. Attacks develop in childhood: frequency lessens with age. Attacks can be associated with myokymia. Potassium channel gene mutations in *KCNA1* cause EA1, the channel related to the peripheral neuromuscular potassium channel, attacked by autoantibodies in neuromyotonia (Chapters 10 and 21), which also causes myokymia. Acetazolamide may help in some.

### Episodic Ataxia Type 2 and Others

EA2 is more common than EA1: attacks resemble a vertebrobasilar migraine attack. Episodes generally last hours, having built up over minutes. There is nausea, vertigo and often vomiting, sometimes with a mild headache. Frequency varies: daily, to once every few months. Episodes become less frequent with age. Unlike EA1 a slowly progressive ataxia can also develop. The typical picture is a child or adolescent with odd episodes, whose parent has a progressive permanent ataxia.

EA2 is caused by point mutations, usually of nonsense type, in the calcium channel gene *CACN1A*, the same gene is associated with familial hemiplegic migraine (Chapter 12) and SCA 6. Allelic heterogeneity describes this – where different disorders are caused by different mutations in the same gene. Acetazolamide may help. Prevention of attacks does not reduce the progressive component.

EA3 describes a family with vertigo and tinnitus and EA4 a family with periodic vestibulocerebellar ataxia.

## X-Linked Ataxias and Mitochondrial Ataxia Syndromes

Ataxic syndromes associated with X chromosome mutations are rare.

*Adrenoleukodystrophy*: a variant can produce ataxia. A pyramidal leukodystrophic phenotype with a demyelinating neuropathy is usually present. Serum very long-chain fatty
acids measurement is a useful screening tool.

*Pelizaeus–Merzbacher disease*: this can lead to ataxia in early life. *PLP* gene mutations can
be detected.

*Neuroacanthocytosis* (Chapter 6): ataxia is overshadowed by involuntary movements.
AD, AR and X-linked forms exist. The X-linked form, a.k.a. McLeod's syndrome, is
associated with a specific Kell system antigen. Acanthocytes are present in peripheral
blood.

*Fragile X tremor ataxia syndrome*: FXTAS causes a late-progressive ataxia and cognitive
decline, from an expanded repeat in the *FMR1* gene. Imaging: volume loss in cerebellum, with signal changes in middle cerebellar peduncles.

*Mitochondrial DNA disorders*: see Chapter 10.

## Congenital Ataxias

These early-onset, generally non-progressive disorders are rarely seen in an adult neurology (Table 17.2).

Developmental delay is usually evident. Imaging: This typically shows a small cerebellum. A sign known as a molar tooth – a deep interpeduncular fossa with elongated, thick
and maloriented superior cerebellar peduncles – is seen in Joubert's syndrome.
Developmental non-progressive abnormalities, such as Arnold–Chiari malformation and
Dandy–Walker cysts, may also become apparent on imaging (Chapter 16).

**Table 17.2** Congenital inherited ataxic disorders

| Syndrome | Additional features | Inheritance | Gene defect |
|---|---|---|---|
| Joubert's | Episodic hyperpnoea, abnormal eye movements and cognitive impairment | AR, heterogeneous | AHI1, NPHP1, CEP290 |
| Gillespie's | Cognitive impairment and partial aniridia | Uncertain | No gene or locus known |
| Congenital nystagmus | Macular hypoplasia in some | AR and X-linked | NYS1–6p,NYS2, X-linked and others |
| Congenital hypoplasia and quadrupedal gait | Cognitive impairment and s eizures | AR | 17p |
| Paine's | Spasticity, cognitive impairment and microcephaly | X-linked | None identified |

## Acknowledgement

I am indebted to Nicholas Wood who wrote the ataxia chapter in Neurology *A Queen Square Textbook*, Second Edition on which this summary is based.

## Further Reading and Information

Wood N. Cerebellar ataxias and related conditions. In *Neurology A Queen Square Textbook*, 2nd edn. Clarke C, Howard H, Rossor M, Shorvon S, eds. Chichester: Wiley Blackwell, 2016. There are extensive references.

Free updated notes, potential links and references as these become available:
https://www.drcharlesclarke.com
You will be asked to log in, in a secure fashion, with your name and institution.

# 18

# Restorative Neurology, Rehabilitation and Brain Injury

Chronic disabling conditions are a major part of health care. Damage to the nervous system accounts for about half of all severe disabilities and about one-third of NHS costs. Rehabilitation addresses issues these patients face: most benefit from a goal-focused approach. Goals are achieved via:

- prevention – of avoidable systemic, neurological and psychological complications
- functional compensation – via behavioural adaptation and substitution; in other words, getting round problems
- neural restoration and substitution – making full use of neurological recovery.

Delivery of successful rehabilitation is via a multi-disciplinary team, whose aim is to help patients increase independence, adjust to loss and improve their quality of life.

## Key Aspects

All rehabilitation programmes include:

- multidisciplinary assessment
- definition of problems and goal setting
- treatment delivery
- evaluation/reassessment.

Treatment is delivered primarily by cognitive, physical, occupational, speech and language therapists. Care and nursing support with medical supervision are also important.
There are three natural histories of neurological injury:

- single incident brain and cord damage or acute paralyses such as polio or Guillain-Barré
- deteriorating conditions such as MS, Alzheimer's, MND and Parkinson's
- static conditions such as cerebral palsy.

*Neurology: A Clinical Handbook*, First Edition. Charles Clarke.
© 2022 John Wiley & Sons Ltd. Published 2022 by John Wiley & Sons Ltd.

In the United Kingdom, National Service Frameworks (NSFs) set out requirements to improve services. The Integrated Care Pathway derived from the NSF provides a focus for a multidisciplinary team to define, achieve and audit long-term goals.

Effectiveness of rehabilitation was demonstrated initially following spinal injuries over 70 years ago. Today, audit has shown that well-organised care delivers valuable outcomes, while advances in neurosciences have provided explanations, both for the mechanisms of disabilities and for how treatments work.

## Restorative and Compensatory Approaches, Skill Learning and Task-Related Training

Interventions via task-related strategies are broadly divided into restorative and compensatory.

- Restorative approaches aim to improve function by bringing about an improvement, for example of weakness or dysphasia.
- Compensatory strategies may be external, for example an ankle-foot orthosis or communication aid. Strategies can also improve function by changing behaviour. Compensation may be the best way to overcome a problem.

Task-related training, meaning trying to achieve a specific goal, is also helpful. Skills are mostly performed in an unpredictable environment, a.k.a. open skills – dealing with the unexpected. Many factors can vary during a simple task such as picking up a cup: the cup's location, its orientation, weight, frictional qualities, adjacent objects, availability of sensory cues and drinking, washing and returning the cup to its place. Acquisition of these open skills requires practice – and during therapy, task parameters are changed randomly, to reflect the normal variation of real life. In other words, open skill learning is helped by varying instructions. By contrast, skills performed in a predictable environment, a.k.a. closed skills, benefit from constant and repetitive practice.

During initial skill learning, feedback involves verbal instruction and demonstration, so that the learner can determine what the goals are and how to achieve them. However, too much therapy especially in the later stages can result in reliance on feedback – phasing out feedback avoids this.

The timing of therapy – as soon as possible – is based on evidence that in stroke, there is a window of heightened CNS plasticity between a few days to several weeks following an infarct. Termination of therapy is often recommended when patients reach a plateau. However, this may be partly an effect of adaptation to a therapy programme. Further improvements can follow modification of a programme and/or new tasks. Potential for improvement frequently persists for several years or more.

High intensity of therapy is beneficial. Ways of delivering high-intensity treatment in a cost-effective way include group training and telerehabilitation. Constraint of a non-affected limb can also help. Emerging interventions include automated robotics and mental imagery. Telerehabilitation is important – there are many interactive websites. There must, however, be careful assessment of the contacts made by this vulnerable group.

## Motor Disorders: Therapeutic Interventions

### Bobath and Motor Relearning Programmes

Different physiotherapy approaches have used theoretical assumptions about control of movement and mechanisms underlying recovery. Bobath focussed on the role of afferent information in facilitating movement. Later, biomechanical knowledge resulted in developments such as the motor relearning programme (MRP). The MRP approach emphasises task-specific activities with verbal instructions. The Bobath approach emphasises the need to facilitate manually normal movements that are absent and to normalise tone. Their effectiveness is similar, though much is sometimes made of one or other technique.

### Sensory Facilitation and Other Techniques

Sensory facilitation uses stimuli such as muscle stretch, tactile input and weight bearing to achieve muscle activation. These passive stimuli facilitate muscle responses less than voluntary action: active participation should be encouraged.

With spasticity, the contribution of neural and non-neural components needs to be established. Neural contributions to hypertonia – the increase in stretch reflex-evoked muscle activity – are amenable to drug therapy. Physical interventions focus on the non-neural aspect of hypertonia – increased joint stiffness and tight connective tissue. Maintenance and restoration of muscle length and muscle compliance can be helped by active and passive stretches, standing regimes, splinting, orthoses and optimising posture. Transcutaneous electrical stimulation and specific cutaneous nerve stimulation also help.

Muscle weakness after a stroke is often the result of a primary deficit in central control that results in alterations in motor unit recruitment, firing patterns and inappropriate agonist–antagonist co-activation. Constraint-induced movement therapy (CIMT) following stroke or traumatic brain injury (TBI) means constraining the non-paretic upper limb while performing intensive task-oriented therapy on the paretic limb.

### Balance and Posture

Balance, posture and mobility require integration of visual, vestibular and somatosensory information. Postural stability is a vital prerequisite for many movements: without it the upper limbs are often used to aid balance. Positioning and good seating can improve limb function and prevent progression of scoliosis and prevent pressure sores. A good wheelchair can greatly improve mobility. Compensatory approaches to gait include walking aids and orthoses.

### Treadmills, Functional Stimulation, Cueing, Fitness and Mental Imagery

Treadmill training with body weight support via a harness and robotic-assisted step trainers allows safe, repetitive practice of the entire act of walking. This improves balance.

Functional electrical stimulation (FES) of a peripheral motor nerve can help compensate for muscle weakness. Foot-drop stimulators are available – onset of swing phase is detected either by a heel switch or other device to trigger common peroneal nerve stimulation. Multi-channel FES has also been used to retrain standing, weight transference and gait. Stepping can be induced via common peroneal nerve stimulation, while quadriceps stimulation provides knee control during standing. Such FES systems have been claimed to restore paraplegia cases to independence. However, fatigue, high energy expenditure and abnormal muscle activation due to hypertonia often fail to make these realistic tools.

Cueing: in Parkinson's disease, gait cadence, stride length and velocity are improved. Cues can be either internal, by paying attention to step length, or external, such as auditory or visual cues. Repeated cueing can overcome freezing, festination and falls.

Cardiorespiratory exercise can reverse the effects of immobility in many situations. All adults should perform at least 150 minutes of moderate or 75 minutes of vigorous activity each week, but shorter periods may be a more realistic target. In people with any physical disability, exercise is beneficial. The difficulty is to maintain it. Mental imagery and sensory stimulation techniques are also used to facilitate retraining.

Robotic devices record movement-associated forces, and so the intensity of therapy can be accurately determined. Robotic gait machines can reduce the need for supervision by a therapist. Virtual reality technology provides a virtual three-dimensional visual environment and encourages the patients to picture their disability.

### Speech and Language Therapy and Communication Aids

Normal language is dependent usually on an intact left hemisphere and on networks within and between hemispheres. For instance, naming is served by an extensive infrastructure, vulnerable to damage in many areas – most aphasic patients suffer from anomia. Speech disorders are in Chapter 5, and neuroanatomy outlined in Chapter 2.

Intensity and goal setting are important. Many packages exist, for example: www.aphasiasoftwarefinder.org/.

Transcranial direct current stimulation via scalp electrodes may be helpful.

In some severe aphasia cases, patients may not be able to mount much of a vocabulary; gesture therapy can help those who may have intact semantics and non-verbal communication skills. Many aids are available, for example via www.sense.org.uk.

### Hemianopic Visual Loss and Restorative Therapies

The commonest causes of hemianopia are stroke, TBI and a tumour. There are about 80 000 people with hemianopia in the United Kingdom. The field defect rarely improves spontaneously after 6 months and affects many activities of daily living.

There are several approaches to treatment. Eye movement retraining can be helpful. Web-based therapies such as www.readright.ucl.ac.uk and www.eyesearch.ucl.ac.uk are designed for home use. Other techniques include NovaVision Visual Restoration Therapy (VRT) and Neuro-Eye Therapy.

### Cognition, Environment and Compensatory Strategies

Neuropsychological interventions involve a phase of education and explanations for patients and their carers. This provides a vocabulary for symptoms that may be unfamiliar. Intervention comprises training in the use of compensatory strategies with the aim of restoring specific impairments.

Environmental manipulation include the provision of a quiet, distraction-free space, breaking down tasks into their components, with monitoring and feedback. Such modifications may be simple, but they can improve an individual's abilities. Assistive technologies for cognitive deficits include memory aids such as the NeuroPage system that uses automated text messages to send reminders.

### Restorative Approaches, Executive Function and Retraining

Restorative approaches aim to recover a lost function through retraining and practice. Attention training is based on the premise that attentional abilities can be improved through discipline. Memory re-training is based on the link between our normal encoding and retrieval processes. Training focuses on visual imagery and/or acronyms or rhymes to aid recall.

Executive function means the set of cognitive abilities necessary for behavioural regulation – the ability to initiate and stop actions, plan and execute and deal with the unexpected. These skills are necessary for the ability to empathise, to recognise emotions and the mental states of others. Personality changes and inappropriate social behaviours, such as disinhibition and indifference, are common. Modifications are essential for resumption of social roles.

Executive and social cognition deficits are frequently present after brain injury. Goal management training (GMT) is one method, the focus of which is to teach the patient to pause, assess, monitor and adjust goals in order to stay on target.

It is also important to consider the person's psychological status. Even mild residual problems can constitute a significant insult to a person's sense of self. Whatever rehabilitation strategy is used, psychological support is essential to assist the patient, their family and carers to come to terms with any enduring changes and to recognise a new post-injury identity.

# Specific Problems

## Spasticity and Ataxia

The impact of spasticity is varied. On one level it may be useful to allow standing when weakness would preclude it, but it can also cause pain and lead to long-term problems such as pressure sores and contractures. As spasticity increases, walking becomes slower, falls more frequent and the ability to transfer or propel a wheelchair reduced. Poorly managed spasticity has long-term consequences. Muscle shortening and tendon contractures lead to restriction of passive movement, physical deformity and cause difficulties with hygiene, dressing, positioning and seating. Pressure sores may increase spasticity and spasms to cause a vicious circle. Early identification of these issues enables timely intervention.

Education of the individual, their family or carers and techniques such as stretching and/or standing are vital. Drugs are also helpful. Those most commonly used are baclofen, tizanidine, benzodiazepines, dantrolene, gabapentin, pregabalin and cannabinoids. The cannabinoid nabiximols (Sativex) has been licensed and is popular. Botulinum toxin type A is widely used. Botox injections most commonly given are medial popliteal blocks to aid spastic foot drop or obturator nerve blocks, either in ambulatory patients with scissoring gait or to improve perineal hygiene and seating posture in those with contractures.

Intrathecal therapies should be considered if oral drugs and physical measures are not tolerated. Small dosages of intrathecal baclofen via a pump are effective. Intrathecal phenol is a cheap and near-permanent solution, but it is reserved for those with no functional movement in their legs, who have lost bladder and bowel function and have impaired leg sensation. Ataxia is challenging to manage (Chapter 17). Movement disorders are discussed in Chapter 6.

## Pain

Pain may be secondary to mechanical factors. Back pain is common in wheelchair users. Pain relief should include local measures such as heat pads and TENS, though drugs may be necessary – initially, NSAIDs and simple analgesics. Shoulder pain is common following stroke. Prevention includes support of the flaccid arm and careful handling techniques to avoid traction injury and sometimes electrical stimulation. Neuropathic pain, pain in MS and central post-stroke pain are discussed in Chapter 23.

## Bladder, Bowel and Sexual Dysfunction

Bladder and bowel dysfunction are common (Chapters 16 and 25). Urinary incontinence after stroke and TBI is usually caused by disruption of inhibition of bladder contractility, with detrusor hyper-reflexia. Detrusor hypo-reflexia and retention can also occur. Occasionally, frontal lobe damage causes inability to suppress the urge to void.

Bowel dysfunction can be distressing and can occasionally lead to pseudo-obstruction. Usually, individuals complain of constipation and/or urgency, rather than incontinence.

Sexual dysfunction, often overlooked (Chapter 25), is common after stroke and TBI and in all neurodegenerative conditions. Psychosexual counselling is helpful. In males, sildenafil, tadalafil and vardenafil have reduced the need for invasive techniques such as intracavernosal injection. Women complain of vaginal dryness and difficulty reaching orgasm; lubricating gels can be helpful. Sildenafil may help some women.

## Fatigue

Fatigue is particularly troublesome following TBI and stroke. Quality of life measures identify this as a major issue. Fatigue can limit education, employment and social opportunities. CNS stimulants are best avoided. Modafinil and 3,4-diaminopyridine are sometimes used. Graded exercise, as part of an agreed goal-directed programme, is probably the most helpful, but it is hard to persuade people that to become tired can overcome fatigue. Cold water immersion therapies are sometimes helpful, if they can be tolerated.

## Dysphagia

Effective dysphagia management, to prevent its attendant risks of dehydration, malnutrition, aspiration and chest infections in the context of single incident or deteriorating neurological conditions, is vital. Dysphagia occurs in some 80% of stroke patients. Aspiration is a common cause of chest infection and death. Video-fluoroscopy and endoscopy increase the reliability of clinical assessment.

## Neuropsychiatric and Endocrine Problems

Neuropsychological problems are common in any physical illness. In neurological disorders, additional factors relating to lesion location may be relevant, for example damage affecting frontal–subcortical circuits predisposing to depression. Disordered mood may be complicated after TBI by organic cognitive and behavioural problems, language disorders, confusion or agitation. Depression is under-recognised and under-treated. Anxiety disorders, including obsessive-compulsive, panic and post-traumatic stress, are frequent. Psychosis and suicide are more common in people who have had a TBI.

Endocrine replacement, the result of hypothalamic-pituitary axis dysfunction, is necessary in some cases following severe TBI and can occur following blast injuries. Specialist investigation is essential.

## Single Incident Brain Injury

Stroke and TBI are the commonest causes of acquired single incident brain injury. They involve different populations – most stroke cases are over 65, while TBI affects a younger population. The costs and economics of such brain injuries are major. In the United Kingdom, the annual costs of direct and informal care and lost productivity due to strokes have been estimated at over £7.0 billion – and more after TBI.

Immediate care guidelines and neurosurgical/ITU management following both stroke and head injury are well established and discussed elsewhere. Rehabilitation during the first few weeks addresses prevention of systemic and neurological complications. Later, rehabilitation focuses broadly on skill learning, to reduce dependency, on social and work-related roles, re-entry into the community and issues of life quality.

### Stroke

Stroke – usually a residual hemiparesis – is a common cause of severe physical disablement. Motor impairment is the commonest evident disability, but there are many other issues. At 12 months post-stroke only half of hemiplegic patients have achieved independence in personal care. One-third are depressed. Over half need help with housework, meals and shopping, and many lack a meaningful activity during the day.

Organised early inpatient and later community-based rehabilitation are firmly established. Aspects of care common to acute and rehabilitation Stroke Units include:

- Medical, nursing and therapy assessments
- Recognition and treatment of hypoxia, hyperglycaemia and infection
- Swallowing assessments and avoidance of urinary catheters
- Early mobilisation
- Goal-orientated multi-disciplinary care
- Discharge planning and involvement of carers.

### Traumatic Brain Injury

Following TBI, the physical aspects of rehabilitation are similar to stroke, but long-term disability frequently follows more from cognitive, affective and behavioural impairments in a younger population with a longer life expectancy. This is reflected in the prevalence of TBI survivors in the homeless and in prisons. In the community, TBI cases often require more supervision than physical care, and needs tend to persist.

## Clinical Scales

Various measurements are in use to try to predict outcome following TBI. Each has values and limitations. The practical problem is that for the individual, rather than the group, it is impossible to predict late outcome following TBI until long after the injury. Accurate and considered early diagnosis is essential – on the one hand to identify issues that may not be immediately apparent in those damaged, and on the other to avoid labelling a minor head injury case as brain damaged – a common error. The term mild TBI should be avoided unless there is clear evidence of brain trauma with enduring effects. An outcome-dominated approach (see below) is one approach in the multidisciplinary management of TBI. Some rating scales are mentioned briefly here, and whilst their authors tried to provide data of value, the scales are neither linear nor, in most cases measurements or predictors of overall outcome.

### Glasgow Coma Scale and Post-Traumatic Amnesia Duration

The GCS helps to grade cases in A&E and especially for assessing deterioration. Claims that this correlates well with prognosis are less helpful. Those with a GCS of 3–8 are usually in stupor or coma, but this bears little relation to individual outcome.

Generally, with post-traumatic amnesia duration:

- 10 days PTA usually implies enduring cognitive problems but does not always preclude return to a former job.
- 4 weeks PTA usually precludes a return to a previous employment but not to an altered work role
- 3 months PTA usually precludes a return to regular paid work but not to voluntary work or community independence.

### 'Mayo' Classification

This study used multiple parameters, rather than a single indicator. Some 1500 head injury cases were divided into three:

- Moderate–severe (Definite) TBI – for example those with a defined lesion on imaging
- Mild (Probable) TBI – for example a skull fracture or PTA of less than 24 hours
- Symptomatic (Possible) TBI – for example no loss of consciousness but headache and/or dizziness.

There were difficulties with data collection and interpretation:

- Glasgow Coma Scale and loss of consciousness information was absent in nearly 75%
- Post-traumatic amnesia assessment was absent in over 50%
- CT brain imaging was not carried out in almost 50%
- In the Symptomatic (Possible) group, most had suffered no brain injury, despite the potential TBI label.

### Annegers Post-Traumatic Epilepsy Data

A population of over 4500 head injury cases was divided into mild, moderate and severe and assessed for late post-traumatic epilepsy.

Mild: PTA < 24 hours
Moderate: PTA > 24 hours
Severe: skull fracture, intracranial haematoma, contusion and diffuse axonal injury (DAI).

Outcome data referred to epilepsy alone. Cumulative probability of a seizure following a severe TBI is of the order of 15% at 15 years. Following a mild TBI, there is little increase above the incidence of a seizure in the general population.

### Role of Imaging
MRI is of value in the confirmation of TBI and recognition of unsuspected TBI. However, MRI is of little value in measurement of outcome. There is also an assumption that abnormalities on MR cortical imaging are invariably followed by cognitive/behavioural impairment:

- MR changes in the brain white matter are common in the symptomless population with increasing age. Specialist neuroradiological opinion must be sought before imaging changes are assumed to be typical of brain injury.
- Normal MRI: it is exceptional for MR brain imaging to be normal when there has been a brain injury likely to cause enduring cognitive/behavioural impairment on an organic basis. This is not to say that some neurone damage cannot occur following even minor brain injuries – experimental animal data supports this.
- DAI: this devasting brain injury that follows rotational and severe acceleration/deceleration has specific imaging characteristics. A minority view is that DAI is more common than is generally thought and is a cause of the behavioural complaints that follow a blow to the head, with normal standard MR imaging.
- Hypothalamic-pituitary dysfunction can rarely be diagnosed by imaging following TBI: specialist endocrine assessment is required.

### Overall Outcome Assessment of TBI
In the aftermath of a head injury, it is essential to assemble all the evidence – clinical history, GCS, PTA, imaging and in particular a detailed neuropsychological assessment – before concluding that an injury to the brain is the cause of enduring symptoms. Grading on any basis can be misleading. Some broad categories are summarised:

- No firm evidence of TBI following appraisal of the history, imaging and neuropsychological assessment. Patients should not be told that they have suffered a brain injury. Some have complaints covered by the term mild neuro-cognitive disorder, which implies either organic or non-organic features. The term post-concussion syndrome has been dropped from DSM-5.
- Evidence of TBI from the history and imaging, with defined mild neurocognitive/behavioural impairment. These cases are typically self-caring and able to return to their former employment. There is a modest increase in post-traumatic epilepsy.
- Evidence of TBI from the history, and imaging, with evident severe neurocognitive/behavioural impairment. Cases may be able to return to some supervised employment. Residual cognitive problems typically involve speed, attention, memory and executive function, often accompanied by irritability, impulsivity and verbal aggression, triggered by anxiety – from difficulties in problem solving with increases in environmental demand.
- Evidence of TBI from the history, and imaging, as above, with severe neurocognitive/behavioural impairment. Such cases require long-term care in form.
- Persistent low awareness states, often requiring feeding and 24-hour care. There is increasing realisation that in some of these cases, responsiveness can be limited more by failure of motor outflow rather than a failure of understanding, even years after injury.

*Dementia*

It is sometimes suggested that there is an increase in dementia following a TBI, even of mild degree. This difficult issue requires qualification:

- Dementia is common in the ageing population, and there is a tendency to assign a cause without a clear evidence base.
- If the volume of brain substance is reduced, for example by a previous TBI, the onset of a neurodegeneration such as Alzheimer's will tend to be more evident.
- One detailed study of over one million people of whom over 130 000 had suffered a TBI indicated a small increase in dementia following TBI but with a distinctly low hazard ratio of 1 : 1.2.
- Neuropathological changes of Alzheimer's are not caused by TBI.

## Service Delivery

Elements of the delivery of rehabilitation include:

- problem definition
- inter-disciplinary assessment
- treatment planning and delivery
- evaluation and reassessment.

Interdisciplinary assessment identifies contributing problems. Take, for example a brain and spinal injury case with a sacral pressure sore. Contributing factors include immobility, incontinence, under-nutrition, lack of insight, low mood and spasms/spasticity, aggravated by constipation and incomplete bladder emptying, and pain from the sore.

- Tone problems are helped by a pressure-relieving cushion
- Nutrition can readily be improved
- CBT and/or an antidepressant helps depression
- A bulk laxative helps constipation and may well help the bladder.

This analysis needs nursing, psychology, medical, OT and physiotherapy support.

One framework for classifying and communicating an individual's difficulties is The International Classification of Function, Disability and Health. Disabilities result from:

- Impairments – losses of body functions/structures
- Activity limitations
- Participation restrictions.

The level of functioning is a complex product of interactions between medical conditions and contextual factors. Contextual factors mean:

- Social and physical environmental factors – social attitudes, access to buildings and legal protection
- Personal factors – gender, age, health conditions, social/family background, religion, education, behaviour pattern, self-esteem, stigma and how a disability is experienced.

It will also be obvious that the way in which a disability has been caused will have a profound effect – an injury caused by one's own fault is perceived very differently to being struck down on zebra crossing. Similar injuries have different outcomes.

## Goal Setting

Having identified the capabilities, disabilities and priorities, the next step is a goal-orientated treatment plan.

Goal origin – self-set or assigned goals – is important. There are four key intervention points:

1) goal intention: definition of practical, attainable goals, the aim being to achieve self-sufficiency
2) specific goal setting – the target and time constraints
3) carrying out the goal-related activity, specifying who does what and when, with plans to overcome problems
4) appraisal, feedback and reward.

## Outcome Measurement

Evaluation of rehabilitation examines process and/or functional outcome. Funding providers often request such evidence. Achievement of a goal is one measure, but one difficulty is that a goal is unique to the individual and thus hard to measure for a group.

Disease-specific measures are another approach, such as the Parkinson's disease questionnaire-39 (PDQ-39) or the MS impact scale (MSIS), the disabilities of the arm, shoulder and hand (DASH) questionnaire and the General Health Questionnaire.

Several measures of outcome are used. The Barthel index (BI) is an ordinal, descriptive scale 1–20. This correlates well with clinical impression and with general ADL. But it is not possible to compare scores from two different scales, e.g. the BI and functional independence measure (FIM), which measure the same construct. Evaluation of service quality is helped by having an Integrated Care Pathway that maps the interventions that should occur during a specific episode.

## Vocational Rehabilitation

Vocational rehabilitation aims to overcome barriers faced by an individual with a disability. This involves:

- Retraining
- Capacity building, e.g. increasing exercise tolerance
- Return to work management, e.g. graded return
- Disability awareness – awareness of how society and individuals perceive people with a disability and its stigma
- Symptom management, e.g. awareness of the roles of OTs and physiotherapists, and counselling
- Adjustments at work – e.g. access and seating.

Employers need to consider:

- Changing recruitment and selection procedures.
- Modifying work premises, e.g. making ramps, modifying toilets.
- Changing job design, work schedules or other work practices, e.g. swapping duties among staff, permitting people to work from home or regular breaks for those with fatigue.
- Modifying equipment, e.g. the provision of voice-activated software for those with upper limb problems or an amplifier-adapted telephone for the hearing impaired.
- Providing training, e.g. induction programmes for staff with a disability and co-workers who ensure staff with a disability can gain access to training.

Ask about work, the impact of work on the disease and the disease upon work. Discuss disclosure, and if agreed, provide support, explaining the needs to an employer. Identify if the individual has access to an occupational health department and inform patient and employer of the terms of the Equality Act.

The UK Equality Act defines that disabled people should not be treated less favourably than others for a reason related to their disability. Employers have to make reasonable adjustments for disabled people. Criteria are broad:

- Whether or not the patient has an illness or disability which is expected to last over 1 year or is a progressive illness.
- Whether the condition affects either the kind of or the amount of work they can do.
- Whether the impact of the condition substantially limits their ability to carry out normal day-to-day activities.

Other practical measures include:

- Making an individual aware of the role of Disability Employment Advisors (DEAs) and the Access to Work scheme. DEAs provide specialist support for those wishing to move into employment or retain an existing job in the event of disability and are based in Jobcentre Plus. The Access to Work scheme provides funding for costs that an employer may incur because of an employee's disability, most commonly used to provide support with transport costs. Other support can be provided such as a powered wheelchair at work, adapted desks, specialist software and adaptations to premises.
- Supporting people who decide to decrease their hours, or retire, by signposting access to benefits and financial advice and providing support with identifying other forms of occupation.

## Acknowledgements

I am most grateful to Richard Greenwood, Diana Caine, Ulrike Hammerbeck, Alexander Leff, Diane Playford, Valerie Stevenson and Nick Ward for their contribution to *Neurology A Queen Square Textbook* Second Edition on which this chapter is based.

# Further Reading, References and Websites

Annegers J, Hauser WA, Coan SP, Rocca WA. A population-based study of seizures after traumatic brain injuries. *N Engl J Med* 1998; 238: 20–24.

Fann JR, Ribe AR, Pedersen HS, Fenger-Grøn M, Christensen J, Benros ME, *et al*. Long-term risk of dementia among people with traumatic brain injury in Denmark: a population-based observational cohort study. *Lancet Psychiat* 2018; 5: 424–431.

Glasgow Coma Scale. The Glasgow structured approach to assessment of the Glasgow Coma Scale, 1974. http//:www.glasgowcomascale.org (accessed 26 August 2021).

Greenwood R, Caine D, Hammerbeck U, Leff A, Playford D, Stevenson V, et al. Restorative neurology, rehabilitation and head injury. In *Neurology A Queen Square Textbook*, 2nd edn. Clarke C, Howard R, Rossor M, Shorvon S, eds. Chichester: Wiley Blackwell, 2017. There are extensive references.

Malec J, Brown AW, Leibson CL, Flaada JT, Mandrekar JN, Diehl NN, *et al*. The Mayo classification system for traumatic brain injury severity. *J Neurotrauma* 2007; 24: 1417–1424.

https://www.gov.uk/government/publications/quality-standards-for-supporting-people-with-long-term-conditions

World Federation for NeuroRehabilitation: http://www.wfnr.co.uk

Free updated notes, potential links and references as these become available: https://www.drcharlesclarke.com
You will be asked to log in, in a secure fashion, with your name and institution.

# 19

# Toxins, Physical Insults, Nutritional and Metabolic Disorders, Unregulated Drugs

Many aspects of medicine, mostly rarities for a general neurologist, are covered in this chapter.

## Heavy Metals, Chemicals and Natural Toxins

### Heavy Metals

Toxicity, typically via mitochondrial damage, tends to be cumulative.

#### Lead: Neuropathy and Encephalopathy

Lead binds to erythrocytes and becomes widely distributed. In adults, a mainly motor poly-neuropathy develops, first affecting the arms, with wrist drop and wasting. Pain can be prominent. Lead encephalopathy causes headache, constipation and fatigue, and then confusion, stupor and seizures. In children, lead can cause learning difficulties. A blue line, a.k.a. lead line, can form at the gingival margin. Investigations: hypochromic microcytic anaemia with erythrocyte basophilic stippling; high blood lead, high uric acid and protoporphyrins and low $\gamma$-amino-laevulinic acid.

#### Mercury: Tremor and Encephalopathy

Poisoning follows either ingestion/inhalation of inorganic mercury – the liquid metal used in thermometer, barometer and battery production or long ago in hat making, when mercuric nitrate was used to cure felt. Tremors develop, with ataxia, weakness, cognitive change and, eventually, stupor/coma. Organic methylmercury, an industrial effluent in Minamata Bay in Japan, was ingested by fish and thus by man and animals. This caused a human encephalopathy in the 1950s and some deaths.

#### Arsenic: Polyneuropathy and Encephalopathy

Inorganic arsenic was once in herbicides and timber preservatives and is now used in glass and microchip production and can be ingested via herbal medications. Odourless and tasteless, arsenic has been questioned as contributing to the deaths of Napoléon Bonaparte and Simon Bolívar. Acutely, vomiting, abdominal pain and diarrhoea progress to

*Neurology: A Clinical Handbook*, First Edition. Charles Clarke.
© 2022 John Wiley & Sons Ltd. Published 2022 by John Wiley & Sons Ltd.

encephalopathy and coma. Chronic exposure causes weight loss, alopecia, white horizontal nail striations, a.k.a. Mees' lines, and polyneuropathy. Arsenic can be detected in hair, nails and teeth. Anaemia with basophilic stippling, pancytopenia and myoglobinuria can occur.

### Manganese and Aluminium: Encephalopathy

Manganese toxicity can follow dust inhalation in steel manufacturing or exceptionally with incorrect parenteral nutrition. Acute exposure can lead to encephalopathy, a.k.a. manganese madness, and chronic exposure, though rarely, to a form of parkinsonism, a.k.a. manganism.

Metallic aluminium usually causes no toxicity. Inhalation of aluminium dust possibly causes an encephalopathy. Dialysis dementia (Chapters 20 and 26) was caused in part by aluminium compounds in dialysis fluids used in the past.

### Thallium: Polyneuropathy and Encephalopathy

Thallium, now banned in pesticides, has been used as a poison. Features are abdominal cramps, vomiting, diarrhoea, alopecia, Mees' lines and a painful polyneuropathy. Thallium can be detected in blood, urine and hair.

### Tin and Bismuth Encephalopathy

Organic forms of tin, particularly triethyl tin, are toxic and can cause an encephalopathy. Bismuth, used in dressings, peptic ulcer treatment and to bulk stools, can exceptionally cause an encephalopathy.

## Solvents and Chemicals

Inhalation of many solvent vapours can cause progressive cognitive, motor and cerebellar deficits. Many are used as recreational drugs.

### Toluene

Toluene, a.k.a. methyl benzene, is a hydrocarbon used in paints, glues and petrol. Poisoning follows glue-sniffing and industrial processes. Toluene crosses the blood–brain barrier readily, to cause demyelination, neuronal damage and also a neuropathy. Inhalation gives some euphoria but can cause headache and vomiting. Long-term exposure causes tremor and encephalopathy. Established damage in glue sniffers rarely improves.

### Trichloroethylene, Tetrachlorethylene, Ethylene Oxide, Xylene, Styrene, Acrylamide, Acrylonitrile, Methyl Bromide, Allyl Chloride and Methyl Chloride

These chemicals used widely in petrochemical and building industries cause a variety of encephalopathies, neuropathies, cranial neuropathies and optic nerve disease. Substantive problems are rare but have come to prominence after incidents, such as with methyl bromide, the cause of deaths in a Royal Navy submarine in World War II.

### Cyanide

Cyanide is rapidly lethal – either as the colourless gases hydrogen cyanide and cyanogen chloride or as crystalline sodium or potassium cyanide. Cyanide blocks cellular respiration enzymes. When inhaled or ingested, cyanide can cause coma and seizures within seconds.

Prolonged intake of low levels of cyanide, such as consuming improperly processed cassava roots – a food source in parts of Africa – can lead to weakness and encephalopathy. Poisoning can occur with smoke inhalation, which probably contributed to deaths in the Grenfell Tower fire in London in 2017. Hydrogen cyanide, a component of the gas Zyklon B, was one method said to have been preferred (by the staff) in Auschwitz for mass extermination during World War II. Hydrogen cyanide has also been used for judicial execution in the United States, and potassium cyanide pills for suicide. And see Konzo. Management: smoke inhalation should be treated with immediate respiratory support and hydroxycobalamin. Blood cyanide levels of 0.5–1 mg/L are mild. Those greater than 3 mg/L generally cause death.

## Methyl Alcohol (Methanol)
Methanol is an industrial solvent and a by-product of ethanol distillation. It is also abused. Toxicity can cause encephalopathy and optic neuropathy.

## Nitrous Oxide
Toxicity from nitrous oxide, a.k.a. laughing gas, occurs very rarely with prolonged general anaesthesia or following abuse. Nitrous oxide disrupts $B_{12}$-dependent pathways. A condition similar to subacute combined degeneration (Chapter 26) can develop.

## Organophosphates
Many pesticides contain organophosphates (OPs). These inhibit cholinesterases, to produce salivation, lacrimation, diarrhoea and urinary frequency. Chronic exposure, a.k.a. sheep dippers' flu, causes headache, rhinitis, pharyngitis and myalgia that resolve over 3 weeks. Muscle weakness occasionally leads to respiratory failure; encephalopathy can occur. There remains controversy about very low levels of OPs, for example in aircraft cabin air – these are generally believed to be harmless.

## Carbon Monoxide
Carbon monoxide (CO), a colourless, odourless gas, is produced by incomplete combustion. It can be inhaled via car exhausts and incorrectly installed heaters and flues. CO binds to haemoglobin preferentially, to form carboxyhaemoglobin, leading rapidly to hypoxaemia. Carboxyhaemoglobin also inhibits oxidative phosphorylation in mitochondria. Mild exposure causes headache, dizziness and confusion. Progressive breathlessness can develop rapidly, with stupor, coma, seizures and cardiac arrest. Cases may have pink–red skin or cyanosis. Coma is followed by death in about 25%. Some survivors have cognitive impairment and/or extrapyramidal features: initial choreiform movements develop into progressive tremor and parkinsonism. Chronic low-level CO poisoning – headache, fatigue and dizziness – is contentious. Prevention: good building practice, chimney maintenance and CO alarms.

## Natural Toxins

### Marine Toxins
Many are unaffected by cooking, freezing or salting. They can be divided into:

- *Ingested*: elaborated by microorganisms – ciguatera, puffer fish, shellfish and scombroid.
- *Contact*: jellyfish, sea urchins, sea anemone, venomous fish and stingrays.
- *Envenomation toxins*: sea snakes and cone snails, whose neuropeptides aim to kill prey.

***Ciguatera*** Ciguatera poisoning follows eating various reef fish, such as barracuda and snapper, mostly in the Indian Ocean, Pacific and Caribbean between latitudes 35° N and S. Fish consume a dinoflagellate that elaborates ciguatoxin that activates voltage-gated sodium channels. Poisoning: vomiting, cramps and diarrhoea, perioral, limb and trunk paraesthesiae. Mild forms resolve within several days. Cranial nerve palsies, a polymyositis and a rapidly progressive polyneuropathy can rarely develop.

***Tetrodotoxin*** Tetrodotoxin (TTX) occurs in liver and ovaries of various puffer fish, a delicacy (*fugu*) in Japan, toad fish and some crabs. This dangerous toxin blocks voltage-gated Na channels. Onset is with numbness of the lips and tongue and facial and limb paraesthesiae. Vomiting, bradycardia, paralysis and death can follow.

***Scombroid*** Scombroid poisoning occurs worldwide and is caused by bacterial degradation that liberates histamine in tuna, mackerel and other fish that have not been cleaned or frozen promptly. Onset resembles anaphylaxis with pruritus, tachycardia, severe throbbing headache, erythema, urticaria, paraesthesiae and palpitation. Though dramatic, this is almost always self-limiting.

***Shellfish, Contact and Envenomation Toxins*** Most shellfish poisoning is caused by infection – diarrhoea, vomiting and prostration can be dramatic but are usually self-limiting. Less frequently, saxitoxin is the cause, a heat-stable toxin concentrated within shellfish. This blocks voltage-gated Na channels. There is a rapid onset of paraesthesiae, particularly periorbital, limb and respiratory muscle weakness. Outbreaks occur in Europe and elsewhere that can lead to a ban on shellfish harvesting.

Contact and envenomation toxins, such as those from jellyfish contain various small polypeptides, phospholipids, glycoproteins and amines that also act largely by blocking voltage-gated Na channels.

## Snake Venoms

Venom from snakes of the *Elapidae* family – the cobra, banded krait and sea snakes – contains bungarotoxins and proteolytic toxins that cause initially local pain, swelling and erythema around the bite. Over the next 12 hours neuromuscular junction blockade, muscle fasciculation and hypotension develop. Snake bites generally cause death because of their systemic effects.

## Spider Venoms

Female *Latrodectus* spiders that include the Black Widow produce latrotoxin that triggers massive presynaptic neurotransmitter release from the neuromuscular junction. Intense pain around the bite can be followed by abdominal muscle and limb spasms. These spiders are widely distributed but are not native to northern Europe. Despite their notoriety, *Latrodectus* bites can be exceedingly unpleasant, though rarely fatal. Female widows are also known to eat their male consorts.

Funnel-web spiders, a.k.a. atracids, native to Australia, produce potent toxins that open voltage-gated Na channels to produce a surge of catecholamines and acetylcholine.

Wandering males are the usual culprits. Bites are painful – piloerection, sweating, spasms and extreme hypertension can follow, followed by hypotension, cerebral oedema and occasionally death. Immediate treatment can be lifesaving; an antivenom prepared from the Sydney funnel-web spider is used.

### Scorpion Venoms
All scorpions elaborate toxins, but the majority do not pose a serious threat. There is intense local pain, followed occasionally by hypotension, fasciculation and progressive weakness. Scorpion venom is used in the pharmaceutical industry and highly valued (>£5 k/litre). Scorpions are a delicacy in Shandong, China.

### Tick Paralysis
Tick toxins from the Rocky Mountain wood tick, the American dog tick and an Australian tick *Ixodes holocyclus* can rarely cause a rapid weakness of ocular, bulbar and limb muscles.

### Fungal Poisons
Fungal poisons are diverse. Some of the *Amanitaceae* family such as the fly agaric (*Amanita muscaria*) contain toxins that act at GABA, glutamate and acetylcholine receptors. The high fatality rate with the Death Cap (*Amanita phalloides*) is caused by amatoxin. This inhibits mRNA synthesis and leads to hepatic and renal damage. Psilocybin mushrooms, a.k.a. magic mushrooms, are widely used hallucinogens.

*Lathyrism*   Lathyrism occurs where the chickling pea/grass pea *Lathyrus sativus* is eaten and endemic in parts of Bangladesh, India and Ethiopia – overconsumption of this generally nutritious legume is implicated. β-N-oxalylamino-L-alanine (BOAA) is an agonist of glutamate receptors. Degeneration occurs in the cortex and pyramidal tracts, with a spastic paraparesis and/or polyneuropathy. Lathyrism can be prevented by leaching grass peas with water.

A related toxin, β-methylamino-L-alanine (BMAA), occurs in cycad palm fruit and may be implicated in the ALS–parkinsonism–dementia complex amongst the Chamorro people of the Mariana islands.

*Konzo*   Konzo occurs in epidemics in East and Central Africa. Children and young women develop symmetrical spastic paralysis and optic nerve lesions. It is possibly associated with dietary cyanide following poorly prepared cassava.

*Hemlock*   *Conium maculatum*, a flowering plant in the carrot family, is native to Europe and widely distributed. It resembles both carrot and parsley. Various piperidine alkaloids are highly poisonous. The alkaloid coniine acts directly on nicotinic acetylcholine receptors and produces paralysis similar to curare. Hemlock was used to poison condemned prisoners in ancient Greece. Socrates took hemlock to kill himself after his trial.

*Subacute Myelo-Optico Neuropathy and Tropical Myeloneuropathy*   Subacute myelo-optico neuropathy (SMON) occurred in Japan mainly in the 1960s. It may have been caused by the antiparasitic drug clioquinol.

Tropical myeloneuropathy describes **s**yndromes with nutritional and/or toxic causes including malnutrition, cyanide intoxication from cassava and lathyrism. A particular epidemic in

Cuba was associated with optic neuropathy, deafness, dorsolateral myelopathy, bulbar weakness and axonal neuropathy. This seemed to be associated with poor diet, tobacco, alcohol and excessive sugar, but an imported toxin from a country nearby has been questioned as the cause.

## Radiation

Radiation occurs naturally at low intensity. Increased levels are caused by occupational or therapeutic radiation and nuclear weapons. UV, infrared, microwaves, radio waves and laser radiation do not cause ionisation. Ionising radiation is produced by high-energy waves that can break chemical bonds, causing DNA damage and mutations – by $\alpha$ particles, electrons, neutrons or protons.

- Alpha particles – two protons and two neutrons – are produced by uranium, radium and polonium. This radiation is usually blocked by paper or clothing but toxic when ingested or inhaled.
- Beta particles are high-energy electrons emitted from isotopes of strontium 90, used to generate X-rays and radiotherapy. Toxicity also occurs with ingestion.
- High-energy neutrons are produced with nuclear fission and are a serious radiation hazard following a nuclear blast or if a reactor damaged.
- Proton exposure also occurs naturally from cosmic radiation.

Nuclear radiation affects first rapidly dividing tissues – skin, bone marrow and gut.

Late toxicity following accidental, therapeutic or deliberate exposure to radiation follows, in organs with slowly dividing cells such as the CNS, kidney and liver, causing radiation necrosis. A delayed complication is malignancy, particularly thyroid, breast and leukaemia. The story of Lucky Dragon 5, the Japanese fishing boat caught in fallout in 1954 from the US Bikini Atoll hydrogen bomb drop, and the Chernobyl disaster in 1986 make grim reading. Therapeutic irradiation is discussed in Chapter 21.

## Lightning and Electrical Shocks

Each year in the United Kingdom, some 50 people are struck by lightning with about three fatalities. Electric shocks at work or at home kill about 30.

### Lightning

It is cloud-to-ground lightning that causes injury. The prelude to a strike, familiar to many mountaineers, is the build-up of atmospheric charge – buzzing of ice axes, skin tingling and hair on end. Immediate evacuation from a summit or a ridge is essential, if feasible – one does not have long.

- Direct strikes are the most damaging when the head is struck.
- Side flash occurs when a nearby tree is struck, and when lightning strikes the ground a shock can be felt up the legs.
- Most indoor strikes are minor – current dissipates along wiring.

It is unusual for lightning to damage aircraft, cars or ships because vehicles act as Faradic cages – the container shields its contents from external electric fields.

### High-Voltage (>1000 V) and Low-Voltage Injuries

Low-voltage injuries that follow a shock at home are rarely severe. High-voltage injuries usually affect those whose occupations bring them into contact with power lines or electrified rails. Kite flying, angling and parachuting are potential risks. High voltages cause most deaths.

### Injury from Lightning and Electric Shock

This can be:

- Immediate and transient
- Immediate and permanent
- Delayed and/or progressive
- Via trauma – for example head or spinal injury.

Confusion, amnesia, paraesthesiae and limb weakness are common transiently. Keraunoparalysis (*kerauno*, Greek = thunderbolt), a.k.a. Charcot paralysis, is short-lived lower limb paralysis that usually resolves over hours.

Mechanisms of more permanent damage are a mixture of thermal and non-thermal effects. CNS haemorrhage, gross and petechial and myelin breakdown occur. Cerebral oedema, stroke due to arterial or venous sinus thrombosis, seizures, extrapyramidal syndromes and cord lesions can follow – and rhabdomyolysis, renal failure and a compartment syndrome can occur. Fern-shaped skin burns can follow lightning – discolouration can persist for years. Cataracts can follow electrical injuries. Delayed and/or progressive complaints such as chronic regional pain may occur, typically when there is litigation.

## Heat, Cold, Diving and High Altitude

### Heat Stroke

A core temperature exceeding 40 °C (104 °F) causes this serious condition, which occurs following prolonged exertion during hot weather or too much clothing such as wet suits. Viral illness, obesity, dehydration, alcohol, cocaine and amphetamines may contribute.

There is tachycardia, hypotension, dehydration, multi-organ failure and stupor. Vague weakness, nausea, cramp and headache can pass unrecognised. Coma carries a high mortality.

### Hypothermia, Frostbite and Non-Freezing Cold Injury

A core temperature <35 °C (95 °F) defines hypothermia. Primary hypothermia is caused by cold and/or immersion, typically at sea, in remote areas or in unheated buildings. Secondary hypothermia is failure of thermoregulation, e.g. with hypothyroidism or a hypothalamic lesion. Hypothermia causes bradycardia resistant to atropine. With mild primary hypothermia, there is intense shivering, confusion, lethargy, poor coordination, dysarthria and sluggish reflexes. Severe hypothermia (<28 °C) causes rigidity, areflexia and coma. At core temperatures <20 °C the EEG can be flat, and the patient unresponsive with fixed pupils. Management: rescue casualties at sea horizontally, if possible. On land, huddle. In hospital, prevent arrhythmias. Ensure adequate oxygen. Rewarm slowly with warm IV fluids. Cases can appear dead, but hypothermia has also neuroprotective effects – some recover completely.

Frostbite, typically of the fingers, toes and nose/ears is the damage that follows when tissue freezes. Non-freezing cold injury (NFCI) describes persistent painful neurovascular symptoms, usually in the feet, following exposure to low temperatures, usually below 15 °C but above freezing. Symptoms can be permanent. Secondary Raynaud's may develop. NFCI has been a problem in the United Kingdom in soldiers of Afro-Caribbean origin.

## Diving and Decompression Sickness (DCS)

Effects of diving relate to high pressure or decompression. Barotrauma occurs when divers descend below 100 m, breathing helium and oxygen mixtures. This can affect the middle/inner ear, sinuses, teeth or gut causing headache, face and ear pain, vertigo, hearing loss and abdominal pain. Direct CNS injury causes tremor, myoclonus, hyperreflexia and cognitive disturbance. Decompression sickness (DCS): nitrogen dissolved in tissues at depth is released as gas bubbles – DCS, a.k.a. the bends, usually develops within 2 hours of surfacing.

- DCS type I: limb and joint pain.
- DCS type II: cardiorespiratory and CNS problems.

Cerebral DCS can lead to headache, gait disturbance, fatigue, diplopia and/or visual loss. There can be hemiparesis, aphasia, hemianopia, encephalopathy and coma. There is brain oedema, haemorrhagic infarction, axonal degeneration and demyelination. Spinal cord DCS can cause a thoracic myelopathy. DCS requires urgent hyperbaric oxygen: most resolve, but residual deficits occur in some.

## High Altitude: Acute Mountain Sickness, Cerebral and Pulmonary Oedema

Acute mountain sickness (AMS) is common in unacclimatised people who ascend rapidly to 2500 m and higher and is usually self-limiting. Headache, fatigue, dizziness, insomnia and vomiting can be prevented by slow ascent – ideally gaining height above 2500 m at 300–500 m/day and carrying little. Acetazolamide, the carbonic anhydrase inhibitor, is widely used for prevention, but a trial dose at sea level is helpful – some do not like the tingling the drug causes. Dexamethasone, analgesics and antiemetics can also be helpful when symptoms are severe. A few cases develop the complications of cerebral and pulmonary oedema, usually >3500 m.

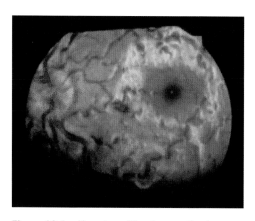

Figure 19.1 Abrupt papilloedema, retinal oedema and venous congestion on Mount Everest. *Retinal photo:* Dr Charles Clarke.

On a 6000-m peak, there is c. 50% of sea-level oxygen; arterial $pO_2$ is c. 50 mmHg. Brain perfusion increases even at 3500 m and can lead to cerebral oedema. Onset is usually with headache and ataxia, cognitive problems and/or hallucinations. Papilloedema (Figure 19.1) and focal signs follow with stupor, coma and death. Sudden cerebral oedema can develop unpredictably at extreme altitude, usually >7000 m.

Investigations are usually impractical. When MRI has been undertaken, brain swelling and sometimes oedema of the splenium of the corpus callosum (Figure 19.2) has been noted. Retinal haemorrhages are also common at >5000 m but rarely cause symptoms or visual loss. They usually resolve spontaneously (Figure 19.4). At autopsy cerebral oedema, ring haemorrhages and arterial and venous thrombosis are seen (Figure 19.3).

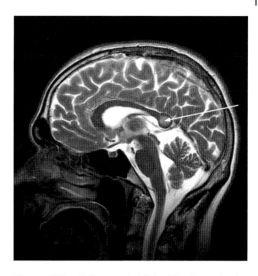

**Figure 19.2** Splenium in high-altitude cerebral oedema. *Source*: Courtesy of Dr S. Wong.

High-altitude pulmonary oedema causes a dry cough, dyspnoea, crackles in the lung bases and occasionally pink frothy sputum.

A high index of suspicion for these emergencies is essential. Descend as soon as is feasible – most deaths occur when the casualty remains at high altitude. Treatment: dexamethasone, oxygen and/or hyperbaric oxygen via a portable chamber.

Stroke and transient ischaemic attacks occur more commonly than expected – related also to dehydration and polycythaemia. Chronic mountain sickness (Monge's disease) is also well described.

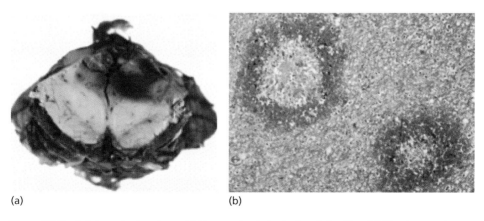

(a)

(b)

**Figure 19.3** Fatal cerebral oedema. (a) Haemorrhagic brainstem infarction. (b) Ring haemorrhages. *Source:* Courtesy of the late Professor Donald Heath.

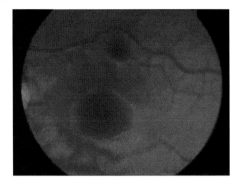

**Figure 19.4** Symptomless retinal haemorrhage on Mount Everest. *Retinal photo:* Dr Charles Clarke.

## Space Travel

Few major neurological problems have been encountered by astronauts. However, vestibular disturbance, weight loss, leg oedema, anaemia, muscle atrophy and negative calcium balance are well recognised. Vestibular reconditioning may be needed on return to earth.

### Neurobiological Weapons

Numerous agents have been considered (Table 19.1).

**Table 19.1** Some potential neurobiological weapons.

Bacteria: *anthrax, brucella, francisella tularensis, rickettsiae, typhoid, shigella, cholera, yersinia pestis*

Viruses: e.g. smallpox, viral haemorrhagic fever

Chemicals: hydrogen cyanide, Zyklon B, chlorine, mustard gas, phosgene, dioxin

Nerve agents: e.g. tabun, sarin, soman, cyclosarin, VX (UK 1950s), VR *et al*, e.g novichok (Soviet Union, 1950s)

Toxins: e.g. aflatoxin, botulinum, ricin, tetrodotoxin, saxitoxin, radioactive toxins

## Vitamin Deficiencies and Copper Deficiency

Deficiencies are summarised in Table 19.2.

**Table 19.2** Vitamin deficiencies and neurology.

| Vitamin | Principal features |
| --- | --- |
| A Retinol | Night blindness |
| $B_1$ Thiamine | Cardiac failure (wet beriberi) |
| | Sensory polyneuropathy (dry beriberi) |
| | Wernicke–Korsakoff syndrome |
| $B_3$ Niacin | Pellagra (dermatitis, diarrhoea, dementia) |
| $B_5$ Pantothenic acid | Paraesthesiae |
| $B_6$ Pyridoxine | Polyneuropathy |
| $B_7$ Biotin | Myalgia, nausea, dermatitis |
| $B_{12}$ Cobalamin | Megaloblastic anaemia, subacute combined degeneration, optic atrophy, dementia |
| Folate | Megaloblastic anaemia, foetal abnormalities |

**Table 19.2** (Continued)

| | |
|---|---|
| C Ascorbic acid | Scurvy – defective collagen, bleeding gums, petechiae, corkscrew hair, impaired wound healing |
| D Cholecalciferol | Proximal myopathy, osteomalacia, rickets |
| E Tocopherol | Spinocerebellar degeneration, neuropathy |
| K Phylloquinone | Haemorrhagic problems |

Copper deficiency is an exceedingly rare cause of myeloneuropathy with ataxia – in enteropathies and with total parenteral nutrition.

## Ethyl Alcohol

Ethanol is rapidly absorbed, sublingually and from the gut, and crosses the blood–brain barrier. It is metabolised in the liver and oxidised to acetaldehyde which is cytotoxic. Intoxication is widely tolerated in many societies. The euphoria, disinhibition and reduced psychomotor capacity are well known. Levels >200 mg/dL cause obvious ataxia, dysarthria, vertigo and nystagmus. Higher levels lead to coma, hypotension and respiratory depression.

### Alcohol Withdrawal

In chronic alcoholism, withdrawal can lead to *delirium tremens* (DTs) – tremulousness, confusion, hyperactivity, hallucinations and seizures can continue for some days, with vomiting, tachycardia, hypertension and sweating. Lucidity follows usually with amnesia. Recurrence is common. Withdrawal seizures, a.k.a. rum fits, a Royal Navy term, and generalised tonic–clonic convulsions can occur. Thiamine and glucose help prevent encephalopathy. A quiet well-lit environment is helpful.

### Alcoholic Cirrhosis and Encephalopathy, Wernicke and Korsakoff

Neurological effects of alcohol abuse often run in parallel with alcohol-related cirrhosis, the commonest serious manifestation of which is portosystemic encephalopathy, with tremor, myoclonus and asterixis.

Acquired nutritional thiamine deficiency causes Wernicke's encephalopathy, acutely or gradually, often triggered by an illness: apathy, confusion, ataxia, with encephalopathy over hours, days/weeks progressing to stupor, coma and death. Hallucinations/agitation are also typical.

- Ophthalmoplegia: lateral recti initially, leading to total external ophthalmoplegia.
- Pupils: sluggish response to light +/− light-near dissociation.
- Fundi: small retinal haemorrhages; occasionally optic neuropathy.
- Nystagmus: horizontal and/or vertical. Ataxia: of gait and/or truncal.
- MRI: high T2W in periaqueductal medial thalamus and shrunken mamillary bodies.
- Serum: low thiamine and erythrocyte transketolase activity. CSF: high protein.
- Pathology: haemorrhages – mamillary bodies, thalamus and pons.
- Treatment: thiamine, sedation and supportive care.

Thiamine depletion can also develop in *hyperemesis gravidarum*, with dialysis, IV nutrition, in severe anorexia, following gut surgery and in AIDS.

Korsakoff's syndrome is a severe amnesia, rarely reversible. Patients show striking loss of memory but retain at the onset normal behaviour. Confabulation is typical. With alcoholism, KS is caused by thiamine deficiency. Other causes: multiple infarcts, anoxia, TBI, herpes simplex encephalitis, severe TLE and frontotemporal tumours.

### Cerebellar Alcoholic Ataxia, Dementia and TBI

Chronic ataxia affects males typically and can progress to inability to stand. Cortical atrophy, ventricular dilatation and dementia develop with prolonged abuse. Depression is common; some develop frank psychosis. TBI – contusions and subdural or extradural haematomas are common.

### Neuropathies, Amblyopia, Strachan's, Myopathy, Marchiafava–Bignami and Foetal Alcohol

Axonal polyneuropathy is common, often mild and mainly sensory.

Common compression neuropathies:

- radial nerve – spiral groove a.k.a. Saturday night palsy
- peroneal nerve – fibula head
- sciatic nerve – gluteal region.

Amblyopia: a rarity – see Chapter 14. Strachan's syndrome is a severe painful ataxic sensorimotor polyneuropathy with optic atrophy caused by multiple nutritional deficits.

Myopathy can develop with chronic abuse or following a binge: pain, cramp, swelling and high CK. Rhabdomyolysis can follow. Cardiomyopathy can coexist.

Marchiafava–Bignami syndrome, a rarity, occurs mainly in the Chianti region of Italy - progressive slowing, incontinence, frontal signs and broad-based gait in chronic alcoholics.

Alcohol excess in pregnancy impairs foetal growth, leading to dysmorphic features and microcephaly.

## Malignant Hyperthermia (MH)

This rarity occurs following anaesthesia with halothane, enflurane and isoflurane and/or a muscle relaxant such as succinylcholine. There is fever and rigidity with a high CK level, acidosis and myoglobinuria. Liability is transmitted in an AD fashion – an excitation–contraction coupling abnormality in skeletal muscle. In some, rigidity and hyperpyrexia can develop within 30 minutes. There is similar sensitivity to anaesthetics in some with Duchenne muscular dystrophy, *myotonia congenita*, myotonic dystrophy, central core disease, congenital myopathy and *osteogenesis imperfecta*. With rapid supportive management, recovery is usual.

## Neuroleptic Malignant Syndrome (NMS)

This rare complication of antipsychotic drugs usually begins within 2 weeks of initiating or increasing a neuroleptic. There is typically a severe pyrexia, often >40 °C and progressive encephalopathy. Severe rigidity, rest tremor and dystonia develop. There is tachycardia, tachypnoea, labile blood pressure, skin pallor or flushing and grossly elevated CK. NMS can progress to rhabdomyolysis, renal failure, DIC, shock, seizures and coma. Mortality: about 20%. Stop the neuroleptic; reduce core temperature. Dantrolene is used.

## Serotonin Syndrome and Tyramine Cheese Reaction

SS is a drug reaction usually involving an SSRI. SS is often mild, with tachycardia, shivering, sweating and mydriasis that abates when the SSRI is stopped. Severe forms can progress to hyperthermia, hypertension and encephalopathy. Rigidity, myoclonus, tremor and hyperreflexia can occur. SS occurs with SSRI monotherapy or when there is an interaction between two SSRIs or other drugs that inhibit serotonin re-uptake – for example duloxetine, olanzapine, mirtazapine and venlafaxine.

Tyramine cheese reaction occurs with non-selective MAOIs. Cheese or red wine can lead to hypertension, flushing, headache, vomiting and rarely hyperthermia, DIC and cardiopulmonary arrest.

## Porphyrias

Abnormal synthesis of haem, a precursor of haemoglobin and cytochrome P450 enzymes, characterises these rare conditions. Most are AD inherited.

The most relevant is acute intermittent porphyria (AIP) caused by deficiency of porphobilinogen deaminase. This leads to accumulation of the neurotoxic porphyrin precursors δ-aminolevulinic acid and porphobilinogen.

Many AIP cases remain symptom free throughout life. However, attacks can be triggered by an infection, surgery, the post-ovulation phase of the menstrual cycle or drugs – notably barbiturates and sulphonamides. There are attacks of acute abdominal pain, vomiting, diarrhoea or constipation and confusion, agitation, insomnia and even psychosis, generally commencing in the teens. There can be hypertension, tachycardia, tremor, hyperhidrosis, urinary retention, seizures and hyponatraemia. A polyneuropathy, acute or subacute, can develop. There is no skin photosensitivity. Polyneuropathy follows neurovisceral attacks but can also occur independently. Elevated urine porphobilinogen during an attack is a sensitive indicator of AIP, and this usually remains elevated between attacks. Management: mainly supportive – discuss with a specialist porphyria service. Liver transplantation has helped in some cases.

## Inherited Metabolic Disorders

Many have neurological features (Table 19.3). Discussion is outside the scope of this chapter. It is exceptional for patients with these conditions to present at an adult neurology clinic.

**Table 19.3**   Metabolic disorders - some relevant examples.

| |
|---|
| ***Amino acid metabolism disorders*** |
| Phenylketonuria, homocysteinuria |
| ***Organic acid disorders*** |
| Methylmalonic aciduria |
| ***Urea cycle disorders*** |
| *N*-Acetylglutamate synthase deficiency |
| ***Fatty acid oxidation disorders*** |
| Very long-chain acyl-CoA dehydrogenase (VLCAD) deficiency |
| ***Disorders of carbohydrate metabolism/transport*** |
| GSD V McArdle disease – see Chapter 11 |
| ***Neurotransmitter disorders*** |
| Dopa-responsive dystonia |
| ***Lysosomal storage disorders*** |
| Glycosphingolipidoses – GM1, GM2, Gaucher, Krabbe, Fabry |
| ***Leukodystrophies, leukoencephalopathies*** |
| Nieman-Pick 1,2,3, Alexander, Vanishing white matter disease |
| ***Peroxisomal disorders*** |
| Refsum's disease |
| ***Disorders of phospholipid and glycosphingolipid biosynthesis*** |
| Phosphatidate phosphatase 1 deficiency, AD serine palmitoyltransferase deficiency |

## Unregulated/Illegal Drugs and Drug Abuse

These can be divided broadly into groups (Table 19.4) – but effects frequently fall into more than one category. Whilst called drugs of abuse, serious harm and deaths pale beside alcohol and tobacco. Brief notes follow about some of these widely available compounds. Designer analogues are synthesised to achieve similar effects and navigate around illegality, so no list can be exhaustive.

**Table 19.4**   Unregulated drugs and the nervous system.

| |
|---|
| **Stimulants** |
| *Sympathomimetics* |
| Dexamphetamine (*speed, phet, whizz*), methamphetamine (*crystal meth, meth, ice, glass*), cocaine (*coke, blow, snow, flake*), crack cocaine (*rocks, gravel*) methylphenidate (*kiddy coke, speed*), ephedrine |
| *Serotoninergics* |
| 3,4-Methylenedioxyamphetamine (MDMA, *Ecstasy*), 3,4-methylenedioxy-N-ethylamphetamine (*MDEA, MDE, Eve*) |

**Table 19.4** (Continued)

*Others*

Modafinil, caffeine, nicotine, cathinone (*khat*), methcathinone (*cat, jeff*), mephedrone (*drone, M-CAT, white magic, meow meow*)

**Sedatives, analgaesics and tranquilisers**

*Opiates/opioids*

Morphine, heroin (*smack*), opium, codeine, hydromorphine, fentanyl, carfentanil, pethidine, tramadol

*Cannabis/cannabinoids*

*Barbiturates, benzodiazepines*

*Others*

Methaqualone (*mandrakes, mandies*), gamma-hydroxybutyrate (GHB, *club drug, date rape*), ethanol, methanol

*MPPP, MPTP and parkinsonism*

**Hallucinogens**

*Psychedelics*

Dimethyltryptamine (DMT, Dimitri), other tryptamines, LSD (*acid, tabs, smilies*), psilocybin (*magic mushrooms*), mescaline, ayahuasca

*Dissociatives*

Dextromethorphan, ketamine, methoxetamine, phencyclidine (*angel dust*)

*Deliriants*

Atropine, scopolamine

**Designer drugs – various effects**

MDMA analogues, phenethylamine derivatives (2C drugs), piperazines (BZP, TFMPP), amphetamine analogues, other cathinones, synthetic cannabinoids, numerous others

**Solvents, fuels and gases**

Propane, butane, toluene, freon, nitrous oxide, amyl/isopropyl nitrate and analogues (*poppers*)

**Performance enhancing drugs**

Steroids, erythropoietin (EPO), diuretics, β-blockers, salbutamol

## Stimulants

Dexamphetamine is used in clinical practice. Methamphetamine causes increased alertness, self-confidence, euphoria, extrovert behaviour, loss of appetite, tremor, dilated pupils, tachycardia and hypertension. Paranoid delusions, hallucinations and violence can occur. Massive overdose leads to convulsions, hyperthermia, rhabdomyolysis and intracerebral haemorrhage.

Cocaine is a common stimulant – snorted, taken parenterally or smoked as crack. Moderate doses are associated with mood elevation, increased alertness and enhanced performance, but paranoia, delusions, hallucinations, seizures, choreoathetoid movements and agitation can develop rapidly. Chronic abuse can lead to progressive neuropsychiatric features, visual and auditory hallucinations and rarely to encephalopathy.

Methylphenidate (Ritalin) was once widely used by medical staff on night shifts. It can rarely cause an amphetamine-like reaction, seizures and intracerebral haemorrhage.

Ecstasy induces euphoria, wakefulness, sexual arousal and disinhibition, but it can cause an acute toxic reaction with headache, hypertension, hyperpyrexia, seizures, rhabdomyolysis and cerebral oedema, herniation and death. Ecstasy causes a massive serotoninergic discharge that can resemble schizophrenia. Many substances have been combined with Ecstasy.

Khat is a plant from East Africa and surrounding regions. Leaves are chewed – they contain cathinone, an amphetamine-like stimulant. Toxic effects include anorexia, tremor, tachycardia, hypotension and respiratory arrest. Methcathinone is a derivative. Mephedrone is a synthetic stimulant of the same class.

### Stroke and Other Complications of Stimulants

Crack cocaine is the commonest cause of drug-related stroke – about half of all cases and commonly in middle cerebral artery territory. Imaging shows asymptomatic subcortical white matter lesions in both crack and cocaine users.

Ischaemic stroke can occur for other reasons – hypertension, vasoconstriction, dissection and infective endocarditis. Haemorrhagic stroke and vasculitis can also occur with amphetamines and cocaine. Other effects of stimulants include seizures, hyperthermia, rhabdomyolysis, myocardial infarction and cardiac arrhythmia. Cocaine and amphetamines also cause vocal and motor tics, chorea, an acute torticollis and oromandibular dyskinesia.

### Sedatives, Analgaesics and Tranquillisers

Heroin and morphine are usually administered IV but can be snorted, smoked or injected subcutaneously (skin popping). Injections are often contaminated.

The effects of heroin are an initial analgesic effect and then the 'rush' with euphoria before drowsiness and sometimes hallucinations. Pruritus, dry mouth, nausea, vomiting, constipation and urinary retention can occur. Small pupils are typical. Respiratory depression and hypoxic–ischaemic brain injury can follow. The immediate effects can be reversed with naloxone, the antidote that should be given to anyone with a suspected opiate overdose.

In coma, compression of peripheral nerves can follow – common peroneal, ulnar or sciatic. Rhabdomyolysis can develop. Repeated intramuscular injections can lead to focal fibrosis with contractures. An acute myelopathy can occur with heroin and/or sensorimotor neuropathy. Inhalation of heroin pyrolate, particularly if contaminated by heating the drug on foil, can cause a toxic encephalopathy. Stroke is secondary to an infective vasculitis or the effect of a mycotic aneurysm.

Withdrawal from opioids leads to craving, restlessness, irritability and autonomic symptoms – sweating, lacrimation and rhinorrhoea. There may be piloerection, abdominal cramps, diarrhoea and coughing.

Fentanyl and carfentanil (especially) are vastly more potent than morphine.

Marijuana can be smoked, eaten or injected. It is widely used to induce a sense of relaxation, euphoria and depersonalisation. In high doses there can be hallucinations, paranoia, aggression or sedation. Synthetic cannabinoids are widely available.

Barbiturates have actions that are similar to alcohol. Intoxication leads to slurred speech, gait ataxia, coma, hypotension, hypothermia and eventually respiratory depression. When barbiturates are withdrawn acutely there may be irritability, tremor, tachycardia and a reduced seizure threshold. It may be necessary to reinstitute the barbiturate.

Benzodiazepines induce a comfortable sensation of idleness, but in excess there is drowsiness and confusion, leading to stupor and coma. The effect of an acute overdose can be reversed by flumazenil, a specific antagonist, but this is short-lived. Chronic use leads to dependence. Withdrawal symptoms develop within 24 hours of cessation of short-acting benzodiazepines – irritability, increased sensitivity to light and sound, tremor, tachycardia and delirium.

### MPPP, MPTP and Parkinsonism

A neurotoxin methylphenyltetrahydropyridine (MPTP) undoubtedly causes a largely irreversible parkinsonian syndrome. The MTPT story is that in 1976 a US chemistry graduate BK synthesised illegally and used desmethylprodine (1-methyl-4-phenyl-4-propionoxypiperidine, a.k.a. MPPP, an analogue of pethidine, a.k.a. meperidine). This MPPP contained MTPT as a major impurity. BK developed parkinsonism. He died some 18 months later from a cocaine overdose. In 1983, four people in California developed parkinsonism having used MPPP contaminated with MPTP.

### Hallucinogens

Dimethyltryptamine (DMT, Dimitri) is found in several plants that can be smoked or snorted. It is a component of ayahuasca, the traditional South American plant preparation.

Lysergic acid diethylamide (LSD) alters perception, mood and thought. Acute effects cause dizziness, blurred vision, nausea and weakness. There is often euphoria, depersonalisation, distortion of time and bizarre effects, including arousal and depression that can lead to accidents or even suicide. Chronic abuse can lead to cerebral infarction and cognitive change.

Ketamine has euphoric and hallucinogenic properties. Large doses can lead to coma. Prolonged use can lead to psychosis, agitation, bizarre behaviour and catatonia.

Phencyclidine is taken orally, nasally or by inhalation and causes euphoria. Catatonia and psychosis can develop with chronic abuse.

### Solvents, Fuels and Gases

Lighter fluids, varnishes and paint thinners contain organic solvents such as toluene. Inhalation can produce a rash around the mouth and nose. There are feelings of exhilaration and giddiness, sometimes with hallucinations. Long-term exposure causes a toxic encephalopathy with progressive impairment of coordination and cognition.

## Acknowledgements, Further Reading and Personal References

I am most grateful to Robin Howard, Jeremy Chataway, Mark Edwards, Simon Heales, Robin Lachmann, Alexander Leff and Elaine Murphy for their contribution to *Neurology A Queen Square Textbook* Second Edition on which this chapter is based. Michael Hayle contributed substantially to the section on unregulated drugs.

Howard R, Chataway J, Edwards M, Heales S, Lachmann R, Leff A, *et al.* Toxic, metabolic & physical insults to the nervous system and inherited disorders of metabolism. In *Neurology A Queen Square Textbook*, 2nd edn. Clarke C, Howard R, Rossor M, Shorvon S, eds. Chichester: John Wiley & Sons, 2016. There are many references.

Clarke C. Acute mountain sickness: medical problems associated with acute and subacute exposure to hypobaric hypoxia. *Postgrad Med J* 2006; **82**: 748–753.

Clarke CA, Roworth CG, Holling HE. Methyl bromide poisoning: an account of four recent cases met with in one of HM ships. *Br J Ind Med* 1945; **2**(1): 17–23.

Critchlow S, Seifert R. Khat-induced paranoid psychosis. *Br J Psychiatry* 1987; **150**: 219–222.

European Monitoring Centre for Drugs and Drug Addiction. https://www.emcdda.europa.eu.

Harris JB, Blain PG. Neurotoxicology: what the neurologist needs to know. *J Neurol Neurosurg Psychiatry* 2004; **75**(Suppl III): 29–34.

Langston WJ. The MPTP story. *J Parkinsons Dis* 2017; **7**(Suppl 1): S11–S19.

Wabe NT. Chemistry, pharmacology, and toxicology of khat: a review. *Addict Health* 2011; **3**(3–4): 137–149.

Warrell DA. Venomous animals. *Medicine* 2012; **40**: 159–163.

Also, please visit https://www.drcharlesclarke.com for free updated notes, potential links and other references. You will be asked to log in, in a secure fashion, with your name and institution.

# 20

# Consciousness, Coma, Intensive Care and Sleep

The areas summarised are consciousness and coma, neurological aspects of intensive care, severe traumatic brain injury and sleep disorders.

## Definitions of Consciousness and Coma

To be conscious means to be aware of both self and environment. Its components are:

- Arousal, meaning alertness
- Cognition – comprehension, expression of learning, memory, emotion and sensory input.

Arousal reflects integrity of the ascending reticular activating system and brainstem, while cognition is cortical. Coma means unrousable unresponsiveness that can follow either damage to both cerebral cortices, the brainstem and its projections or metabolic changes. Damage to one hemisphere does not by itself cause stupor or progress to coma.

## States of Impaired Consciousness

The spectrum from normality to coma is shown in Table 20.1.

**Table 20.1** The vocabulary of altered consciousness.

| | |
|---|---|
| Clouding | Impaired attention, distractible, irritable, slow thought |
| Acute confusion | Bewildered, disorientated, impaired comprehension |
| Delirium | Disorientated, irritable, +/− visual hallucinations |
| Obtundation | Mental blunting, apathy, drowsy, little interest in surroundings |
| Stupor | Similar to deep sleep, arousal only by vigorous, repeated stimuli |
| Coma | Unrousable unresponsiveness. Eyes closed (usually). Stimuli: no response |
| Vegetative state | Appears awake but no evidence of awareness |
| Minimally conscious state | Low level responses – after, for example, emergence from coma |
| Locked in | Consciousness and cognition preserved but not evident: see below. |
| Akinetic mutism | Slowed or absent movements +/− paralysis: see below. |
| Psychogenic | Various states: e.g. fugues, NEAD, deliberate. |

*Neurology: A Clinical Handbook*, First Edition. Charles Clarke.
© 2022 John Wiley & Sons Ltd. Published 2022 by John Wiley & Sons Ltd.

**Table 20.2**   Coma + meningism +/- lateralising signs: examples.

| | |
|---|---|
| Infection | meningitis, encephalitis, malaria, HIV, abscess |
| Vascular | subarachnoid haemorrhage |
| Tumour | mass lesion, malignant meningitis |

## Stupor and Coma: A Practical Approach

Following emergency triage, consider the diagnosis in the broadest terms.
   First, answer two questions (Table 20.2)

- Meningism? If present, meningitis is a possibility – and minutes count.
- Are there lateralising signs? If so, a focal brain lesion is likely.

   The stuporose or comatose patient with neither meningism nor lateraling signs (Table 20.3) is the commonest and familiar A&E presentation. Many of such cases will be recognisable immediately from the history or presenting features. Coma of wholly unknown cause is uncommon.

**Table 20.3**   Coma without meningism and without lateralising signs.

| | |
|---|---|
| Drugs | Sedatives, anaesthetics, alcohol, etc. |
| Seizures, epilepsy | Convulsive and non-convulsive status epilepticus, post-ictal coma, non-epileptic (NEAD) status |
| Hypoxia–ischaemia | E.g. encephalopathy following cardiac arrest |
| Respiratory failure | Hypoxaemia, hypercarbia |
| Electrolyte disturbances | Hyponatraemia, hypernatraemia; hypocalcaemia, hypercalcaemia; rarities – hyper/hypomagnesaemia |
| Diabetes mellitus | Hypoglycaemia, ketoacidosis, lactic acidosis, hyperosmolar non-ketotic coma |
| Hepatic and renal failure | Encephalopathy |
| Endocrine failure and overactivity | Panhypopituitarism and pituitary apoplexy, hypothyroidism, hypoadrenalism, Hashimoto's encephalopathy, hyperthyroidism |
| Core temperature | Hypothermia, hyperpyrexia |
| Nutritional | Wernicke's encephalopathy |
| Inborn metabolic | Hyper-ammoniacal states, aminoacidurias, etc. |
| Toxins | E.g. CO, methanol, lead, cyanide, thallium |
| Extrapyramidal | Status dystonicus, neuroleptic malignant and serotonin syndromes |
| Autoimmune | Steroid responsive encephalopathy, encephalitis |
| Others | E.g. porphyria, Reye's syndrome, idiopathic recurrent stupor, mitochondrial disease, hypothalamic lesions, sepsis, malaria, TBI |
| Coma mimics | Catatonia, conversion/psychogenic, malingering |

## Detailed Assessment

- History, from witnesses. Trauma, fever, headache or epilepsy?
- Breath – alcohol, ketones, hepatic or renal fetor?
- Mucous membranes – cyanosis, anaemia, jaundice or carbon monoxide?
- Skull/mastoid/orbital bruising, blood in external auditory meatus? CSF rhinorrhea?
- Otorrhoea or haemotympanum?
- Skin: purpuric/petechial/maculopapular rash – infection? Nailbed splinters (endocarditis)? Bullae – barbiturates? Needle marks – opiates?
- Body temperature: normality does not exclude intracranial infection.
  - Hyperpyrexia: thyrotoxic crisis, heat stroke, Ecstasy, malignant hyperthermia.
  - Hypothermia: accidental, hypothyroidism, hypopituitarism, hypoadrenalism, drugs, alcohol.
  - Profuse sweating: neuroleptic malignant or serotonin syndrome.
- Fundi: diabetes, raised ICP, hypertensive retinopathy, $CO_2$ retention, SAH (subhyaloid blood).
- Blood pressure:
  - hypertension – frequently secondary, e.g. SAH rather than hypertensive crisis.
  - hypotension – shock, hypovolaemia, myocardial infarction, septicaemia.
- Level of consciousness: assess at regular intervals.
- Neurological examination.

### Level of Consciousness: Glasgow Coma Scale

The Glasgow Coma Scale (GCS) is widely used (Table 20.4). Strengths are its brevity and its recognition within all emergency services. However, whilst the shorthand GCS 15/15 implies normality, and 3/15 deep coma, the sequential numbers bear little relation to each other. A notation such as GCS 12/15 [4 + 5 + 3] is sometimes taken to indicate brain trauma or intracranial pathology. The reality is that Confused speech (4) + Localises pain (5) + Eye opening to speech (3) can occur when a normal person is awakened from deep sleep, with alcohol or analgaesia/sedation.

**Table 20.4** Glasgow Coma Scale score.

| Eye opening | Motor response | Verbal |
|---|---|---|
| 4 Spontaneous | 6 Obeys command | 5 Orientated |
| 3 To speech | 5 Localises pain | 4 Confused speech |
| 2 To pain | 4 Withdrawal | 3 Inappropriate words |
| 1 None | 3 Flexion posturing | 2 Incomprehensible sounds |
| | 2 Extensor posturing | 1 None |
| | 1 None | |

## Neurology

Examination in coma is limited. The principles are outlined here.

### Eyelids in Coma
Eyelids are closed, and slow closure follows gentle parting the lids. In psychogenic (faked) coma, there is forceful resistance. The rare 'eyes open coma' can follow a brainstem lesion.

### Pupils in Coma
Equal, light-reactive pupils indicate an intact optic nerve-midbrain tegmentum-IIIrd nerve pathway.

- Normal pupils are typical of a metabolic cause.
- Pupils size fluctuation (hippus): normal phenomenon.
- Ciliospinal (pupillary-skin) reflex – pupil dilation to pain applied to neck/face: normal.
- Horner's syndrome: sympathetic pathway lesions – a lateralising sign.
- IIIrd nerve compression: first a sluggish light response, followed by fixed dilatation.
- Fixed dilated pupils follow brain death and occur in hypothermia. Anticholinergics - atropine, cyclopentolate - also cause dilated pupils.
- Injury, topical or systemic medication can cause asymmetry or even a fixed pupil.
- Mid-position unresponsive pupils: dorsal tectal, pretectal or tegmental lesions.
- Irregular oval, unequal pupils can follow brainstem herniation.

### Eye Movements in Coma
Roving eye movements – slow random lateral movements, conjugate or dysconjugate – occur in light coma, typically metabolic. The eyes may be either dysconjugate, conjugate and midline or deviated. Some dysconjugate deviation is often decompensation of a pre-existing strabismus. In coma, eye movement abnormalities can be masked.

- Start simply: are the eyes symmetrical? If not, this is a potential lateralising sign.
  - Is there a IIIrd nerve palsy, a VIth or internuclear ophthalmoplegia?
  - A complete IIIrd: dilated pupil, ptosis, eye deviation 'down and out'.
  - Internuclear ophthalmoplegia: failure of ADDuction with nystagmus of the ABDucting eye.
  - A VIth nerve lesion: inward deviation and failure of ABDuction.
- Is there horizontal conjugate ocular deviation?
  - With a destructive cortical lesion, the eyes deviate TOWARDS the side of lesion and thus AWAY from a hemiparesis. Others (below) are unusual.
  - Below the pontomesencephalic junction, eyes deviate AWAY from the lesion side and look TOWARDS the hemiparesis – a relative rarity.
  - A seizure can cause intermittent adversive (AWAY from the focus) deviation. Eyes can also deviate TOWARDS the focus in post-ictal gaze palsy.
  - Horizontal nystagmus: an irritative adversive (AWAY from) epileptic focus – usually with eyelids, face, jaw or tongue movements.
- Is there some rarity?
  - Tonic downward deviation: tectal compression – e.g. thalamic or dorsal midbrain haemorrhage.

- Prolonged tonic upward deviation can follow hypoxic–ischaemic damage but may occur transiently in seizures, oculogyric crises or with neuroleptics.
- Intermittent nystagmoid jerks, horizontal or rotatory – mid or lower pontine damage.
- Dysconjugate vertical gaze may be caused by a skew deviation.
- Parinaud's syndrome (dorsal midbrain): loss of upgaze, light-near dissociation of pupils, convergence-retraction nystagmus and eyelid retraction. There may also be accommodation or convergence spasm, oculomotor palsy (III, IV), skew deviation or internuclear ophthalmoplegia.
- Periodic alternating gaze (an absolute rarity) – horizontal deviation for several minutes before alternating – is seen in hepatic encephalopathy.

## Other Cranial Nerves

In light coma, a bilateral blink reflex is usual in response to corneal or eyelash stimulation. An LMN facial nerve or nuclear lesion causes ipsilateral paralysis. A UMN lesion produces contralateral facial weakness but tends to spare the forehead. A facial grimace reflects facial nerve function – this may be asymmetrical. The jaw jerk may be brisk. Vestibulo-ocular reflexes: passive head turning or irrigation rarely gives useful additional information.

## Motor Responses

Assess:

- Resting posture of the limbs and head
- Involuntary and spontaneous movements
- Two characteristic patterns:
  - Decorticate posturing refers to flexion at the elbows and wrists with shoulder adduction and internal rotation and extension of the lower extremities – poor localising value.
  - Decerebrate posturing refers to bilateral extension of the lower extremities, adduction and internal rotation of the shoulders and extension at the elbows. It is usually caused by severe brainstem lesions.

*Tone and Reflexes*   Asymmetry of limb tone is a lateralising sign. Spasticity implies an established lesion. The presence of a unilateral grasp reflex indicates an ipsilateral frontal lobe disturbance. Remember that acute damage to the spinal cord can lead to initial bilateral limb hypotonia.

## Involuntary Movements and Respiration

Tonic–clonic or other stereotyped movements suggest a form of epilepsy or myoclonus. Plucking movements occur in light coma. Respiration slows as coma deepens and abnormal patterns develop:

- Ataxic respiration: an irregular cycle with apnoea may herald respiratory arrest.
- Cheyne–Stokes respiration: smooth waxing and waning of breath volume and frequency separated by periods of central apnoea.
- Apneustic breathing: sustained inspiratory cramps with prolonged pauses at full inspiration.

## Other Coma-Like States

### Locked-In Syndrome

Locked-in implies preservation of consciousness but dissociation between automatic and volitional control. This means that control of volitional respiration, facial, bulbar and limb muscles is lost, but there is preserved awareness. The patient is NOT in coma, obviously. Communication can be achieved through vertical eye and upper eyelid movements, often slow and incomplete, because there is no horizontal gaze, no speech and tetraplegia. There may be involuntary movements – such as ocular bobbing, facial grimacing and automatisms, palatal myoclonus and even laughing and crying.

The most frequent cause is vertebrobasilar occlusion or other vascular or inflammatory reasons for pontine damage. The prognosis for most cases is poor. A severe neuropathy can cause an apparent locked-in syndrome.

### Vegetative State a.k.a. Unresponsive Wakefulness

These severely damaged patients appear to be awake with eyes open but show no evidence of awareness. There are no reproducible responses to stimuli nor of language comprehension or expression. VS cases breathe spontaneously. Pupillary, ocular, gag, cough and swallowing reflexes are typically present. Sleep–wake cycles are preserved and also brainstem autonomic responses. There is incontinence. Inconsistent non-purposive movements – grimacing, smiling and frowning, chewing, noises, grasping and or eye movements may occur. The unresponsive state usually follows coma due to bilateral hemisphere damage. Some functional imaging suggests that stimuli activate the cortex – such unresponsive patients may have some awareness.

### Minimally Conscious State

Patients in a minimally conscious state (MCS) have emerged from coma or a VS. They have low-level behavioural responses – a broad spectrum. Some show consistent awareness of themselves or their environment by making eye contact, turning their heads to sound, feeling pain or following simple commands, making yes/no responses and sometimes intelligible speech or purposeful behaviour.

### Akinetic Mutism

Akinetic mutism describes cases who move little or not at all and who do not speak in the normal fashion. However, their gaze may follow or be diverted by sound. Most motor functions such as facial expressions and gestures are usually absent/reduced, but the patient appears to be awake. They may speak in a whisper slowly, sometimes in single syllables. They are not paralysed but appear to be unable to move normally. No organic condition causes this picture. On recovery, some cases describe that as soon as they attempted to move, a 'form of internal resistance' prevented them from doing so.

### Psychogenic Unresponsiveness

This may be suspected from the history. Sometimes there is coma with a theatrical onset and even pretended paralysis with apparent respiratory failure. Inconsistent volitional responses are typical, particularly on eyelid opening. When the patient's hand is held above their face and then released, it drops next to the face rather than directly on it. Sudden upward and downward gaze with rapid changes are typical. Pupils are normal.

### Brain Death

Brain death (a.k.a. brainstem death) describes the situation when a person on ventilatory life support no longer has brain function but retains a cardiac output. They have fixed dilated pupils. They cannot breathe without support. All ITUs have protocols for recognition/ assessment of detailed criteria and testing, before consideration is given to withdraw support. Diagnosis of brain death has three stages:

The cause must be known and obviously:

- Reversible causes of coma such as hypothermia and drugs must be excluded
- Bedside tests of brainstem function are then undertaken to confirm brain death and to exclude any relevant metabolic derangement.

## Neurological Intensive Care

Neurological intensive care provides supportive treatment for patients with encephalopathies; raised ICP; ventilatory, autonomic and bulbar insufficiency and consequences of neuromuscular weakness (Table 20.5). Myasthenia gravis, Guillain–Barré syndrome, CNS infections, status epilepticus, severe traumatic brain injury (TBI), stroke and hypothermia are typical examples. The ITU of a district general hospital is frequently where many such cases are treated, but specialist neuro-ITU facilities may be available. Some broad principles are outlined – but one overriding factor is important – it is vital, on a general ward to recognise cases who may be at risk. Ventilatory failure is the prime example: the patient may have few complaints as respiration fails – unless you actually measure the vital capacity and assess oxygenation.

The headings of medical care, nursing and therapies are outlined here:

- Medical, ventilatory, anaesthetic and nursing care, skin care, tracheostomy care
- Nosocomial infection and surveillance
- Anticoagulation and recognition of coagulopathy
- Pain control, comfort
- Communication, psychological support, family liaison
- Physiotherapy, occupational therapy, speech and language, swallowing
- Common major issues
  - Failure to waken
  - Weakness and failure to wean from ventilation
  - End-of-life issues
  - Assessment of brain death.

The details of these issues are outside the remit of this chapter.

**Table 20.5** NICU: Examples of conditions supported.

Acute bacterial meningitis, herpes simplex encephalitis, other encephalitides

Metabolic, septic, uraemic, hepatic encephalopathy, hyperpyrexia, hypothermia, drug overdose

Status epilepticus

Acute inflammatory demyelinating polyneuropathy (Guillain–Barré), Miller Fisher syndrome

Myasthenia gravis, prolonged neuromuscular blockade

Anterior horn cell disease, cervical cord lesions

Traumatic brain injury, hypoxic–ischaemic brain injury (HIBI)

Diabetic and hypoglycaemic coma, hyponatraemia, hypernatraemia, cerebral salt wasting, SIADH

Posterior reversible encephalopathy syndrome (PRES)

Botulism, tetanus, rabies, stiff person syndrome, acute intermittent porphyria

## Severe Traumatic Brain Injury (TBI): General Principles

Advanced Trauma Life Support guidelines will be familiar:

- Stabilisation of the airway, breathing and circulation
- Attention to spinal cord trauma
- Neurological assessment
- Many patients with severe TBI develop hypoxia and/or hypotension. These must be recognised and addressed immediately.

Drug recommendations: whilst there are no absolute recommendations for severe TBI, tranexamic acid is widely used and has been shown to reduce the risk of death from mild to moderate TBI when given within 3 hours. Secondary insults – principally hypoxia – that exacerbate neuronal injury are vital to recognise.

Important mechanisms in severe TBI are shearing of grey and white matter and neighbouring vessels. This follows acceleration, deceleration and rotational forces on the brain. Penetrating injuries are less common. Classifications and rating scales are discussed in Chapter 18 and the GCS mentioned above. The aim of intensive care management of the brain-injured patient is to prevent and treat secondary insults, to maintain the patient so that potential for recovery is maximal and to recognise neurosurgical emergencies. The broad headings, for recognition and management, are:

- Diffuse axonal injury, disruption of brain vessels, haemorrhagic contusion, SAH
- Raised ICP and/or herniation – monitoring/decompression
- Systemic hypotension and hypertension
- Hypoxaemia, high carbon dioxide
- Epilepsy
- Coagulation disorders
- Infection.

## Neurosurgical Aspects of Severe TBI

Skull vault fractures when open or depressed require neurosurgical assessment. Base of skull fractures may not be obvious – they can cause periorbital bruising, bruising over the mastoid process (Battle sign), blood behind the tympanic membrane or nasal/ear CSF leak. Most leaks close spontaneously, but bacterial meningitis can supervene. Such fractures may be found only on detailed imaging and are usually managed conservatively.

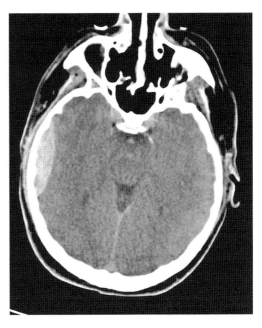

An extradural haematoma (Figure 20.1) is accumulation of blood, often rapid between the skull inner table and the dura. Most EDH follow a skull vault fracture and rupture of the middle meningeal artery or tearing of veins/venous sinuses. There is typically a lucid interval after the injury followed by stupor, an ipsilateral dilated pupil and coma. Immediate imaging followed by surgery can be lifesaving – or in a remote setting, surgery alone. If an EDH case is unconscious before surgery, mortality approaches 20%.

**Figure 20.1** CT – acute extradural haematoma.

With a subdural haematoma, blood accumulates between the inner layer of the dura and the arachnoid either acutely or chronically following a substantial blow to the head, a minor head injury or even sometimes spontaneously. SDH is due to tearing of cortical veins and/or small arteries. In many acute SDH cases, there is also an evident TBI – the patient is stuporose with lateralising signs. Acute SDH can also present with seizures or even TIA-like episodes. A small acute SDH can be managed conservatively, but generally neurosurgical assessment and drainage is necessary. Poor outcomes are likely if there is a severe brain contusion, the SDHs are bilateral or when essential surgery is delayed.

Chronic SDHs are expanding blood clots that can develop many weeks or even months after a head injury that may have been minor and forgotten. Old age, alcoholism, coagulopathy, epilepsy and a ventricular drain are factors that predispose to a chronic SDH (Figure 20.2). Headache is a common symptom that worsens over days or weeks, followed by deteriorating consciousness, focal signs seizures and sometimes papilloedema. Treatment: surgical evacuation.

### Neurological Sequelae of ITU Care

Meticulous attention to day-to-day care in ITU avoids many of the complications of intensive therapy seen in the past. However, in terms of outcome from a neurological

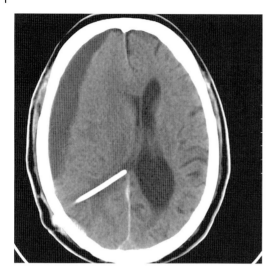

**Figure 20.2** CT – large chronic subdural haematoma with an intraventricular drain.

perspective, several issues stand out. One is the inability to predict accurately cognitive outcome following brain pathology of any cause, an insoluble question but one often asked in relation to the patient in coma. Another is difficulty with respiration during weaning from a ventilator – a complex issue handled usually by an anaesthetist. A third problem is compression of individual peripheral nerves, typically the ulnar and common peroneal – avoided to some extent by nursing attention but sometimes evident with the highest care standards. Recovery following a pressure palsy is usual but not invariable.

***Critical Illness Polyneuropathy and Myopathies*** Critical illness polyneuropathy (CIP) is an acute sensorimotor axonal neuropathy. This develops particularly with hypoalbuminaemia and hyperglycaemia. CIP is characterised by limb muscle wasting, weakness, areflexia and sensory loss – signs impossible to elicit when a patient is in coma. CIP is typically a diagnosis made during recovery. The condition has no clear explanation and is felt to be unavoidable, and whilst self-limiting, prognosis is variable. When CIP has been mild, recovery can be complete. With a severe polyneuropathy, substantial enduring deficits are common.

Myopathies of critical illness also occur. There are three main types:

- Diffuse non-necrotising cachectic myopathy
- Myopathy with selective loss of thick (myosin) filaments a.k.a. critical illness myopathy
- Acute necrotising myopathy of intensive care.

## Sleep and Its Disorders

### Sequence of Normal Sleep

Sleep is divided into stages and cycles defined by its depth, EEG changes, electro-oculogram (EOG) and muscle tone:

- wakefulness
- light sleep
- slow wave sleep (SWS) and
- rapid eye movement (REM) sleep.

After falling asleep there is descent through the stages of deepening non-REM sleep during the first hour accompanied by a gradual slowing of EEG rhythms. The cycle continues, with REM sleep passing directly to light sleep or even wakefulness and then a further descent/ascent sequence to the next REM. This is then repeated several times during the night. The first episode of REM generally occurs after about 60–90 minutes. As these cycles continue during a typical night, the length of time spent in REM tends to increase.

### The Autonomic Nervous System and Sleep

SWS sleep leads to an increase in parasympathetic and decrease in sympathetic tone with a reduction in heart rate, blood pressure, respiratory rate and bowel activity. REM sleep is associated with autonomic instability and fluctuations in heart rate and blood pressure. The muscles of the upper airway relax during all stages of sleep, especially in REM sleep, to cause snoring and a predisposition to airway obstruction that underlies sleep apnoea/hypopnoea. Respiratory failure from neuromuscular weakness is exacerbated during REM sleep. Bladder activity varies – from suppression of the urge to void in many females and younger men, until in older males prostatic symptoms bring about nocturnal frequency. Enuresis, common in boys, usually resolves by the age of 10.

### Regulation of Wakefulness and Sleep

Regulation of wakefulness and sleep depends on neuronal and biochemical interactions involving the cortex, thalamus, hypothalamus and brainstem. Neurotransmitters include those that are either wake promoting such as noradrenaline, acetylcholine, histamine and dopamine or sleep promoting such as melatonin and GABA. Others can be either sleep or wake promoting, for example serotonin. The hypocretin (orexin) system also has critical role in sleep regulation. REM sleep is thought to depend on interaction between REM-inhibiting nuclei (raphe nucleus secreting serotonin and *locus coeruleus* – noradrenaline) and REM-promoting nuclei (laterodorsal and pedunculopontine tegmental nuclei – acetylcholine).

Regulation of the timing of sleep cycles involves two mechanisms:

- Central rhythm generation determined by a circadian oscillator in the suprachiasmatic nucleus of the hypothalamus, influenced by light and melatonin. Oscillations are mediated by the so-called clock genes.
- Independent mechanisms track and respond to the time spent awake. Sleep debt that builds up during long periods of wakefulness depends on the accumulation of postulated somnogens, possibly adenosine, that make one feel tired.

The role of sleep is restorative if incompletely defined. Also, sleep is involved in cognitive processing, such as memory consolidation. Even minor degrees of sleep deprivation have effects on cognition, memory and behaviour.

## Sleep Disorders

It is odd that with many common brain diseases, disorders of sleep are not prominent. However, excessive daytime somnolence (EDS) can follow a TBI or encephalitis and can also be a feature of a neurodegenerative condition, of MS or myotonic dystrophy. Dementia is also sometimes accompanied by disruption of normal sleep patterns with nocturnal wakefulness – a difficult issue for a carer already tired following their efforts by day.

There is one exceptional condition of great rarity: fatal familial insomnia is the prion disease caused by mutation in codon 178 of the prion protein gene. In this strange condition, there is insomnia, loss of SWS, daytime dream-like episodes and enactment, a.k.a. oneiric episodes, cognitive decline and eventually death.

Common sleep disorders and the groups to which they are allocated are summarised in Table 20.6.

## Insomnia

Insomnia is simply a complaint about the duration or quality of sleep, meaning that it is inadequate and non-restorative. Severe insomnia can be lifelong and presumably has a genetic basis. As old age approaches, many who had unbroken sleep in earlier years find that their sleep pattern becomes fitful. Little is known about why this happens – and it remains unexplained why one person can fall asleep within seconds, while for another this takes longer.

Sleep can be disrupted by depression, anxiety, worry, pain, pregnancy, nocturia, respiratory and cardiac disorders. Insomnia can also occur because of other sleep disorders such as restless legs. Other factors contribute: beta-blockers, caffeine, alcohol, cocaine and stimulants. Insomnia has economic and social effects; it also causes depression and can lead to demands for sedatives, and to unregulated drugs.

In many instances, a simple manoeuvre can help insomnia. One aspect of management is to treat the underlying cause such as depression. Also, establish good sleep hygiene with a regular bedtime, avoidance of stimulants, stress and exercise close to bedtime. Regular exercise some hours before bedtime can consolidate sleep. Cognitive–behavioural therapy, either face to face or via many websites, is effective for chronic insomnia. The drugs so widely marketed are agonists at the benzodiazepine site of the $GABA_A$ receptors. Many have effects other than sedation, such as muscle relaxation, antiepileptic and anxiolytic effects, but they also can cause memory and behavioural disturbances and ataxia. Some drugs have more specific actions (e.g. zolpidem and zopiclone) by targeting specific $GABA_A$ subtypes. Sedative antidepressants such as mirtazapine, trazodone and amitriptyline are also used. Melatonin can also be helpful.

**Table 20.6** Common sleep disorders.

| |
|---|
| Insomnia |
| Obstructive sleep apnoea/hypopnoea |
| Hypersomnias of central origin – narcolepsy, cataplexy |
| Circadian rhythm sleep disorders |
| Parasomnias |
| Sleep-related movement disorders |
| Isolated symptoms, normal variants |
| Other sleep-related disorders – epilepsy, TBI, extrapyramidal syndromes |

## Obstructive Sleep Apnoea/Hypopnoea

Obstructive sleep apnoea/hypopnoea syndrome (OSAHS) is a common cause of daytime somnolence. It also causes nocturnal sleep disturbance, unrefreshing sleep, difficulty in concentration and nocturnal choking. Sleep apnoea refers to a cessation in airflow during sleep >10 seconds. Hypopnoea is >50% reduction in airflow associated with oxygen desaturation >4% or arousal. More than five apnoeas/hypopnoeas per hour (apnoea/hypopnoea index, AHI) are significant. AHI 5–15/hour represents mild, AHI 15–30/hour moderate and AHI >30/hour severe OSAHS.

Obstruction of the upper airway is usually between caudal soft palate and epiglottis. This is worsened anyway during sleep by collapse of the upper airway. This is exacerbated by obesity, a narrow palate, crowding of the oropharynx and jaw/facial anomalies.

Patients have difficulty falling asleep, loud snoring, stridor, coughing spells and restlessness. There may be prolonged apnoea. Severe sleep apnoea is associated with morning headache, impaired cognition, nocturia and even *cor pulmonale*.

### OSAHS Management

The first line is weight reduction, sleep hygiene and avoidance of alcohol, nicotine, caffeine and sedatives in the evening. CPAP by nasal or face mask is effective. This improves sleep architecture, oxygenation and the symptoms of sleepiness, impaired cognition and mood. Mandibular advancement splints are also used. Surgery (e.g. uvulopalatopharyngoplasty) rarely has a role. Tracheostomy may be necessary in patients with incipient *cor pulmonale*.

## Hypersomnias of Central Origin

### Narcolepsy

Narcolepsy is the commonest central hypersomnia. The peak age of onset is 15–25 years. It is rarely familial. The symptoms are excessive daytime somnolence (EDS), with irresistible sleep attacks at inappropriate times. Other symptoms are cataplexy, sleep paralysis, hypnogogic hallucinations, disrupted sleep, including REM behavioural disorder and short periods of automatic behaviour. Secondary symptoms include poor concentration. Narcolepsy has an impact on relationships, education, employment, driving, mood and quality of life.

### Cataplexy

Cataplexy describes brief episodes of muscle weakness with emotion – laughter, anger or surprise. There is a partial or complete loss of muscle tone. In its mild form, cataplexy leads to transient bilateral ptosis, head droop, slurred speech and/or dropping things. Cataplexy may be severe enough to cause falling. The episodes are brief, lasting seconds or minutes, but they may be followed by a sleep episode or occur recurrently *(status cataplecticus)*. Cataplexy is present in many with narcolepsy and can predate it.

### Possible Pathophysiology

Narcolepsy is associated with abnormalities of the hypocretin–orexin neurotransmitter system. Low or undetectable levels of CSF orexin/hypocretin are found in most. This has led to one hypothesis that there is hypocretin deficiency from neuronal loss in the hypo-thalamus, and in most, there is an autoimmune condition. Narcolepsy is associated with anti-tribble homolog 2 autoantibodies (TRIB2, a protein found in hypocretin secreting neu-rones). There may also be a narcolepsy variety – hypocretin resistance with abnormal hypo-cretin dynamics and overproduction of hypocretin. Narcolepsy can also very rarely occur with a tumour, encephalitis, following TBI and MS.

### Investigations and Management

Polysomnography is used to investigate other causes of EDS including obstructive sleep apnoea, periodic limb movement disorder and REM-related behaviour disorder; however, all are more common in people with narcolepsy. The Multiple Sleep Latency Test can be used to confirm the diagnosis. Narcolepsy is a life-long condition, with implications. People with narcolepsy are required to declare the diagnosis to the DVLA. Regular noctur-nal sleep habits and attention to sleep hygiene help to minimise EDS, and planned naps can help. Drug treatments include modafinil, methylphenidate, pitolisant and dexamphetamine.

Cataplexy often resolves with improvement in nocturnal sleep and daytime somnolence, and symptoms tend to improve with age. Treatments include tricyclic antidepressants (clo-mipramine), fluoxetine and other antidepressants such as venlafaxine. Sodium oxybate is also used.

### Hypnogogic/Hypnopompic Hallucinations, Sleep Paralysis and Automatic Behaviours

These hallucinations are brief vivid dream-like episodes that occur at sleep onset (hyp-nogogic) or on awakening (hypnopompic) and are often frightening – brief visual, tactile or auditory events that can continue for several minutes. Sleep paralysis is the inability to move on waking. Respiratory muscle activity continues. There is persistence of REM-related atonia in the waking state. The paralysis can be associated with a hypnic hallucina-tion of someone pressing on the chest or choking. Short periods of automatic behaviour occur on wakening, characterised by absent-minded behaviour and nonsense speech or writing, reflecting the intrusion of sleep into the awake state. All are common in narcolepsy and cataplexy.

### Primary (Idiopathic) Hypersomnia

This rarity is EDS without cataplexy or nocturnal sleep disruption that usually starts in adolescence. Aetiology is unknown. There is occasional familial incidence. Prolonged nocturnal sleep times are also the rule – the person often sleeps through an alarm clock. Sleep drunkenness is common in the morning – the person is disorientated, con-fused, slow, unsteady and sleepy. EDS is unaffected by prolonged nocturnal sleep or frequent naps. Primary hypersomnia can be associated with low levels of CSF orexin/hypocretin.

### Idiopathic Recurring Stupor

Idiopathic recurring stupor is an extraordinary rare syndrome – episodes of entirely iso-lated stupor and/or coma lasting hours to days with no obvious precipitating factor or cause and complete recovery. The condition sometimes responds to the benzodiazepine antagonist flumazenil, raising the possibility that endogenous benzodiazepine agonists are involved.

### Recurrent Hypersomnia (Kleine–Levin Syndrome)

This is a rare sleep disorder – episodes of severe hypersomnia with cognitive and behavioural disturbances. Confusion, derealisation, apathy, compulsive eating, aggression and hypersexuality occur, usually in male adolescents.

### Circadian Rhythm Adjustment Disorders: Shift Work and Jet Lag

Intrinsic circadian rhythms maintain our daily sleep–wake cycle, set by daylight duration and influenced by social activity. A mismatch between this intrinsic cycle and the environment leads to insomnia and EDS. This occurs typically with changes in time zones (jet lag) and with unfamiliar nocturnal shift work. Melatonin may help. Circadian rhythm disorders also occur with neurodegenerative conditions and in schizophrenia.

### Delayed/Advanced Sleep Phase Syndrome

This is a rare distinct and enduring inability to fall asleep or remain asleep at a conventional time. Advanced sleep syndrome (early to bed and early to wake) has been putatively associated with mutations in clock genes. Stimulants, hypnotics or alcohol tend to make matters worse. CBT and/or melatonin helps some.

## Parasomnias

Parasomnias are undesirable and sometimes bizarre physical events during sleep, classified as non-REM and REM, i.e. by the sleep state when they arise.

### Non-REM Parasomnias

These childhood phenomena include sleep walking, night terrors and confusional arousals. They usually resolve after a year or two. Sleep walking is common in children, typically in the first third of the night. The child may be either calm or agitated. Repetitive behaviour and occasionally eating may be a feature. Episodes usually last several minutes. It is often disruptive to wake the child who is often confused. To steer them gently back to bed is usually the best remedy.

Sleep terrors are disturbing but benign. They can start with a scream, and the child is both inconsolable and amnesic for the event when they awake. Often, the child reports being attacked and remains in a state of terror for a few minutes. Treatment: usually reassurance – for the parents.

In children and sometimes in adults, confusional arousals are characterised by partial awakening, movements in bed, thrashing about or inconsolable crying. Behaviour is often inappropriate and may be aggressive. Episodes are usually brief. Confusional arousals can rarely be associated with metabolic and toxic encephalopathies and hypersomnias. Complex actions may be carried out during a non-REM parasomnia including sexual acts (sexsomnia), sleep eating, driving and violence. These may be of forensic importance, if the situation described is credible.

### REM Sleep Parasomnias

REM-related parasomnias include nightmares, sleep paralysis and REM sleep behaviour disorder. Nightmares are frightening dreams, as we all know. Hypnagogic hallucinations (see above) are part of narcolepsy but may also occur in isolation. Sleep paralysis may also be isolated. Episodes are frightening but harmless and triggered by sleep deprivation.

REM sleep behaviour disorder (RBD) is characterised by loss of normal atonia during REM sleep and thus abnormal motor activity and behaviour, such as dream enactment and aggression. Duration: seconds to minutes. RBD occurs in male patients over 60 and is associated with neurodegenerative disorders, narcolepsy, cerebrovascular disease and rarely MS. RBD may develop for months or years before evidence of neurodegeneration. RBD may also emerge during withdrawal from alcohol or sedatives. Antidepressants can sometimes induce it. Clonazepam is an effective treatment. Melatonin may help. Safety measures are important to avoid injury.

### Other Parasomnias

In exploding head syndrome, there is the sensation of a noise bursting within the head. This sometimes seems to be provoked by benzodiazepines or their withdrawal. Another rare problem is a hypnic headache that tends to occur at a constant time each night, typically in those over 60 years. A diffuse mild headache wakes the patient.

Catathrenia (sleep groaning) occurs during REM sleep. The sound can be high pitched. The patient is usually unaware, but this often disturbs a companion. Bruxism is grinding or clenching teeth during sleep, common in children.

Faciomandibular myoclonus is a distinct benign syndrome of focal myoclonic jerks mainly during non-REM sleep.

## Sleep-Related Movement Disorders

### Restless Legs Syndrome and Periodic Limb Movements of Sleep

Restless legs syndrome (RLS) affects 5–10% of people over 60. F>M. Criteria:

- An urge to move the legs, usually with uncomfortable dysaesthesiae
- An urge to move or sensations that worsen during inactivity
- The urge is partially or totally relieved by movement
- The urge to move or sensations are worse at night.

There is difficulty getting to sleep and disturbed sleep and usually a chronic course. Periodic limb movements (PLMs) of sleep are associated. RLS may be idiopathic or secondary to iron deficiency, pregnancy, uraemia or other neurological conditions such as a neuropathy and spinal cord disease.

RLS is difficult to relieve completely. Measure iron stores, and treat if ferritin is low. Alcohol, caffeine and smoking avoidance may help. Ropinirole, pramipexole and rotigotine are licensed in the United Kingdom; pregabalin, gabapentin and benzodiazepines are also used. Antipsychotics and antidepressants sometimes exacerbate RLS.

PLMs of sleep are also common over 60. Movements commonly affect the legs – dorsiflexion of toes, ankles and sometimes hips. Severe cases have more than 50 per hour.

## Transition Disorders – Normal Variants

Sleep–wake transition disorders are common and normal. Hypnic jerks (sleep starts) and nocturnal leg cramps occur in healthy individuals. Visual, auditory or somatosensory sleep starts can also occur. In non-REM sleep, small flickering movements a.k.a. sleep myoclonus can occur. In some, their amplitude and frequency increase – sometimes called fragmentary myoclonus.

## Other Sleep-Related Disorders

### Epilepsy and Sleep

It can be hard to distinguish sleep-related paroxysmal events from nocturnal epilepsy. Epilepsy has a complex association with sleep. Certain seizures are more common during sleep such as some frontal lobe seizures that occur from light non-REM sleep. Rarely, nocturnal seizures may be the only manifestation of epilepsy. Nocturnal frontal lobe seizures are brief, stereotypical, cluster and occur at any time of night. Many cases of episodic nocturnal wanderings are possibly seizures or post-ictal confusion. Rarely, non-convulsive status epilepticus can occur during SWS, particularly in children. Lack of sleep can precipitate a seizure, especially in the idiopathic generalised epilepsies.

### Traumatic Brain Injury and Sleep

Sleep–wake disturbances are common after a severe TBI, particularly EDS and increased sleep need. Reduced hypocretin has been found in some patients. Fatigue can also be seen after a severe TBI, and sometimes following minor injuries, with anxiety and depression. Modafinil can be tried but is rarely helpful. Melatonin, CBT and light therapy can be used.

### Extrapyramidal Disease and Rhythmic Movement Disorder

In extrapyramidal disorders, particularly idiopathic Parkinson's disease, Huntington's, Tourette's syndrome and torsion dystonia, involuntary movements may persist during sleep.

Rhythmic movement disorder (*jactatio capitis nocturna*) describes rhythmic head or limb oscillations, head banging or body rocking – typically just before sleep and/or in light sleep. They are most common in young children with cognitive impairment. Complications include scalp and body wounds, retinal petechiae, callus formation and even subdural haematoma. Behavioural therapy may help.

## Acknowledgements, Further Reading and Personal References

I am most grateful to Robin Howard, Sofia Eriksson, Nicholas Hirsch, Neil Kitchen, Dimitri Kullmann, Christopher Taylor and Matthew Walker for their contribution to Neurology *A Queen Square Textbook* Second Edition on which this chapter is based.

Howard R, Eriksson S, Hirsch N, Kitchen N, Kullmann D, Taylor C, et al. Disorders of consciousness, intensive care neurology & sleep. In Neurology A Queen Square Textbook,

2nd edn. Clarke C, Howard R, Rossor M, Shorvon S, eds. Chichester: Wiley Blackwell, 2016. There are many useful references.

Hopkins A, Clarke C. Pretended paralysis requiring artificial ventilation. *BMJ* 1987; 294: 961–962.

Also, please visit  https://www.drcharlesclarke.com for free updated notes, potential links and other references. You will be asked to log in, in a secure fashion, with your name and institution.

# 21

# Neuro-Oncology

Primary CNS tumours account for about 2% of all cancers in adults and 20% in childhood. In adults, over half are hemisphere gliomas. In adolescence, brainstem and cerebellar tumours are more common – germ cell tumours and astrocytomas – and in mid-life, meningiomas and pituitary adenomas. In later life, high-grade gliomas and metastases are typical.

Survival: brain malignancies are responsible for more years lost than many other cancers and have a high case fatality ratio. For adults with a brain malignancy, 25% will die from this. For high-grade IV astrocytomas, 5-year survival remains less than 5% and has improved little in the past decade. With benign tumours such as meningiomas, many survive for decades or are cured.

The cause of almost all primaries remains unknown. Ionising radiation, either following radiotherapy or exceptionally nuclear explosions, is one risk factor. Cranial radiotherapy even at low doses increases meningioma and glioma risk. HIV is associated with primary CNS lymphoma (PCNSL).

Brain tumours also occur with genetic neurocutaneous syndromes – neurofibromatosis (optic nerve glioma, meningioma and vestibular schwannoma), tuberous sclerosis (subependymal giant cell astrocytoma) and von Hippel–Lindau (VHL) syndrome (haemangioblastoma). There are also rare familial syndromes, for example Li–Fraumeni syndrome (glioma) and Cowden's disease (dysplastic cerebellar gangliocytoma a.k.a. Lhermitte–Duclos disease).

## Clinical Features

Any mass lesion has the potential to produce a focal deficit, headaches, seizures and raised intracranial pressure. Low-grade tumours are infiltrative, less destructive and tend to present with seizures alone.

There are no features unique to a brain tumour. Imaging may well be the first pointer. Even then, tumour mimics on both CT and MRI can be confusing – high-grade glioma mimics include brain abscesses, tumefactive MS, TB and toxoplasmosis; low-grade mimics include cortical dysplasia, viral encephalitis and neurocysticercosis. Liaison with neuroradiology is vital.

*Neurology: A Clinical Handbook*, First Edition. Charles Clarke.
© 2022 John Wiley & Sons Ltd. Published 2022 by John Wiley & Sons Ltd.

## Headache

Whilst it is exceptional for a brain tumour to present with headache alone, tumours can produce headache, either by their mass effect, meningeal distortion and vasogenic oedema or by blockage of CSF pathways. The latter is seen typically with posterior fossa and intra-ventricular tumours. Intra-tumoural haemorrhage can cause a severe headache with reduced consciousness.

Severity of headache is not helpful – indeed, most severe headaches are caused by primary headaches such as cluster. With tumours, headaches are present in under half and are similar to tension-type headaches or migraine in most. Brain tumour headaches tend to be made worse by bending down in around one-third, unlike tension-type headaches, but postural headaches occur in migraine. Nausea and/or vomiting are present in under half. Early morning headache is uncommon though frequently cited. What singles out a brain tumour is either a change in a prior headache pattern or its gradual evolution, with features such as a focal deficit, seizures or with a posterior fossa tumour ataxia and vomiting.

## Seizures and Focal Deficits

Seizures may be partial, a pointer to the tumour origin and/or generalised. There is an inverse relationship between tumour grade and seizures: low-grade tumours such as oligo-dendrogliomas and gangliogliomas tend to cause seizures. There is little association between seizures and behaviour of an underlying tumour – for example, return of seizures after a period of freedom does not invariably indicate recurrence.

Focal deficits are usually progressive. However, sudden stroke-like presentations and TIA-like events occur – caused either by intra-tumoural haemorrhage or presumed vascular changes. Progressive focal deficits occur typically in patients with high-grade tumours, such as glioblastoma and metastases. A parasagittal tumour, typically a meningioma, can present with a spastic paraparesis or monoparesis.

## Brainstem/Cerebellar, Cognitive and Behavioural Symptoms

Vertigo, poor balance and/or diplopia are common with posterior fossa tumours. In cerebello-pontine angle (CPA) tumours, such as a vestibular schwannoma, unilateral hearing loss is usually an early symptom – before trigeminal, facial nerve and brainstem compression. Depression of the corneal reflex occurs early, before evident trigeminal sensory loss. Pineal and tectal plate tumours can present with Parinaud's syndrome (Chapter 14) and hydrocephalus.

A minority present with failing cognition, depression, delusions, personality change or dementia. Specific cognitive deficits such as aphasia, alexia and acalculia can occur.

## Endocrine, Visual and Olfactory Symptoms

Patients with pituitary and hypothalamic tumours can present with endocrine disturbances, and visual failure but rarely with epilepsy. In children, hypothalamic and thalamic tumours can cause failure to grow as expected, with emaciation, a.k.a. – a diencephalic syndrome. Precocious puberty, particularly in boys, can be caused by a glioma, pineal or germ cell tumour. Anosmia (Chapter 13) can follow olfactory nerve compression by an orbital plate mass.

## Imaging

MR imaging is now routine. Appearances of common tumours are shown in Figure 21.1, and the reader is referred to public sources (see References). Contrast enhancement is seen with highly vascular such as a meningioma (Figure 21.2) or in an intra-axial tumour such as a lymphoma (Figure 21.3).

Physiological imaging, spectroscopy and f-MRI can help distinguish grades and monitor growth but are primarily research tools.

## Tumours: The Multidisciplinary Approach

Effective management requires many skills – clinical neurology, neuroradiology, neuropathology, neurosurgery, radiotherapy, oncology, specialist nursing, general practice and palliative care. Quality of life assessment, the wishes of the patient – that may change over time – the needs and observations of family and carers are also pivotal. One advance is frank discussion of the outlook that has tended to replace attitudes of the past.

### Neurosurgery

Surgery remains important – for stereotactic biopsy, debulking and tumour resection in some cases. However, in a highly malignant tumour, radical resection is inappropriate. Techniques include image-directed biopsy and stereotactic or frameless neuronavigation. Neuroendoscopy for skull base, pituitary and parasellar tumours has enabled extensive operations to be less invasive.

### Radiotherapy and Chemotherapy

CT slices are fused with MRI data to define the precise volume to be irradiated. Appropriate shielding gives a steep dose gradient to avoid irradiation of normal brain. Total doses are usually 45–60 Gy, in daily fractions. Stereotactic radiotherapy/radiosurgery are refinements – for benign brain tumours,

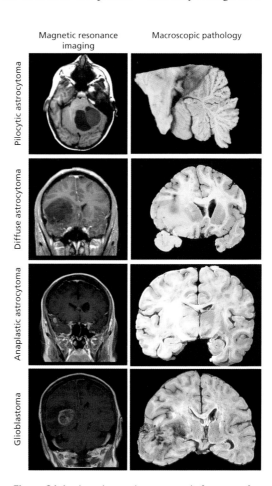

**Figure 21.1** Imaging and macroscopic features of gliomas Grades I–IV.

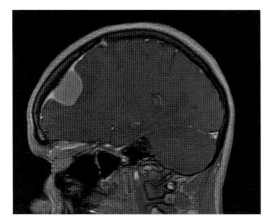

**Figure 21.2** Frontal meningioma. MR T1-enhanced image.

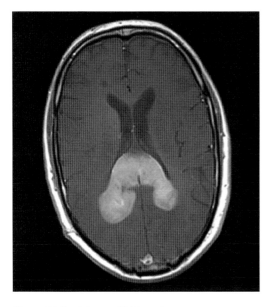

**Figure 21.3** Primary CNS lymphoma.

such as a pituitary adenoma, meningioma and vestibular schwannoma. Chemotherapy for gliomas is chiefly with temozolamide.

**Classification and Grades**

The WHO 2016 classification lists over 120 CNS tumour types based on histology. The principal tumour types are shown in Table 21.1.

The histogenesis of cancers, molecular mechanisms and genetic components are outside the scope of this chapter. The essential histology of common astrocytomas is outlined in Figure 21.4.

The four WHO grades are:

Grade I – low grade, without nuclear or cellular atypia
Grade II – atypia alone
Grade III – atypia and mitosis
Grade IV – atypia, mitosis, vascular proliferation and necrosis.

**Diffuse Astrocytomas and Oligodendroglial Tumours**

The most common primary brain tumours are high-grade hemisphere gliomas – Grade IV glioblastoma, a.k.a. *glioblastoma multiforme* (GBM), gliosarcoma (a histological variant) and Grade III anaplastic astrocytoma. GBM is the most frequent in older people in a temporal, parietal or frontal lobe. Typical GBM histological features include poorly differentiated, pleomorphic cells with nuclear atypia, brisk mitotic activity, necrosis and/or microvascular proliferation.

**Surgery, Radiotherapy and Chemotherapy**
Gliomas infiltrate the surrounding brain. A biopsy is essential but surgical cure impossible. Indications for debulking are raised intracranial pressure and/or focal deficits. In a few, a second debulking resection is considered.

**Table 21.1** Nervous System Tumours – from WHO Classification

| | |
|---|---|
| ***Diffuse astrocytomas and oligodendroglial tumours*** | ***Meningiomas*** |
| Diffuse astrocytomas and oligodendroglial tumours, *glioblastoma multiforme* (GBM, IV), gliosarcoma (IV), anaplastic astrocytoma (III), diffuse astrocytoma (II), anaplastic oligodendroglioma (III), oligodendroglioma (II) | Fibrous, psammomatous, clear cell, anaplastic (malignant) |
| ***Other astrocytic tumours*** | ***Mesenchymal non-meningothelial tumours*** |
| Pilocytic astrocytoma (I), grade II astrocytoma | Haemangioblastoma, lipoma, chordoma, chondroma, chondrosarcoma, lipoma, many others |
| ***Ependymal tumours*** | ***Lymphomas*** |
| Ependymoma (I, II), anaplastic ependymoma (III) | Diffuse large B-cell CNS lymphoma, HIV-related CNS lymphoma, intravascular CNS lymphoma |
| ***Choroid plexus tumours*** | |
| Choroid plexus papilloma (I) and carcinoma (III) | |
| ***Neuronal and mixed neuronal–glial tumours*** | ***Germ cell tumours*** |
| Dysembryoplastic neuroepithelial tumour (DNET, I), gangliocytoma (I), ganglioglioma (I), central neurocytoma | Germinoma, choriocarcinoma, teratoma |
| ***Pineal region tumours*** | ***Tumours of the sellar region*** |
| Pineocytoma (I), pineoblastoma (IV) | Pituitary tumours, craniopharyngioma (I) |
| ***Embryonal tumours*** | ***Metastatic brain and spinal tumours*** |
| Medulloblastoma (IV) | Many systemic cancers |
| ***Cranial and paraspinal nerve tumours*** | ***Other mass lesions*** |
| Schwannoma (I), neurofibroma (I), malignant peripheral nerve sheath tumour (II–IV) | Dermoids, epidermoid cysts, colloid cysts, Rathke's pouch cysts, neuro-enteric cysts, optic pathway glioma |
| | ***Primary Spinal Cord Tumours and Spinal Metastases*** |

Radiotherapy is standard palliative management. In Grade IV gliomas with little deficit, radiotherapy improves survival by 5–6 months. Occasionally, radiosurgery is used for small nodular recurrences.

Temozolomide chemotherapy with radiotherapy increases survival by some months, with occasional unexpectedly longer responses. *Pneumocystis carinii* pneumonia can be a problem. This surgery/radiotherapy/chemotherapy regime is now standard. Relapses are sometimes treated with further chemotherapy. Carmustine wafers, carboplatin and taxol are sometimes used. Anaplastic oligodendrogliomas and other Grade III tumours have a slightly better prognosis than GBM.

## Other Astrocytic Tumours

Low-grade gliomas (Grades I and II) occur in children and young adults with a peak incidence in the second and third decades. The most common is the pilocytic astrocytoma (Grade I),

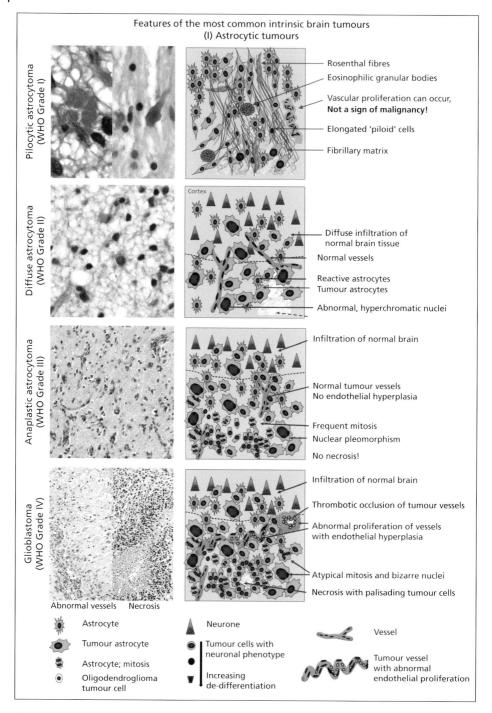

**Figure 21.4** Histological features of Grade I–IV astrocytomas.

which has a predilection for the cerebellum and midline structures – hypothalamus, thalamus, optic chiasm and brainstem. In adults, these tumours also grow in the cerebral hemispheres, usually cystic with nodular or ring enhancement. Resective surgery has a 10-year survival over 90%, with or without focal radio- and chemotherapy.

Grade II gliomas tend to transform to a higher grade. For a Grade II glioma, survival is 5–7 years for an astrocytic tumour, and 10–15 years for oligodendroglial.

## Ependymal Tumours and Choroid Plexus Tumours

Ependymomas arise most frequently in the fourth ventricle and occasionally in the cervical region or *conus medullaris*. They are most common before the age of 20.

Typically of Grades I or II, histological features are pseudorosettes. Imaging: an intraventricular, lobulated mass. Total resection can sometimes be achieved.

Choroid plexus tumours are either papillomas or carcinomas. In childhood, a cauliflower-like mass grows in the trigone of a lateral ventricle. In an adult, they occur predominantly in the fourth ventricle.

## Neuronal and Mixed Neuronal-Glial Tumours

These rarer tumours present typically with seizures and can usually be treated with surgery alone. Dysembryoplastic neuroepithelial tumours (DNETs) are Grade I, typically in the cortex. Thinning and remodelling of overlying bone is present in about half, reflecting their slow growth. Gangliogliomas and gangliocytomas (Grade I) are slow-growing tumours usually within a temporal lobe. Central neurocytomas (Grade II) grow within a lateral ventricle. Obstructive hydrocephalus is common.

## Pineal Region Tumours

These include pineocytoma and pineoblastoma. Features are determined by the proximity of the quadrigeminal plate, midbrain, third ventricle and cerebellar vermis:

- Obstructive hydrocephalus: headache, vomiting and obtundation
- Parinaud's syndrome: vertical gaze palsy, light-near dissociated mid-point pupils, loss of convergence and convergence–retraction nystagmus (Chapter 14)
- Ataxia: cerebellar involvement.

Treatments: surgery, irradiation and chemotherapy. There is a high morbidity with pineal region surgery and poor prognosis with high-grade tumours.

## Embryonal Tumours

Medulloblastomas (IV) originate from the cerebellum external granular layer and usually arise in the cerebellar midline in children. Clinical features include gait ataxia, headache, vomiting, hydrocephalus and papilloedema. Treatment: surgery, craniospinal irradiation and chemotherapy.

## Cranial and Paraspinal Nerve Tumours

Schwannomas are benign tumours of Schwann cells (Chapter 20). The commonest location is in the cerebellopontine angle (CPA), but they can occur on any cranial nerve, on spinal roots and peripheral nerves. Neurofibromas tend to encase nerve roots and can be fusiform, whereas Schwannomas are typically round. The rare malignant peripheral nerve sheath tumour is invasive.

Vestibular schwannomas, a.k.a. acoustic neuroma, cause hearing loss, tinnitus and vertigo. Assume that unilateral sensorineural hearing loss or tinnitus might be caused by 'an acoustic' until proven otherwise. Headaches can be prominent when patients develop obstructive hydrocephalus with a substantial tumour, typically larger than 4 cm. Bilateral schwannomas occur with NF2 – a defective tumour suppressor gene on chromosome 22q12.2. Other manifestations – peripheral neurofibromas, meningioma, glioma and juvenile posterior subcapsular lenticular opacities – can be present. Management depends on age, size and tumour growth rate and comorbidities. In younger patients, microsurgical resection is usual. There are various radiotherapy/radiosurgery options.

## Meningiomas

Meningiomas are common well-demarcated extra-axial tumours that grow slowly and usually do not infiltrate brain. They originate from meningothelial cells, most abundant in the arachnoid villi. They are most common in the elderly, F > M. The commoner varieties are meningothelial, fibroblastic and psammomatous – abundant whorls with calcification. Most are Grade I. Grade II and Grade III (anaplastic meningioma) have mitotic activity and recur.

Meningiomas can be spherical, well-circumscribed, craggy/irregular or infiltrating *en plaque* lesions. They arise within the parasagittal area, convexities, sphenoid wing, *tuberculum sellae*, olfactory groove, tentorium, foramen magnum and elsewhere. On CT, over half are hyperdense without contrast; some 20% calcify. Hyperostosis indicates the site of attachment to the meninges. On MRI, they can be isointense to cerebral cortex and sometimes difficult to detect without contrast. Vasogenic oedema is often disproportionate to tumour size. Linear enhancement can extend along the adjacent dura – the dural tail. Recurrences are rare after radical excision. Radiotherapy is given when excision is impractical. Spinal meningiomas tend to arise dorsally in the thoracic region, mainly in women.

## Mesenchymal, Non-Meningothelial Tumours

Haemangioblastomas are cystic, vascular tumours, typically in the posterior fossa. They tend to cause raised intracranial pressure and/or cerebellar dysfunction. Polycythaemia occurs in 10% from tumour production of erythropoietin. They may also arise within the cord, sometimes with a cavity and syringomyelia. Rarely, they are supratentorial. Haemangioblastomas are most commonly associated with VHL syndrome (Chapter 26).

Resection is generally possible and curative. Radiotherapy is used for any residual tumour.

Chordomas arise from embryonic notochord remnants at any point along the neuraxis – skull base and clivus, vertebral column and sacrum. They invade bone and occasionally metastasise. Chondromas and chondrosarcomas are also rare tumours – they arise from embryonal cartilaginous remnants, commonly in the petro-occipital synchondrosis.

## Lymphomas

Primary CNS lymphomas (PCNSLs) account for about 3% of brain primaries. The immuno-suppressed and HIV-positive are at risk, but PCNSLs have also increased in the immunocompetent population. PCNSLs are dense patternless masses that infiltrate adjacent brain. Most are of B-cell type and multifocal. A PCNSL usually presents as either solitary or multiple supratentorial masses with raised pressure, focal signs and seizures. Rarely, the lymphoma invades brain vessels – intravascular lymphoma. PCNSLs can also develop in the meninges. Ocular lymphoma with visual loss can predate the appearance of intracranial disease.

Diagnosis is usually suspected from imaging – one or several homogeneously enhancing or ring-like masses, typically periventricular. Stereotactic biopsy is usually needed. Serum LDH is often greatly raised.

Treatment: high-dose methotrexate with whole brain radiotherapy. In some HIV-negative patients under 60, there is a 5-year survival around 50%, but in most the outlook is gloomy.

## Germ Cell Tumours

Germinomas are rare tumours, predominantly of childhood. They are largely midline and grow in the pineal and third ventricular regions.

Metastatic brain choriocarcinoma can present as intracerebral haemorrhage in women of childbearing age. Occasionally, these highly malignant tumours can be cured by chemo- and radiotherapy.

Intracranial teratomas are rare childhood tumours. They occur exceptionally in adults.

## Tumours of the Sellar Region

The sellar and parasellar regions are sites of many disease processes (Table 21.2). Pituitary tumours account for most – about 10% of all intracranial neoplasm.

Benign pituitary adenomas are typical, but some invade the capsule, dura and/or the sphenoid and cavernous sinus. Carcinomas are rare. Microadenomas are less than 10 mm on MR. Cells are defined by their histological, hormonal and immunological characteristics. Acidophilic and chromophobe cells produce prolactin, GH or TSH. Basophilic cells produce ACTH, LH or FSH. Most adenomas are functionally inactive and typically chromophobe. Of those that secrete hormones, c. 70% secrete prolactin, 15% GH and 5% ACTH.

**Table 21.2** Sellar region lesions.

Pituitary tumours, craniopharyngioma

Meningioma, germ cell, granular cell tumours

Gliomas – hypothalamic, optic pathway

Lymphoma, ependymoma, metastases

Rathke's pouch cysts, epidermoid/dermoid cysts

Empty sella, lymphocytic hypophysitis

Aneurysm: carotid, anterior communicating artery

Sarcoid, GPA, Histiocytosis X

Bacterial/fungal abscess, TB, syphilis

Pituitary adenomas present typically to a neurologist with mass effects – chiasmal compression, headaches and/or endocrine problems. Macroadenomas cause various bitemporal hemianopias and/or optic nerve lesions. Oculomotor palsies and V nerve lesions develop if the adenoma extends into the cavernous sinus. Extension into a temporal lobe can occasionally cause epilepsy. Rarely, hydrocephalus and/or erosion through the sella with CSF rhinorrhoea occurs. Internal carotid artery compression can lead to cerebral ischaemia. Hypothalamic invasion causes hypersomnolence, autonomic dysregulation and diabetes insipidus.

**Pituitary Apoplexy**

Pituitary apoplexy follows haemorrhagic or ischaemic infarction, often from an unrecognised adenoma – the tumour outgrows its blood supply. There is sudden headache, meningism, vomiting, visual loss, ophthalmoplegia, visual field defect and sometimes coma. CSF is haemorrhagic. Predisposing factors: pregnancy, postpartum haemorrhage, trauma, diabetic ketoacidosis, radiotherapy, post-angiography and occasionally following bromocriptine. Steroids are required urgently. Surgery may be necessary. Panhypopituitarism usually follows and requires treatment.

**Pituitary Tumour Management**

Treatment in a specialist unit aims to normalise hormone secretion and prevent visual loss and other deficits. Trans-sphenoidal surgery is used for macroadenomas causing chiasmal compression. GH-secreting tumours can be treated initially with the GH receptor antagonist, pegvisomant, or somatostatin analogues such as octreotide and lanreotide. Prolactinomas are treated with dopamine agonists such as cabergoline and bromocriptine. Radiotherapy is an effective adjunct.

**Craniopharyngioma**

These are slow-growing benign extra-axial parasellar cystic tumours. Cysts, sometimes multiple, contain thick proteinaceous material and can extend in any direction – into the hypothalamus, basal cisterns, third ventricle, CPA, posterior fossa, foramen magnum or frontal region. Presentation is usually as a slow-growing mass, but there can be a sudden onset, either because of increase in volume or rupture – with a chemical meningitis and/or ventriculitis. Common features are headaches, visual failure and endocrine dysfunction. Secondary hypothalamic involvement can lead to obesity. Radical cure is the exception – cysts are multiple and adherent. Radiotherapy may be helpful.

## Metastatic Brain and Spinal Tumours

See below, in Neurological Complications of Cancer and Spinal Metastases.

## Other Mass Lesions: Dermoids, Epidermoid Cysts, Colloid Cysts, Rathke's Pouch Cysts, Neuro-Enteric Cysts, Optic Pathway Glioma

- Dermoids arise from inclusion of ectodermal tissue during neural tube development. Dermoid cysts contain hair follicles, sweat glands and sebaceous glands. They arise in the posterior fossa and present with local mass effects or rupture to cause a granulomatous meningitis.
- Epidermoid cysts arise in the CPA or middle cranial fossa and cause mass effect, facial pain and cranial nerve lesions. Removal of an epidermoid can be impossible because they spread along the cranial nerves.
- Colloid cysts tend to grow in the third ventricle and may block the foramen of Monro – drop attacks and hydrocephalus.
- Rathke's pouch cysts arise in the sellar region.
- Neuroenteric cysts arise in the cord or brain.

### Optic Pathway Glioma

Optic pathway gliomas (OPGs) are rare astrocytomas that arise typically in children. Half have NF1. They cause gradual visual loss. The common histology is a pilocytic astrocytoma. OPGs in adults are rare and tend to be highly aggressive.

Treatment: for children with NF1, chemotherapy is usual, to delay the need for radiotherapy. Vincristine and carboplatin are used. For adults, radiotherapy and palliative surgery are rarely helpful.

## Primary Spinal Cord Tumours and Spinal Metastases

Primary cord tumours (Figure 21.5) are relatively rare and are usually astrocytomas or ependymomas and low-grade, either of the cervical cord or the *conus* (ependymomas). Other primary tumours are meningiomas, schwannomas arising from a spinal nerve root and lipomas, either intramedullary or extramedullary. Features are combinations of nerve root entrapment at the tumour level, such as girdle pain, and cord compression – para- or tetraparesis. MRI is usually diagnostic.

Radical surgery is usual for extramedullary tumours via laminectomy. Extensive approaches are sometimes required, for example for dumb-bell schwannomas via thoracotomy. Radiotherapy is usually given for malignancies. Chemotherapy is of little value.

Spinal metastases are common, commonly with bone invasion, but sometimes with extradural deposits and/or, rarely, intramedullary spread. Frequently, there is rapidly progressive paraparesis. Speed is of the essence in minimising permanent weakness. If the patient has a severe paraparesis with lost sphincter function for more than 12 hours, the results of decompression are poor. If a spinal metastasis is suspected, imaging should be immediate, and specialist advice sought.

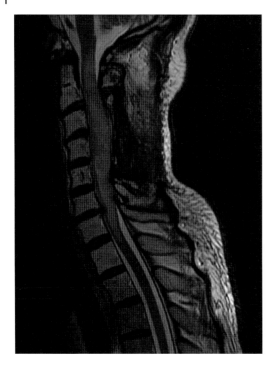

**Figure 21.5** Intramedullary cervical cord glioma. MR T2W.

# Complications of Radiotherapy and Chemotherapy

Radiotherapy-induced neurotoxicity follows treatment of many tumours. Acute and early-delayed toxicity improve spontaneously and/or with steroids. Late-delayed toxicity is irreversible.

## Acute Radiation Toxicity and Early-Delayed Toxicity

Common acute effects are alopecia, scalp erythema, fatigue, headache, nausea and vomiting. Neuronal toxicity underlies the lethargy. In early-delayed toxicity there is a longer period of lethargy and somnolence lasting up to 3 months. Worsening of pre-existing deficits and seizures can occur – usually reversible with steroids and/or time.

## Late-Delayed Toxicity, Radiation Necrosis, Optic Neuropathy and Other Effects

Late-delayed effects include cognitive decline – from leukoencephalopathy, vascular damage and necrosis. These can become apparent between 6 months and possibly up to 20 years following radiation. Necrosis, typically 6–24 months after radiation, can mimic tumour recurrence radiologically.

Optic neuropathy following radiation of sellar and parasellar lesions is a late-delayed complication. Other radiation effects:

- Cataract, chiasmal and pituitary damage
- Secondary tumours
- Vascular disease
- Myelopathy, radiculopathy and plexopathy.

## Chemotherapy

Many drugs are neurotoxic and cause neuropathy and encephalopathy. A pure sensory neuropathy is commonly associated with vinca alkaloids, taxol and cisplatin. Oxaliplatin causes a reversible syndrome – painful dysaesthesiae on contact with cold, and laryngo-spasm, probably a reversible sodium channelopathy. Motor neuropathies are occasionally seen with suramin and vincristine. Many chemotherapies can cause an encephalopathy with seizures and confusion. The most notable is the combination of methotrexate and cranial irradiation – an irreversible leukoencephalopathy. Ifosfamide used mainly for sarcomas can also cause an encephalopathy.

# Neurological Complications of Cancer (NCCs)

The majority of NCCs are caused by direct invasion or metastatic spread, usually evident clinically and/or with imaging. Any malignancy can spread within the neuraxis. Invasion or compression occurs when a tumour or draining lymph node is in contact with a nerve, nerve root, cord, meninges or brain. Tumour invasion of a nerve root can cause severe pain; previous radiotherapy tends to cause painless radiculopathy. Growth along nerve sheaths can also occur. Examples are multiple cranial nerve palsies with nasopharyngeal carcinoma, and lymphoma, brachial plexopathy from breast cancer and T1 radiculopathy with Horner's syndrome with apical lung cancer (Pancoast's syndrome).

Metastases in the CNS are commonly terminal events, but some tumours are resectable – an isolated posterior fossa metastasis is an example.

Malignant meningitis, a sinister complication of any cancer, usually occurs in the late stages but occasionally presents with no known tumour. Tumours that commonly cause MM are lung and breast cancer, melanoma and leukaemia/lymphoma. MM presents with cerebral, cranial nerve, spinal and/or radicular features. Initial symptoms are often vague: nausea, drowsiness, confusion and odd numb skin patches. Papilloedema can occur and occasionally a meningitic syndrome.

MRI shows changes in most MM cases – coating of the brainstem, cerebellar folia or the cord, with linear or nodular meningeal deposits. Communicating hydrocephalus can develop. CSF cytology is useful. Treatment is palliative; survival – a matter of months.

## Indirect and Secondary NCCs

There are numerous rare NCCs. Whilst a general neurologist may see these seldom, it is important to appreciate their biological importance and that some are immune mediated.

- Toxic and metabolic encephalopathy
- Stroke – cerebral haemorrhage, venous sinus thrombosis, coagulopathy/hyperfibrinogenaemia and antiphospholipid syndrome
- Non-bacterial thrombotic endocarditis
- CNS infections – cryptococcus, listeria, toxoplasma, aspergillus and nocardia
  Paraneoplastic neurological disorders – autoimmune attack triggered by tumour antigens. Various antineuronal antibodies have been found.
  - Lambert–Eaton myasthenic syndrome (LEMS)
  - Encephalomyelitis, sometimes with rigidity
  - Limbic encephalitis, brainstem encephalitis
  - Subacute cerebellar degeneration
  - Opsoclonus-myoclonus
  - Sensory neuronopathy (dorsal root ganglionopathy)
  - Dermatomyositis/myositis

- Chronic gastrointestinal pseudo-obstruction
- Paraneoplastic retinal degeneration
- Necrotising myelopathy
- Progressive subacute motor neuronopathy
- Primary lateral sclerosis-like condition
- Paraneoplastic sensory neuronopathy
- Acute necrotising myopathy
- Other neuropathies – sensory, motor, autonomic, CIDP-like neuropathy, Guillain–Barré-like and vasculitic
- Myasthenia gravis – with thymoma
- Neuromyotonia
- Neuralgic amyotrophy.

## Acknowledgements, Further Reading and Websites

I am most grateful to Jeremy Rees, Robert Bradford, Sebastian Brandner, Naomi Fersht, Rolf Jäger and Elena Wilson for their contribution to *Neurology A Queen Square Textbook* Second Edition on which this chapter was based.

Davies E, Hopkins A, Clarke C. Malignant cerebral glioma I: survival disability and morbidity after radiotherapy. II: perspective of patients and relatives on the value of radiotherapy. *BMJ* 1996; 313: 1507–1517.

Louis DN, Perry A, Reifenberger G, von Deimling A, Figarella-Branger D, Webster K, et al. The 2016 World Health Organization classification of tumours of the central nervous system: a summary. *Acta Neuropathol* 2016; **131**: 803–820. DOI: 10.1007/s00401-016-1545-1.

Rees J, Bradford R, Brandner S, Fersht N, Jäger R, Wilson E. Neuro-oncology. In *Neurology A Queen Square Textbook*, 2nd edn. Clarke C, Howard R, Rossor M, Shorvon S, eds. Chichester: John Wiley & Sons, 2016. There are numerous references.

https://www.nhs.uk/conditions/brain-tumours/
https://www.cancerresearchuk.org/
https://radiopaedia.org. The online collaborative radiology resource.

Also, please visit https://www.drcharlesclarke.com for free updated notes, potential links and other references. You will be asked to log in, in a secure fashion, with your name and institution.

# 22

# Neuropsychiatry

Neuropsychiatrists and neurologists usually confer for one of three reasons:

- Neurological symptoms with no organic cause, such as convulsions, apparent dystonia or paralysis, sensory loss, amnesia, blindness and dysphonia, known as functional neurological disorders (FNDs).
- Psychiatric symptoms with a neurological disease. Depression is common. Suicidal ideation must be recognised.
- Behavioural change and concern about a disease such as dementia.

Here, a summary of the mental state examination precedes the main relevant psychiatric conditions. Both need to be understood.

## Mental State

These are the headings with which one can usually decide whether abnormal behaviour is a feature, consequence or imitator of a disease and formulate a diagnosis.

### Appearance and Behaviour

Important clues:

- *Clothing and personal care*: self-neglect – depression, psychosis or dementia.
- *Behaviour:* agitation and distractibility – psychosis, delirium and dementia. Abnormal movements – for example tremor, chorea or a tic.
- *Activity level*: retardation or excitability – depression or mania.
- *Appropriateness*: disinhibition and inappropriate crying/laughing.

### Speech

- *Quantity:* reduced in depression and dementia
- *Rate:* rapid in mania and slow in depression
- *Tone:* monotonous in depression

*Neurology: A Clinical Handbook*, First Edition. Charles Clarke.
© 2022 John Wiley & Sons Ltd. Published 2022 by John Wiley & Sons Ltd.

- *Rhythm:* normal intonation and rhythm – lost in psychosis
- *Volume:* loud in mania; quiet in depression.

### Mood and Affect

Subjective statements are obvious – '. . .down . . .low. . .or sad' or 'I'm high/wonderful'. Objectively, the patient may *appear* depressed, manic or euthymic (normal). Affect – mood variation – is reactive in euthymia, flat/unchanging in depression or can be labile/exaggerated.

- *Anhedonia*: inability to enjoy things – depression.
- *Sleep*: hypomanic patients need little sleep. Depression causes early morning waking.
- *Appetite*: weight loss – common in depression.
- *Energy and libido*: reduced in depression and elevated in mania.
- *Suicidal ideation*.

### Thought

- *Speed of thinking*: increased in mania with flight of ideas and slowed in depression.
- *Ordering of thoughts*: disrupted in both organic disease and psychosis. Perseveration, in frontal lobe damage and thought block (abrupt cessation) in psychosis.
- *Psychotic, formal thought disorder:* abnormal transitions in thought processes – derailment (shifting off the point); tangential (related, but off the point); knight's move thinking (illogical shifts).

### Thought Content

- *Delusions*, firmly held false beliefs – persecutory, grandiose, nihilistic, hypochondriacal and bizarre. Delusions occur in schizophrenia, depression/psychosis and mania, and in temporal lobe attacks, dementias and Parkinson's.
- *Abnormalities of possession* (thought insertion, withdrawal and broadcasting) – beliefs of being under control of an outside force.
- *Obsessional thoughts* are ideas perceived as coming from within (cf. hallucinations and delusions), but the patient is unable to prevent their intrusion. They may be compelled to carry out ritualistic acts, such as washing.

### Perceptions

*Illusions*: false perceptions, misinterpretation of the surroundings.
*Hallucinations*: perceptions, believed to be true, but without any external stimulus. Visual hallucinations are typical of an organic cause – delirium, dementia and Parkinson's.
*Auditory hallucinations* are typical of primary psychotic illnesses. Some with schizophrenia experience command hallucinations – voices command them to cause harm. In psychotic depression, voices indicate worthlessness/guilt; in mania, God's voice can be heard.

*Pseudohallucination*: usually visual; object(s) seen but recognised as unreal – faces on curtains but realising that they are not there.

*Depersonalisation*: distorted sense of self – a patient describes feeling outside their body.

*Derealisation*: distorted sense of reality – looking on the world from the outside rather than being in it. Persistence suggests a dissociative or anxiety disorder. Both can occur transiently, in a partial seizure, and *déjà vu*, the abnormal feeling of familiarity.

## Cognition and Insight

*Cognition*: impairment is usually evident in conversation.

*Insight*: does the patient believe symptoms are a sign of illness?

*Specific*: anosognosia with a parietal lesion.

*General*: in dementia and psychosis – has insight been lost?

## Formulation

Summarise the history and mental state: try to make a diagnosis.

### Risk Management

Consider: is the patient at risk from the following?

*Lack of Insight*   Lack of insight is common in dementia. Risks include wandering, leaving the gas on, continuing to drive when it is unsafe and not taking medication.

*Suicidal Ideation and Behaviour*   Suicidal thoughts should be identified: to enquire about them does not increase suicidal behaviour. Risks are increased with past suicide attempts, with chronic illness, older age, unemployment, isolation, drug and alcohol dependence. Distinguish between a considered wish to die, vague thoughts in that direction and active plans.

*Agitation and Aggression*   Hallucinations or delusions are frightening. De-escalation techniques – a quiet environment, standing back to give space, speaking slowly and listening – come first. Medication: use if this fails. Lorazepam – a useful first choice and/or an antipsychotic.

# Mental Health and Capacity Acts

Legal frameworks protect people who cannot make decisions. Any doctor – and many others – should be able to assess and document Capacity. There are no required qualifications. Capacity is issue specific – someone can agree to a blood test but not about major surgery. To have Capacity, someone must be able to:

- understand relevant information
- weigh up the pros and cons of their decision

- retain information long enough to make that decision
- communicate that decision.

Capacity is assumed, unless someone has a disorder that affects decision-making. Legal frameworks also protect patients, and others, from harm – usually this requires the psychiatric team.

## Definitions and Diagnoses in Psychiatry

Reference to DSM-5 may be helpful.

### Personality Disorders

Personality disorders are 'associated with ways of thinking and feeling about oneself and others that significantly and adversely affect how an individual functions in many aspects of life'. Various types are recognised, often with features of more than one.

- *A*: (odd/eccentric): paranoid, schizoid and schizotypal personality disorders.
- *B*: (dramatic, emotional/erratic): antisocial, borderline, histrionic and narcissistic personality disorders.
- *C*: (anxious/fearful): avoidant, dependent and obsessive–compulsive personality disorders (OCPDs).

Each is a set of traits, pervasive, maladaptive and present from young adulthood. We all have some of these features; margins are vague. It is important to recognise newly acquired changes, for example the antisocial personality disorder characterised by callousness and disinhibition. If these develop *de novo*, they can indicate fronto–temporal neurodegeneration. Typical, less-defined changes develop in MS, such as emotional lability, and apathy in Parkinson's. Traumatic brain injury can lead to many personality changes.

Functional neurological symptoms – see below – tend to develop in the context of a personality disorder. Borderline, a.k.a. emotionally unstable, is characterised by difficulty maintaining relationships, instability and impulsivity, self-harm and anger. OCPD, a.k.a. anankastic personality disorder, is characterised by perfectionism and persistence with fruitless behaviours, often with difficulty in expressing emotion (alexithymia).

### Obsessions and Compulsions

Obsessive–compulsive Personality Disorder describes a person's rigid way of thinking about how the world should be. They view that their way is correct. OCPD differs from Obsessive–Compulsive Disorder (OCD).

OCD cases tend to be anxious, and preoccupied - often realising that their behaviours are irrational but unable to resist them, for example, compulsive repetitive washing to prevent contamination. OCD is common and many of us have some minor features.

Compulsive behaviours, without the rigidity of OCPD and the pathological anxiety of OCD, can also occur as separate phenomena. Compulsive behaviours are common in

Tourette's. Complex motor tics are difficult to distinguish from compulsions: both are preceded by an urge, and both result in stereotyped actions/movements. However, compulsions, unlike motor tics, are usually goal directed, such as tidying or perfecting something. Compulsions can also occur in Parkinson's with dopamine agonists – impulse control disorder (ICD).

## Anxiety

Anxiety is characterised by fear, with physical symptoms reflecting autonomic overactivation – palpitation, dyspnoea or throat constriction (*globus*). Tremor, dizziness and paraesthesiae (from hyperventilation) can be prominent. When anxieties are triggered by certain events, they are classified more specifically, for example as post-traumatic stress disorder (PTSD) – after a life-threatening experience, or Social Anxiety Disorder – meeting new people or performing to the public.

Neurological disorders themselves provoke anxiety. The common disorders are panic disorder, which is triggered, and generalised anxiety disorder, in which symptoms are free floating and pervasive – triggers are no longer obvious. Patients may be referred to a neurologist because anxiety is accompanied by fatigue, poor concentration or because general anxiety or panic disorder is misinterpreted – as complex partial seizures, a vestibular disorder, MS or a movement disorder. Over-diagnosis of physical disease is frequent.

## Mood

Mood changes are common, sometimes in reaction to a diagnosis, to disability or pain. In some conditions, mood disturbance appears to be a reflection of how **a** disease process interacts with the brain systems that mediate emotion and cognition, as in epilepsy, Parkinson's and MS. In pseudobulbar palsy, dramatic changes in expression occur, such as excessive laughing and crying – without a psychiatric cause.

### Depression

Depression is both a colloquial and specific term. People use depression to mean transient lowering of mood (dysphoria) in response to circumstances. Unstable mood is a feature of borderline personality disorder.

When depression is of sufficient severity to affect quality of life, it becomes specific. Disorders of mood are classified as depressive or bipolar. Major depression refers to persistent low mood, anhedonia, sleep and appetite disturbance. Persistent Depressive Disorder (dysthymia) can lead to pseudodementia – cognitive impairment with depression that can resemble true dementia. Impairment generally improves with treatment.

### Mania and Hypomania

Mania is excessive heightening of mood; hypomania is less dramatic. In both, there is a sense of increased well-being, euphoria, racing thoughts, pressure of speech and diminished sleep. In mania, there is also thought disorder with rhyming speech, punning/wordplay, grandiose delusions and auditory hallucinations. In mania, dysphoric mood often follows a period of elation, with irritability or aggression. Bipolar disorder, much overused, means depression alternating with hypomania/mania. Cyclothymic refers to a mild bipolar disorder.

### Psychosis

This means loss of contact with reality. Hallucinations and delusions are frequent. Thought disorder can occur. Psychosis occurs primarily in mental illnesses, such as schizophrenia. Psychosis can also arise in neurodegenerative disorders and in delirium. People with epilepsy can become psychotic with seizure activity (peri-ictal or ictal psychosis) or between attacks.

The form of hallucinations and the content of delusions point to the nature of a disorder. In organic psychoses, hallucinations are usually visual. Patients see animals, people or vivid, frightening scenes. Tactile hallucinations – ants crawling (formication) occur in alcohol withdrawal and with cocaine. Olfactory or gustatory hallucinations occur in complex partial seizures. Auditory hallucinations usually point to schizophrenia or major affective disorder. One exception is epilepsy: interictal psychosis (Chapter 8) can occasionally resemble schizophrenia.

Psychosis can arise with severe depression, with a critical voice indicating guilt/worthlessness. Nihilistic delusions are also typical – part of the body has become dysfunctional, rotten or has even disappeared (Cotard's syndrome). In mania, delusions are usually grandiose.

Specific misidentification delusions can be seen in schizophrenia, dementia and following brain injury:

- The Capgras delusion: replacement of a familiar person by an imposter.
- The Fregoli delusion: the delusion of doubles. Two people are the same person in disguise.
- Reduplicative paramnesia: the belief that one is in a familiar place, such as at home, while admitting this is also located elsewhere.

### Catatonia

This rare state occurs in both psychiatric and neurological conditions – in schizophrenia, severe depression and in forms of encephalitis. The patient is mute, with bizarre motor abnormalities. Catatonic posturing means an unusual position held for a long duration; a limb can be moved passively to a position that is then maintained, a.k.a. waxy flexibility. Immobility can be interspersed by purposeless hyperactivity – catatonic excitement. At its most severe, in catatonic stupor, persistent rigidity, immobility and resistance to passive movement (a.k.a. *gegenhalten*) can progress to lethal catatonia – autonomic instability, hyperpyrexia and high CK. This resembles the neuroleptic malignant syndrome.

### Benign Sleep and Waking Phenomena

During transition from wakefulness to sleep (hypnagogic) or vice versa (hypnopompic), phenomena are common, without any suggestion of psychiatric or neurological disease. These include noises – bumps in the night, one's name being called out or fragments of speech. Whilst experienced from without, and they can be frightening, insight is swiftly regained. Visual phenomena – shapes, people, smells and sensations of being touched also occur. See also Chapter 19.

# Functional Neurological Disorders

One problem is that the word Functional, used to label such cases, has a clear meaning to those who deal with them, but little to others before the term is understood.

## Functional: Terminology and Background

The dictionary definition of functional begins:

- *of, or having a special activity, purpose or task; relating to the way in which something works or operates. 'There are important functional differences between left and right brain...'*
- *designed to be practical and useful, rather than attractive '... the house is functional and simple...'.*

We use functional for something different, to mean that the nervous system is NOT functioning normally despite there being no known disease.

Functional neurological disorders (FNDs) is the term used to explain features that are NOT due to damage to or disease, defined briefly here:

- One or more symptoms of altered voluntary motor or sensory function.
- Evidence of incompatibility between symptom(s) and a neurological or medical condition.
- Symptom(s) or deficit(s) are not better explained by another medical or mental disorder.
- Symptom(s) or deficit(s) cause significant distress/impairment, in social, occupational or other areas. . ..or warrants medical evaluation.

For well over a century FNDs were considered to be caused by psychological events. The term *conversion* was coined by Freud, to explain that the mind defended itself, against psychic pain by converting, unconsciously, emotion into physical symptoms. *Conversion disorder* then became incorporated into medicine. However, whilst a causative stressor may have been at work, there is little evidence to support this in most FNDs. Various pejorative/emotive terms described these phenomena, such as hysteria – or worse. Functional Neurological (Symptom) Disorder has no connotations. About one fifth of referrals to neurology clinics have an FND. Many have had an FND at some time.

## Diagnosis of FNDs

Neurologists elicit signs that indicate clearly, to them, that a problem is not organic – giveway weakness or bizarre patterns of sensory loss. In the past, the tendency was to refer to a psychiatrist, on the basis that there was a psychiatric disorder. This had drawbacks. First, the FND is a neurological diagnosis. Secondly, most of these cases do not have psychiatric illness or psychopathology. Thus, both sides were uncomfortable – psychiatrists were dealing with unfamiliar physical symptoms, and neurologists felt out of their depth.

FND can be present in isolation or as part of a disorder involving other systems, such as the bowel. Former labels included Briquet's syndrome and somatisation disorder. DSM-5 also uses Somatic Symptom Disorder to describe similar phenomena and, importantly, accepts that organic and non-organic problems can coexist. Two FNDs are mentioned here. There are many more in all specialities.

### Functional Seizures

About one fifth referred to an epilepsy clinic have functional seizures; apparent status epilepticus is often diagnosed as functional, eventually. Female:Male 4:1. Personality disorder and anxiety are common and, unlike other FNDs, a story of physical or sexual abuse. Attacks are given many different labels; the commonest now is non-epileptic attack disorder (NEAD).

NEADs either resemble generalised tonic–clonic seizures or blank spells – the patient lies motionless and uncontactable. Seizures are more likely to be non-epileptic if:

- either the prodrome or seizure itself lasts more than 5 minutes
- the eyes are closed and resist passive opening
- there are side-to-side head movements.

NEADs also occur with features typical of epilepsy, such as tongue biting, urinary incontinence, auras, confusion and apparent status, so these are poor discriminators. Injuries are also seen, typically cuts or bruises but occasionally fractures.

During an attack, the patient is conscious, though may appear unconscious. Afterwards, patients often describe that they were aware but felt detached, as in depersonalisation/derealisation, and unable to speak.

NEADs can be unrecognised panic attacks. This is especially so if the patient does not describe subjective fear but displays autonomic symptoms such as tremor and depersonalisation/derealisation. Apparent NEADs can also be syncope, with myoclonic jerks.

One discriminator is a normal EEG, during an attack. However, frontal seizures can generate bizarre movements with a normal EEG. Following a generalised tonic–clonic seizure, the serum prolactin level can be raised for 10–20 minutes; however, this too is unreliable. Failure to respond at all to anti-epileptic drugs, with frequent attacks, should raise questions.

### Functional Fixed Dystonia

Dystonia means sustained, often painful contraction of muscle groups, with involuntary movements or postures. Dystonia can be functional. Fixed dystonia is an extreme form – an abnormal posture becomes permanent. There is often a history of a minor physical injury, followed by abnormal movements.

For example, dystonia can begin with finger flexor contraction, moving to the wrist and further. In a leg, the foot becomes inverted. The patient walks on the lateral border of the foot or even on the dorsum or cannot walk at all. Dystonia can spread even to the other leg. The patient cannot move the limb voluntarily. Attempts at passive movement are met with resistance. Patients can become dissociated from the limb – they feel that it is not part of them. Joints can become ankylosed. They sometimes request amputation, and on occasion this is carried out – usually by a surgeon unfamiliar with this area of psychopathology. Paradoxically, whilst functional dystonia exists, many labelled initially as functional turn out to have an organic basis – the converse of the situation in epilepsy.

Whilst there is no doubt that functional dystonia exists, many labelled initially as functional turn out to have an organic basis – the converse of the situation in epilepsy.

### Other Diagnoses

Factitious Disorder, Munchausen's Syndrome, faking and even malingering must be considered (see DSM-5). FND should be diagnosed with extreme caution where there is blame attached and in any medicolegal case.

### Management: FNDs

When confronted with the notion that there is no organic condition, many are reluctant to accept this and feel offended. However, a clear explanation is frequently sufficient to reduce symptoms. CBT is the cornerstone. Inpatient therapy may help, with an approach similar to rehabilitation for an organic disorder. Drugs are of little value.

## Dissociative Disorders

Dissociation – a word from psychoanalysis – denotes separation of memory, sense of identity or sense of reality from consciousness. A precipitant can be psychological trauma. Dissociative disorders define the behavioural expression of these phenomena – what they look like. Dissociative disorders present as amnesia, fugue or depersonalisation/derealisation.

### Dissociative Amnesia and Fugues

Dissociative amnesia, a.k.a. psychogenic amnesia, denotes inability to recall important personal information, usually related to a psychologically stressful event. There is usually preservation – of comprehension, of environmental information and performance of learned skills.

Fugue denotes wandering – the patient appears to behave normally in a goal-directed manner but with no recollection of events and can be confused about their identity. A new identity may be adopted. A dissociative fugue can last hours to days. Similar events can be seen in epileptic automatism, but episodes are transient, and the state of altered consciousness obvious; behaviour is purposeless. In transient global amnesia (Chapters 5, 6), the patient is aware, but they cannot remember preceding events. They retain their sense of personal identity.

### Depersonalisation/Derealisation Disorder

These two states usually occur together. Patients describe feelings of disconnection from their body or not being fully inside their body, or out-of-body experiences. These are most unpleasant and pervasive. There are risks of suicide.

## Neurology and Psychiatry

Each neurological disease is associated with its own pattern of psychiatric disorder. The focus here is limited to epilepsy and disorders of movement, in part because we have some indication of the neurobiology that creates both psychiatric and organic problems.

## Epilepsy and Psychiatry

### Pre-ictal, Ictal and post-ictal Disorders

Pre-ictal depression and mood lability can occur for hours to days – usually alleviated by the seizure.

Ictal symptoms occur in complex partial seizures. Even when they precede a tonic–clonic seizure, and labelled an aura, they are ictal, usually from a frontotemporal lobe focus. Patients describe intense fear, transient depersonalisation/derealisation, *déja vu*, a taste or smell, often accompanied by transient staring, lip-smacking or plucking movements.

Post-ictally, the most common features are delirium and psychosis. Post-ictal delirium usually presents with confusion and withdrawal. Agitation/hyperactivity is less common. During delirium the patient needs to be kept safe; nothing further is usually necessary. If delirium persists, non-convulsive status and other causes should be considered.

Post-ictal psychosis typically occurs with temporal lobe attacks: a cluster of seizures is followed by a lucid interval of several hours to days. During this interval, unusual behaviour such as lethargy, irritability and restlessness may occur. Psychosis then emerges, with visual and/or auditory hallucinations and delusional beliefs, often of a religious or paranoid nature. Patients can be aggressive, violent and at risk to themselves and others. Violent and impulsive suicide is sometimes a feature. An occasional case can remain psychotic for months.

*Inter-ictal Disorders*   The most common is depression, particularly linked to temporal lobe epilepsy. Also, following neurosurgery for epilepsy, depression can develop *de novo*.

The major depressive symptoms – pervasive low mood and disturbances of sleep and appetite – are well recognised. In addition, a group of symptoms has been labelled inter-ictal dysphoric disorder. This is a state of irritability, anergia, depressed mood, insomnia, atypical pain and anxiety, sometimes with intermittent euphoria.

Depression can be treated with CBT and an antidepressant. SSRIs lower the seizure threshold less than tricyclics.

Inter-ictal psychosis is also recognised. This typically develops long after the onset of seizures. It is also termed the schizophrenia-like psychosis of epilepsy. Though a major problem, there is a better preservation of personality than in schizophrenia itself.

*Forced Normalisation in Epilepsy*   This refers to the observation that psychosis or depression or agitation can emerge when an EEG becomes normal, and/or when seizures come under control. If seizures return, there is usually an improvement in psychosis – described by the odd term alternative psychosis.

*Personality Changes in Epilepsy*   The prevalence of a personality disorder is higher in people with epilepsy than in the general population. In addition, there are behavioural traits said to be seen with epilepsy, especially temporal lobe epilepsy. Certain features are grouped together – Gastaut–Geschwind interictal behaviour syndrome. These include stickiness of thought, hypergraphia – compulsive and excessive writing, hyper-religiosity and decreased libido. The syndrome is controversial and its elements coexist rarely, if at all.

***Psychotropic Effects of Anti-Epileptics*** Anti-epileptic drugs also have psychotropic effects. For example, depression has been attributed to tiagabine, topiramate and felbamate. Drugs that promote GABA tend to be sedative and anxiolytic, such as pregabalin, gabapentin and valproate. Those that inhibit glutamate tend to be activating, such as lamotrigine. Topiramate may possibly increase the risk of psychosis.

## Movement Disorders and Psychiatry

Parkinson's, Lewy Body Dementia (LBD), multisystem atrophy (MSA), progressive supra-nuclear palsy, Wilson's disease, Huntington's and Tourette's are disorders of movement that have distinct neuropsychiatric features.

### Parkinson's Disease

Anxiety, depression, apathy, psychosis and dementia are well-recognised features of Parkinson's. Anxiety and depression tend to present early; dementia appears late.

One way of thinking about the neuropsychiatry of Parkinson's is to consider what is postulated about Lewy pathology – that it begins in the medulla and olfactory bulb. From there, the pons, midbrain, limbic cortex and neocortex become involved. Motor symptoms correlate with Lewy body pathology in the *substantia nigra*. It is likely that psychiatric symptoms develop as pathology affects systems that regulate cognition, mood and behaviour.

One difficulty with depression in Parkinson's is that there is an overlap with features such as reduced facial expression and psychomotor slowing. Depression is more frequent in Parkinson's disease than in other disabling conditions. About one-quarter of those with Parkinson's take antidepressants.

***Depression in Parkinson's*** First, are there practical issues at home that can be addressed? Optimisation of levodopa therapy is needed, especially for those whose mood dips as the dose is wearing off. If this strategy does not help, SSRIs or SNRIs are used, in the first instance. MAOIs are absolutely contraindicated in Parkinson's. In severe depression, ECT can be effective, though this is now little used.

***Anxiety in Parkinson's*** Anxiety frequently accompanies low mood. Anxiety can be intense, especially at night. Similar to depression, a link between anxiety and reduced dopaminergic neurotransmission should be considered when marked anxiety is interspersed with periods of calmness and normality. Treatment principles for depression apply; in other words, optimisation of levodopa/dopamine agonists, followed by antidepressants.

***Apathy in Parkinson's*** Apathy has many features in common with depression and is often comorbid with it and with cognitive impairment. A distinguishing feature of pure apathy is impaired motivation without low mood. Apathy may be a predictor of dementia in Parkinson's.

***Psychosis in Parkinson's*** Visual hallucinations are common – people or animals move, usually in the periphery. Another sensation is a presence, usually of a person, outside the visual field, a.k.a. an extracampine hallucination. It is often assumed that because hallucinations in Parkinson's occur in treated patients they are medication induced. Psychosis was seen before the levodopa era. Visual illusions are also common – objects seem to merge into living things – and also pseudohallucinations – the patient is aware that an object is not real. Reduction in dopaminergic therapy is the management of choice but hard to achieve. Rivastigmine and clozapine may help.

***Cognitive Impairment in Parkinson's*** About 50% of Parkinson's cases develop dementia. Main predictors are age, severe motor impairment, early visuospatial problems and low speech output. Executive dysfunction is also seen reflecting reduced dopaminergic input into non-motor cortex. Executive dysfunction alone that may improve with levodopa does not predict dementia.

***Impulse Control Disorder in Parkinson's*** Dopamine receptor agonists such as ropinirole have an unusual adverse effect – the development of ICD. Features such as gambling, overspending, inappropriate sexual behaviour and overeating emerge, largely in men. Another compulsion is punding – a behaviour originally goal directed, such as sorting clothes, that becomes senseless and repetitive. ICD occurs typically in men with young-onset Parkinson's. Management: try to stop the dopamine agonist.

### Psychiatry and Other Movement Disorders

Similar to Parkinson's, LBD and MSA are α-synucleinopathies associated with movement disorders. In LBD, pathology is prominent in the cortex – there is dementia, with visual hallucinations.

In MSA, pathology involves the brainstem autonomic nuclei and cerebellum – with ataxia, there are bladder problems and blood pressure instability. Frontal executive deficits occur in MSA, but dementia is rare.

Progressive supranuclear palsy (PSP) is a tauopathy involving amine and cholinergic neurotransmitter nuclei – *substantia nigra*, *locus caeruleus* and raphe nuclei, basal ganglia and oculomotor complex. This explains the range of symptoms – parkinsonism with oph-thalmoplegia, executive dysfunction, and apathy, mood lability, disinhibition and compulsive behaviour.

In Wilson's disease, rigidity, dystonia and choreoathetosis are accompanied by cognitive impairment, personality change, depression and even psychosis.

In Huntington's disease, psychiatric problems develop early, even before chorea. There are personality changes – irritability, aggression and disinhibition. Depression is common, and suicide an issue. Paranoid psychosis occurs.

Tourette's is an abnormality of GABA and/or dopamine synaptic function with motor and vocal tics. Tics are characterised by the build-up of an urge to perform them, which can be partially resisted. Obsessive–compulsive behaviours emerge in the late teens. Rituals of hand washing seen in OCD are not common. Instead, there is arithmomania – the need to count actions/objects and a compulsion for symmetry and order. Self-injurious tics occur – punching or eye poking – and touching can be directed at strangers. Tic suppression may be helped with dopamine receptor antagonists, in particular aripiprazole and risperidone. Obsessive–compulsive behaviour may be helped by an SSRI.

### Electrical Stimulation Effects
Deep Brain Stimulation (DBS) is an established treatment for many motor problems. However, there is a small increased risk of suicide following DBS, and cognitive decline has been reported.

### Neuropsychiatry and Other Conditions
Two other associations are mentioned briefly here. MS is common. Minor head injury sequelae are controversial.

### Psychiatry and MS
Psychopathology can develop in white matter disorders – MS and the leukoencephalopathies.

In MS, the main neuropsychiatric problem is disturbed cognition. This occurs early and can be detected in many patients when tested formally. Speed of information processing, working memory and attention are affected.

Depression, agitation, anxiety and irritability are common, often associated with inflexible thinking. Mania is also more common in MS than in the population. In more general psychiatry practice, of possible relevance to the pathology of the neuropsychiatry of MS, deep white matter lesions are seen on MR imaging more in bipolar disorder and treatment-resistant depression than in the general population.

Severe depression is a side effect of β-interferon treatment. Suicide is a distinct risk.

A state of euphoria and eutonia – the sense of well-being – was once felt to be common or even specific for MS. It was postulated that this might be a pseudobulbar effect in which mood and affect are disconnected, leading to denial of illness severity. An alternative explanation is that a minor degree of dysarthria, so common in MS, gives an impression of being joyful.

### Minor Head Injury
The neuropsychiatric features of severe TBI are discussed in Chapter 18.

Following a minor head injury, recovery over several weeks is usual, but some patients have enduring symptoms for months or years. Headaches, dizziness, fatigue, noise sensitivity and poor concentration are typical. Post-concussion syndrome, implying brain trauma, and even mild TBI are terms sometimes used when there is no evidence of neuronal damage. DSM-5 now uses the broad, if vague term neurocognitive disorder. These complaints are felt by many, but not all, to be psychological in origin, especially in legal cases.

## Acknowledgement and Further Reading

I am most grateful to Professor Eileen Joyce for her contribution to *Neurology A Queen Square Textbook* Second Edition on which this chapter is based.

**Further Reading**

DSM-5. *Diagnostic & Statistical Manual of Mental Disorders*, 5th edn. Washington, DC: American Psychiatric Association, 2013.

Joyce E. Neuropsychiatry. In *Neurology A Queen Square Textbook*, 2nd edn. Clarke C, Howard R, Rossor M, Shorvon S, eds. Chichester: John Wiley & Sons, 2016. There are useful references.

Also, please visit https://www.drcharlesclarke.com for free updated notes, potential links and other references. You will be asked to log in, in a secure fashion, with your name and institution.

23

# Pain

In neurology, we often emphasise that accurate anatomical diagnosis is essential for management. With pain, that primary diagnosis is only the beginning of the problem because characteristics of pain are generally not disease specific. For example, neuropathic limb pain can occur with peripheral neuropathy, syringomyelia or follow cerebral infarction. A diagnosis does not inform us about the nature of pain.

## Definitions

Pain is 'an unpleasant sensory and emotional experience associated with actual or potential tissue damage or described in terms of such damage'. This accepts that pain can be perceived with potential damage and includes its emotional component. Also, associations of pain are situational; some are even perceived as pleasant – forms of massage, exercise or eating a chilli. However, pain is generally unpleasant, especially when one has no control over it.

Pain can be either:

* nociceptive or
* neuropathic, a.k.a. neurogenic.

Nociceptive pain is entirely familiar – an injury or damage activates nociceptive neurones in an intact nervous system.

Neuropathic pain is harder to define – 'pain arising as a consequence of a lesion or disease affecting the somatosensory system' and qualitatively different from nociceptive.

With nociceptive pain, the pain we all know, the nervous system returns to normality. With neuropathic pain, the system is changed – consider post-herpetic neuralgia (PHN) or post-stroke pain.

Neuropathic pain is either peripheral or central. We need to try to explain how a peripheral lesion such as trauma or shingles can become dominated by central mechanisms.

Allodynia is pain from a normally innocuous stimulus:

* mechanical – light touch or
* thermal – warmth/cooling.

*Neurology: A Clinical Handbook*, First Edition. Charles Clarke.
© 2022 John Wiley & Sons Ltd. Published 2022 by John Wiley & Sons Ltd.

Hyperalgesia is sensation perception at an increased intensity.

Both allodynia and hyperalgesia can be subdivided:

- static – light pressure
- punctate – a pinprick or
- dynamic – light brushing.

Hyperpathia is a decreased or altered threshold for perception, features of neuropathic pain. A stimulus may not be felt initially, but when sustained, there is explosive pain, a reflection of central sensitisation.

Dysaesthesia is any unpleasant abnormal sensation, spontaneous or evoked. Abnormal pains, such as tactile allodynia, fall within this. Dysaesthesia need not be painful, such as sensations of insects crawling on the skin.

## Neuropathic Pain Mechanisms – Sodium and Calcium Channel Expression

In neuropathic pain, neurones develop increased excitability to produce allodynia or hyperalgesia. Explanations on the basis of ion channel changes following peripheral nerve injury include up-regulation, down-regulation, translocation and gain of function of individual voltage-gated channels.

Voltage-gated Na channels are divided into subgroups by their reaction to tetrodotoxin (TTx), puffer fish neurotoxin.

- $Na_v1.7$ and $Na_v1.8$ (both TTx resistant) influence nociception.
- Drugs that block Na channels, such as lidocaine, help neuropathic pain.
  Mutations of the *SCN9A* gene ($Na_v1.7$ channel) occur in three rare disorders:
  - a loss-of-function mutation in Congenital Insensitivity to Pain
  - a gain-of-function mutation in Primary Erythromelalgia and in
  - Paroxysmal Extreme Pain Disorder.

Calcium channel activation is also essential for neurotransmitter release:

- Activation of N-type Ca channels reduces hypersensitivity to stimuli.
- L-type Ca channels: cannabinoid receptor agonists exert analgesic effects through inhibitory action. The $\alpha_2\delta$-1 subunit that exhibits up-regulation in dorsal root ganglia and dorsal horn neurones is one site of action of gabapentin/pregabalin.
- Transient receptor potential (TRP) ion channels occur in nociceptive primary afferent neurones.
- Activation of TRPV1 – by noxious heat/capsaicin and TRPA1 – noxious cold/mustard oil – causes burning sensations. Following nerve injury, these ion channels increase within small sensory nerve fibres, the potential mechanism for cold hyperalgesia, possibly relevant in non-freezing cold injury where mild cold generates pain of a burning quality.
- Activation is also expressed in non-nociceptive Aβ fibres – a putative mechanism for mechanical allodynia.

## Sensitisation and Wind-up

Central sensitisation describes hyperexcitability of nociceptive neurones involved in allo-dynia and hyperalgesia, for example in the dorsal horn. Hypersensitivity occurs because of CNS changes, even if initiation was peripheral. Wind-up – as in a spring – describes the increasing response of dorsal horn neurones to repetitive C-fibre volleys.

## Excitation

Glutamate is the principal excitatory neurotransmitter released in the dorsal horn in response to noxious stimuli. Glutamate acts on the *N*-methyl-D-aspartic acid (NMDA) receptor, a key element in central sensitisation. Once activated, a feedback loop maintains sensitisation. Ketamine reduces sensitisation.

Following nerve injury, reorganisation occurs around termination of Aβ afferents These afferents sprout and terminate in lamina II of the dorsal horn rather than their usual deeper location. This provides another explanation for tactile (mechanical) allodynia.

## Inhibition

GABA and glycine are inhibitory neurotransmitters within the cord. Decreased GABA and loss of GABA receptors in the dorsal horn occur in peripheral nerve injury.

The endogenous opioid system is also affected by nerve injury, with loss of μ receptors in the DRG and dorsal horn, accompanied by increased synthesis of cholecystokinin, an opi-oid antagonist – one explanation for ineffectiveness of opioids in neuropathic pain. By contrast, endogenous cannabinoids appear unaffected by peripheral nerve damage – the rationale for cannabinoids.

## Inflammation, Immune System and Pain

In peripheral nerve injury, chemical mediators are released from macrophages, mast cells and Schwann cells, including tumour necrosis factor-α (TNFα) and interleukins 1β and 6 (IL-β and IL-6), prostaglandins and nerve growth factor (NGF). In the dorsal horn, activa-tion of microglia causes release of pro-inflammatory mediators, increasing hypersensitiv-ity. The parasympathetic system has a role in reducing hypersensitivity.

## Supraspinal Influences

Descending pathways from the periaqueductal grey (PAG) and medulla modulate trans-mission of pain at spinal level, with either facilitation or inhibition. In neuropathic pain, there is a shift towards facilitation.

## Central Pain

How brain and spine lesions produce central pain is uncertain – but broadly, via excitation of damaged pathways, diminution of inhibition or both.

Pain impulses reach the brain via three pathways:

*Spinoparabrachial pathway*: originates in lamina I of the dorsal horn and projects to the brainstem, PAG, hypothalamus and amygdala. This pathway is concerned with pain's emo-tional component.

*Spinothalamic pathway*: ascends in the cord, terminates in the posterolateral thalamus and projects to the sensory cortex – concerned with pain discrimination and localisation.
*Visceral and urogenital pathway*: ascends close to the cord central canal.

Descending inhibitory pathways from cortex, thalamus, hypothalamus and brainstem reach the cord and modulate/reduce spinal nociception:

- Drugs such as SSRIs that enhance the effects of noradrenaline and serotonin, the neurotransmitters that inhibit pain tend to alleviate pain. Conversely, drugs/toxins such as reserpine, para-chlorophenylalanine (PCPA, a.k.a fenclonine) and strychnine that block serotonin and GABA can produce pain.
- Stimulation of cerebral and spinal inhibitory targets alleviates pain.

Descending excitatory pathways – key relay station in the rostro-ventromedial medulla – contribute to hyperalgesia:

- CNS excitation can cause pain.
- Brain stimulation can cause pain.
- Abnormal activity develops in thalamus, midbrain and cord in central pain.
- Pain can occur in an epileptic seizure.
- Anticonvulsants and local anaesthetics alleviate central pain.

Psychological factors – the affective processing of pain, depression and blame are also important.

## Pain in CNS Diseases

### MS, Non-paroxysmal, Paroxysmal and Nociceptive Pain

Pain in MS is common, frequently severe and an example of the diversity of pain within a single disease.
Neuropathic non-paroxysmal pain is the commonest and usually of cord origin. Pain is typically in the legs and trunk with sensations of pressure, constriction and icy feet.
Neuropathic paroxysmal pain is typified by MS trigeminal neuralgia.
Lhermitte's phenomenon – spreading electrical sensations down the back and into the lower limbs provoked by neck flexion is usually painful.
Paroxysmal MS pain can occur – either spontaneously or be stimulus evoked, reflecting the site of a plaque.
Nociceptive pain from spasticity – in advanced MS.

### Parkinson's Disease, Dystonia/Dyskinesia Pain, PAF and MSA

Neuropathic (central) pain in PD is burning/stabbing with tingling, itching, tension and restlessness that can precede motor symptoms. Pain can be more marked on one side and involve the mouth, throat or genitalia. The mechanism is unknown. Levodopa rarely switches it off. Limb pain and stiffness are also common in PD.
Many involuntary movements – tics, Tourette's, torticollis, chorea or dystonia – can give rise to mechanically induced musculoskeletal pain. Other combinations of pain and

involuntary movements occur in painful legs and moving toes, chronic regional pain syndrome (CRPS) and in phantom phenomena.

In pure autonomic failure (PAF) and multiple system atrophy (Chapter 24), intense discomfort, a.k.a. coat-hanger pain, follows ischaemia in paracervical muscles.

## Central Post-Stroke Pain

Neuropathic pain can follow both infarction and haemorrhage. Thalamic pain is a term used frequently, but pain can follow a stroke elsewhere. Central post-stroke pain (CPSP) is the appropriate term.

Some 5% of stroke patients develop some CPSP. There is typically a rapidly improving hemiparesis with enduring hemianaesthesia or hyperaesthesia and/or some hemiataxia, astereognosis and choreoathetosis. There is pain on the weak side.

Weakness may be of any degree. Pain is restricted, generally, within the area of sensory loss. Pain develops within a few weeks of the stroke, but there is some delay – to even months or years. Burning is a frequent quality, and tactile/cold allodynia common. Pain can be of exceptional severity. Kinaesthetic allodynia – pain moving a small joint, a rarity – is pathognomonic.

## Spinal Cord Injury, Syringomyelia and MND

Many cord injury patients have chronic pain. Central pain can occur with a complete cord lesion/severed cord but also with partial cord lesions.

In syringomyelia, dissociated sensory loss follows damage to spinothalamic tracts and painless injuries. Central pain is also common.

In motor neurone disease, pain is aching, cramping, burning, shock-like or indescribable. In some, pain can be a dominant symptom, even when weakness is not advanced.

## Phantom Pain

Whenever a body part is removed, perception of the missing part can persist – the phantom sensation. Phantom pain develops in a missing limb or part of one; phantom teeth, breast, eye and genitalia also occur.

Phantom pain can also occur in an area that has been denervated but not amputated, for example following a brachial plexus avulsion.

Phantom pain can be burning, aching, crushing/gnawing, continuous or intermittent, sometimes with paroxysms – or with cramps, postures and distortions within the phantom. It is worse if the patient feels they cannot move the phantom. The phantom area can shrink and produce curious phenomena – of a hand tucked up under the shoulder or of a finger being enlarged, twisted and painful.

Phantom pain can develop instantaneously or days, weeks, months or years later. It is typically life-long. Resolution does rarely occur – and sometimes after a stroke in the phantom area of the cortex.

Phantom sensations occur regardless of whether the loss was due to trauma or surgical removal. Usually, loss will have been rapid, but similar phenomena occur in leprosy, where tissue loss has been gradual. Phantom phenomena are rarely experienced with congenital absence of a limb or following amputation in childhood.

Explanations include the idea that when there is denervation, changes in the cortex and thalamus develop rapidly – even a single finger ring block causes changes in the cortex within minutes. The area of brain from which input has been deprived is then invaded by innervation from adjacent areas. Shifts in cortical representation are likely to extend following amputation and may account, for instance for a touch on the face being felt in a phantom limb.

Attempts to alleviate a phantom include motor imagery. The patient is asked to mimic with the intact limb the perceived position of the phantom limb. Apparent ability to exert control over the phantom can sometimes help the pain.

Phantom pain differs from local post-amputation pain, where there are both neuropathic and nociceptive pains.

### Painful Legs and Moving Toes

There are movements, of the toes, foot or lower leg. Pain varies from discomfort to the severe and intractable – burning, crushing, cramping or twisting. Movements are usually slow, irregular and with toe fanning/clawing. Movements can be stopped deliberately but resume. They tend to become bilateral. PLAMT is sometimes confused with Restless Legs (Chapters 7 and 20).

### Epilepsy

Pain occurs, if rarely with a seizure:

- Unilateral face, arm or leg pain: seizures originate in the contralateral hemisphere. A parietal tumour can be the cause.
- Headache: distinct from post-ictal headache, an isolated headache or a migraine can be part of the seizure.
- Abdominal pain: a rare feature.

### Fibromyalgia

In fibromyalgia syndrome, a.k.a. muscular rheumatism or interstitial fibrositis, there is widespread muscle pain with no evidence of an inflammatory, fibrositic or autoimmune disorder. Pain could be caused by a state of diffuse central sensitisation, if it is accepted that there is an organic underlying cause. Associations with fibromyalgia include poor sleep with daytime fatigue, headache, irritable bowel syndrome, temporo-mandibular pain and unusual personality traits. A multi-disciplinary approach may be of some help in these cases.

## Peripheral Pain

Pain is conveyed by primary afferent nociceptor neurones activated by mechanical, thermal, tactile and chemical stimuli. These neurones contain thinly myelinated, fast conducting Aδ fibres and unmyelinated, slower C fibres; the former mediate the familiar brief, sharp first pain, and the latter delayed, diffuse and duller second pain. The majority of Aδ and C fibres are polymodal – they react to a variety of stimuli.

C fibres are subdivided into:

- Fibres that express P2X3 purine receptors – one type of ATP-responsive channel – and receptors for glial cell line-derived neurotrophic factor (GDNF). These fibres, sensitive to GDNF, terminate deep into the *substantia gelatinosa* of the cord and are important in mediating neuropathic pain.
- Fibres that contain peptides such as substance P and calcitonin gene-related peptide (CGRP) express the high-affinity NGF receptor TrkA. The fibres terminate superficially in the dorsal horn and mediate neurogenic inflammation. This inflammation sensitises nociceptor endings and produces peripheral sensitisation. These fibres are part of the diffuse visceral afferent system. They also appear to regulate behavioural sensitivity to pain via projections to the hypothalamus and amygdala.

Both groups of C fibres respond to noxious stimulation and express the vanilloid (capsaicin) TRPV1 receptor which transduces noxious chemical and heat (>43°C) stimuli. Noxious cold (<15°C) is mediated by the menthol and other cold receptors. Chemicals such as bradykinin and serotonin, lipids and low pH stimulate other receptors. Mechanical stimuli are also transduced by other receptors, poorly characterised.

These peripheral systems and their central connections can generate pain in many ways:

- *Ectopic discharges*: discharges from damaged and adjacent neurones and Schwann cells generate pain-producing substances.
- *Changes in properties of neurones*: disorders affecting the sensory nerves cause gene up- and down-regulation. For example, the α2δ Ca channel subunit is up-regulated following nerve injury – that may explain how gabapentin helps in neuropathic pain.
- *Loss of sensory neurones*: after peripheral damage, atrophy begins to affect the entire sensory bundle. This loss particularly affects C fibres. The central ends of C fibres atrophy in the dorsal horn and adjacent Aβ fibre terminals may sprout into that area. Innocuous mechanical stimuli become perceived as pain – mechanical allodynia.
- *Central sensitisation* following peripheral sensory nerve lesions takes place in the cord and brain. Central sensitisation is associated with enlargement of the peripheral area where pain is perceived. Sub-threshold stimuli now reach threshold, with an increased response to supra-threshold stimuli and pain via the affected nerve territory, prolonged pain, allodynia and hyperpathia.
- *Disinhibition* is also important, a contrast to these excitatory process. Normally, GABA and glycine mediate inhibit pain. Blocking them can cause pain. Nerve injury causes impaired GABA inhibition in the cord.
- *Microglia and other glial cells* are involved in the immune responses that follow CNS damage – see also Neuropathic Pain Mechanisms.

Trigeminal neuralgia and glossopharengeal neuralgia are covered in Chapter 13.

## Painful Peripheral Neuropathies

Examples include:

- Small fibre neuropathies, inflammatory and vascular disorders – Guillain–Barré, CIDP, diabetes, collagen vascular and vasculitis.
- Infection – HIV, leprosy, varicella-zoster and Lyme.
- Nerve infiltration – sarcoid and cancer.
- Metabolic – diabetes, alcohol, nutritional and vitamin deficiencies, cold injury, peripheral ischaemia and toxic and drug induced – thallium, vincristine (Chapter 19).
- Trauma, including iatrogenic.
- Hereditary peripheral neuropathies.

### Small Fibre Neuropathies

Burning, typically of the feet, is often caused by SFN (Chapter 10), sometimes only detectable on skin biopsy. Causes include:

- Diabetes mellitus
- Connective tissue disorders such as Sjögren's
- Monoclonal gammopathy
- Non-freezing cold injury
- Acquired amyloidosis
- Genetic causes, e.g. SCN9A mutation.

### Guillain–Barré and Neuralgic Amyotrophy

In GBS, pain can be the first symptom, mainly in the back, buttocks and thighs. This is neurogenic and radicular. Pain can be severe, even with mild weakness. It is under-recognised and can persist for several years.

Neuralgic amyotrophy (Chapter 10) is almost always extremely painful. Opioids may be needed. Pain usually subsides over some days or weeks. Steroids are unhelpful.

### Painful Inherited Neuropathies

Inherited neuropathies (Chapter 10) associated with pain include:

- Hereditary sensory and autonomic neuropathy (HSAN) type I
- Fabry's disease – paroxysmal painful symptoms from childhood bear some resemblance to erythromelalgia
- Familial amyloid neuropathies
- Tangier disease
- Erythromelalgia.

## Other Painful Conditions

### Shingles and Post-Herpetic Neuralgia (PHN)

Pain in acute shingles ranges from trivial to excruciating, but it is transient. PHN – pain 3 months after shingles-is common, increasing with the patient's age: 50% at 50, 90% at 90 is a guide. The two patterns of PHN are ends of a spectrum. In one, there is marked sesory loss, paroxysmal pain with some background pain. In the other, sensory loss is less evident, but stimulus-evoked pain – allodynia and hyperalgesia – are severe. Skin biopsies show that PHN patients have fewer cutaneous nerve endings than the pain free cases. There is focal atrophy of the dorsal horn; inflammatory changes therein persist even 2 years after shingles.

### Erythromelalgia

Features of this ill-understood condition are episodes of heat, redness and pain, predominantly in the feet, worse in hot weather. Patients sometimes immerse their feet in cold water. The heat triggering differentiates erythromelalgia from SFNs.

Erythromelalgia can be divided into:

- Sporadic, cause unknown.
- Hereditary – rare AD childhood onset with mutation in *SCN9A* encoding $Na_v1.7$.
- Secondary – to thrombocythaemia, collagen vascular disease, diabetes, calcium-channel blockers, pergolide and bromocriptine, following freezing and non-freezing cold injury.

There appears to be sensitisation of polymodal C nociceptors with abnormally low thresholds, prolonged after-discharges and vascular leakage, but how these cause the episodes remains obscure.

### Complex Regional Pain Syndrome

There is no fully accepted theory relating to CRPS and no definitive investigation. There is a tendency for CRPS to be applied indiscriminately to regional pain that remains unexplained, or for such pain to be labelled as psychiatric or even deliberate. There is a characteristic picture of which this is a dramatic personal example, adjusted to preserve confidentiality.

*A previously fit 32-year-old female sustained a sprained ankle whilst doing PT in a gym. The expected local pain and swelling followed. The ankle was bandaged, and the joint immobilised. However, the pain did not settle but gradually increased over 2 months. Oedema persisted with erythema and later pallor, mottling and coldness. Excessive sweating followed toenail thickening and coarsening of the leg hair.*

*In addition to pain, tactile and cold allodynia emerged and worsened. The foot adopted a fixed posture of plantar flexion and inversion. Two years after the injury, she had a cold, blue, immobile and useless foot that she could not bear to be touched. She perceived the limb as alien. She sought advice from several surgeons, until she found one prepared to amputate the lower leg. Pain persisted in the below-knee amputation stump and continued. She is asking for further surgery. There is litigation against the gym.*

Complex Regional Pain Syndrome was the term proposed in 1995 to replace Reflex Sympathetic Dystrophy (RSD) and causalgia. Causalgia was first coined during the American Civil War to explain the pain suffered by soldiers following amputations.

The term RSD followed a belief that the sympathetic nervous system was involved. Surgical and/or chemical sympathectomy and local anaesthetic blocks became common procedures, now believed to be futile.

The CRPS criteria are shown in Table 23.1

**Table 23.1**  Complex regional pain syndrome.

| **'Budapest Criteria'** | |
| --- | --- |
| A. Continuing pain – disproportionate to any inciting event.<br>B. At least one SIGN in two or more categories below.<br>C. At least one SYMPTOM in three or more categories below.<br>D. No other diagnosis can better explain the features. | |
| Sensory | Allodynia to light touch and/or temperature sensation and/or deep somatic pressure and/or joint movement and/or hyperalgesia to pinprick |
| Vasomotor | Temperature asymmetry and/or skin colour changes and/or skin colour asymmetry |
| Sudomotor/ oedema | Oedema and/or sweating changes and/or sweating asymmetry |
| Motor/trophic | Decreased motion and/or motor dysfunction – weakness, tremor, dystonia and/or trophic changes in hair, nails and skin. |

CRPS is often divided into type I when there is no demonstrable major nerve injury and type II when there is a major nerve injury. This distinction has little value for treatment nor does it contribute to our understanding.

CRPS can develop when there has been no trauma at all, for example following:

- Shingles
- Stroke, shoulder injury, MS and immobilisation
- Electric shock
- Systemic illness such as myocardial infarction
- Guillain–Barré
- Carpal tunnel syndrome and wrist fracture.

Sensory loss is frequently found. Pain is described as being ripped apart, burning, stinging and squeezing. Tactile and cold allodynia occur in about one-quarter, and hyperalgesia and spontaneous pain in most. Abnormalities also point to central mechanisms, such as neglect – reminiscent of a parietal lobe lesion – and perception that the extremity is enlarged.

Vasomotor changes evolve over weeks and months. Early vasomotor instability can produce vasodilatation, a.k.a. warm CRPS – and vasoconstriction, a.k.a. cold CRPS. These can alternate. After months, cold CRPS is usual. Disuse atrophy contributes to reduced blood flow. Sudomotor changes and oedema develop, almost invariably. Paucity of movement is common, but tremor and dystonia also occur.

Dystrophic changes: skin becomes thin and shiny, the digits taper, the nails become thickened, brittle and ridged. Local hair is either lost or becomes coarse. Osteoporosis occurs, but in some cases appears disproportionately severe for disuse alone. Some changes are explicable purely by disuse – think of the appearance of a limb in a cast after a fracture.

The degree of prominence of one of these domains in an individual case suggests perhaps that they are independent. In one, pain can be severe but vasomotor changes trivial, whereas in another the reverse occurs. CRPS varies greatly. Mild CRPS resolves spontaneously and few progress to resemble the case described earlier. However, in order to prevent the severe case, active movement should start early.

There is debate about whether CRPS is primarily neuropathic, or that it becomes neuropathic. Mediators of inflammation account for many of its features. Microneuronography and catecholamine venous blood assays indicate that local sympathetic outflow is reduced. The apparent excessive sympathetic activity is explained by increased sensitivity to local effects of catecholamines. There is no specific treatment. Physical therapies and psychological interventions have roles in rehabilitation.

### Viscerosomatic Disorders: Burning Mouth, Vulvodynia and Visceral Pain

Burning mouth syndrome embraces persistent and unpleasant sensations within the mouth and includes terms such as glossodynia. Women are affected more than men, typically of 50–70 years. Burning sensations are usually bilateral; any area within the mouth and tongue can be affected by persistent variable pain, with dryness of the mouth and altered taste. Examination is normal. Sensory testing suggests an abnormality of small fibre function, possibly a trigeminal neuropathy.

Vulvodynia is vulval pain with painful burning sensations, mechanical allodynia and hyperalgesia. Sometimes there is allodynia only, provoked by touch and pressure. The disorder is multi-factorial, possibly secondary to vulval atrophy, vaginal inflammation or infection.

Visceral pain means pain from activation of nociceptors in the thoracic, pelvic or abdominal organs. These structures are generally sensitive to distension, ischemia and inflammation but relatively insensitive to stimuli that normally evoke pain. Visceral pain is hard to pin down and is often accompanied by emotional problems. Two conditions, classified within gut disorders, are functional dyspepsia and irritable bowel syndrome. Such cases rarely present to a neurologist.

*Paroxysmal Extreme Pain Disorder*   Originally known as familial rectal pain, this rarity consists of pain in the rectum, face and eye, sometimes associated with flushing. Mutations in the voltage-gated sodium channel $Na_v1.7$ are usually present (SCN9A gene).

### Plexopathies

Dorsal root ganglia and proximal sensory roots can be affected by many conditions that cause pain. Three causes of painful plexopathies are:

- Trauma
- Malignancy
- Post-irradiation.

The commonest traumatic brachial plexus lesion is injury following a motor cycle accident in which there has been stretching and/or avulsion of both plexus and extradural/intradural nerve roots. Paradoxically, crash helmets are said to have made these dreadful injuries more frequent, because without head protection the rider was likely to have been killed. Pain following trauma often develops immediately but can develop or increase as months go by. Pain has a severe burning quality.

Metastatic disease, DXT or a primary tumour can infiltrate brachial or lumbosacral plexus to cause severe and unremitting pain.

### Orthopaedic Conditions: Glomus Tumour and Osteoid Osteoma

Glomus tumour is an uncommon benign bone tumour. Some 50% are in the hand – a small blue nodule beneath a nail. Features:

- Severe and continuous pain
- Extreme cold sensitivity
- Extreme tenderness – even slight contact induces exquisite pain.

Diagnosis is straightforward when a tumour is visible. Plain X-rays/MRI: bone erosion. Excision is curative.

Osteoid osteoma: typical features are severe localised pain in a limb, usually worse at night, with short-lived response to anti-inflammatory drugs. The reason for the pain, and its transient relief, is thought to be that fine nerve terminals in this benign tumour are exposed to tumour prostaglandins. The abnormal bone can show up as a radiolucent or radio-opaque nidus and a focal hot spot on isotope bone scanning. Excision is curative.

## Pain Management

Knowledge of the causes of pain focuses on the possible diagnoses. For example, a painful arm following a stroke may be from a frozen shoulder, i.e. local nociceptive pain; or, the frozen shoulder might have led to CRPS. An alternative reason is chronic post-stroke pain (CPSP) – central and neuropathic.

### Drug Treatments

In neuropathic pain, it is frustrating that no drugs are truly effective. This is in contrast to most nociceptive pain – that almost always responds to an opioid, provided the dose is sufficient. However, in neuropathic pain, not only are opioids ineffective, but drugs such as tricyclic antidepressants (TCAs) can be effective in one case but ineffective in another with the same diagnosis. Many drugs are also poorly tolerated.

Generally, even those drugs that have been shown to work do so in a minority. One measure of a drug's worth is the number of patients one needs to treat to achieve >50% pain relief in one. Typical figures are four cases with TCAs, six for SSRIs and seven cases with gabapentin or pregabalin – fairly gloomy. The reasons are poorly understood – possibly genetically determined differences in drug metabolism, or that this variation reflects differences in activation of nociceptive receptors.

#### Antidepressants

The TCAs, typically amitriptyline, have long been used in neuropathic pain of all types. They have several actions – central serotonin and noradrenaline reuptake inhibition and inhibition of voltage-gated sodium channels. All these probably contribute. Selective serotonin and noradrenaline re-uptake inhibitors (SNRIs) such as duloxetine and venlafaxine are both effective, to an extent, and better tolerated than TCAs.

### Antiepileptics

The analgaesic properties of these drugs are probably attributable to two broad mechanisms:

- Blocking of sodium channels – phenytoin, carbamazepine and oxcarbazepine, lamotrigine and lacosamide
- Inhibitory action at the α2δ-1 subunit of pre-synaptic calcium channels – gabapentin and pregabalin.

### Local Anaesthetics and Topical Agents

Drugs such as lidocaine with inhibitory actions at voltage-gated sodium channels are effective in neuropathic pain. Inhibition of neuronal activity by systemic local anaesthetics and anti-arrhythmics such as mexiletine occurs at multiple sites – peripheral neurones, dorsal root ganglia, dorsal horn, medulla and PAG. Surprisingly, a single dose of IV lidocaine can produce analgesia that persists longer than predicted from its kinetics. Lidocaine patches and capsaicin cream are used in post-herpetic and for diabetic neuropathic pains.

### NMDA Receptor Antagonists and Cannabinoids

NMDA receptor antagonists, particularly ketamine, are used in both central and peripheral pain. Ketamine is reasonably safe and can be given IV and sublingually.

Cannabinoids can relieve both neuropathic pain and painful spasticity. Nabilone (synthetic tetrahydrocannabinol, THC) in a capsule and a spray (Sativex), a mixture of THC and cannibadiol, are used. Neuropathic pain appears more responsive to cannabinoids than nociceptive pain.

### Botulinum Toxin

Botulinum toxin has pain-relieving properties in addition to the relief of muscle spasm. Post-herpetic neuralgia and trigeminal neuralgia may be helped. Botox has become widely used in headache therapy.

### Intrathecal Drugs

Baclofen, clonidine, opioids and ziconotide have been used – principally baclofen for spasticity. Phenol has long been used intrathecally to destroy nerve roots in severe spasticity. The evidence bases for these therapies are poor and benefit unpredictable.

### Neuroablative Procedures

Over the past 30 years, there has been a decline in procedures designed to interrupt pain pathways. Apart from local risks of any destructive procedure, painful sensory loss, a.k.a. *anaesthesia dolorosa*, can follow a section of nerve. Destructive procedures are still occasionally performed, for instance dorsal root entry zone lesions for pain from spinal cord or brachial plexus injury. Trigeminal ganglion injection can be helpful in trigeminal neuralgia, and radiofrequency thermocoagulation denervation remains an established treatment.

### Neurostimulation Procedures

Many parts of the nervous system have been stimulated to try to relieve pain. Whilst electrical stimulation was carried out, sometimes in an almost punitive way in the nineteenth century and later, much of the rationale for neurostimulation is based on the 1965 Gate Control Theory of Pain (Chapter 2) – the concept that activation of large diameter afferent fibres might inhibit or gate small diameter, pain-subserving fibres in the dorsal horn and possibly elsewhere. Although controversial, Gate Theory led to largely innocuous neural stimulation techniques and generated great interest in pain modulation.

*Transcutaneous Nerve Stimulation*   TENS involves applying skin electrodes with an interposed gel. Impulses are of variable frequency and intensity, selected by the patient. Stimulation can be continuous or intermittent. Benefit is unpredictable, but TENS sometimes helps. Some pains are made transiently worse, particularly if there is tactile allodynia. Controlled trials are obviously difficult, but TENS is simple, safe and cheap. One suggested mechanism is segmental inhibition at the dorsal horn.

### Peripheral Nerve Stimulation

Implantation of electrodes around a peripheral nerve to obtain pain relief is now rarely undertaken. However, there is a trend for dorsal root ganglion stimulation and pulsed radiofrequency stimulation. Occipital nerve stimulation has also become established in the treatment of intractable headache (Chapter 12).

### Spinal Cord Stimulation

Spinal cord stimulation (SCS, a.k.a. dorsal column stimulation) was also initiated on the basis of Gate Control Theory, with electrodes implanted in the posterior epidural space. The aim is to stimulate the dorsal columns, but this is probably not its only mode of action. Successful stimulation generally produces paraesthesia in the painful territory.

Indications include CRPS, neuropathic nerve root pain and following poor outcome from decompressive spinal surgery. In general, neuropathic pain where the lesion is peripheral responds better than pain of cord origin. SCS has been tried for some visceral pains and for angina.

### Deep Brain Stimulation

This specialised technique originated from two startling observations: in humans, stimulation of the fornix and septal regions during psychosurgery produced analgesia, and in rats, stimulation of the central midbrain grey matter allowed the animals to be operated on without an anaesthetic. The three areas most frequently targeted include the PAG, periventricular grey matter and the somatosensory nuclei of the thalamus. Debate continues about indications for DBS – it is sometimes considered in cases with constant, burning neuropathic pain unresponsive to other measures.

### Motor Cortex Stimulation

This counter-intuitive procedure involves the extradural placement of electrodes over the motor cortex. Pain relief is thought to occur from descending inhibition, in turn mediated by sensory pathways in the motor cortex. Repetitive transcranial magnetic stimulation over the motor cortex has been used to provide analgesia in both central pain and trigeminal neuralgia.

**Other Physical Treatments**

Many forms of physical therapy and massage by osteopaths and chiropractors, physiotherapists, occupational therapists and others can be helpful in chronic pain. Acupuncture is another form of peripheral stimulation.

*Acupuncture*   Acupuncture has been used for millennia. Various techniques are employed:

- Needle stimulation of local points in painful areas, such as for tennis elbow.
- Needle stimulation of distant points, sometimes multiple and along Chinese acupuncture lines. Importance of these precise points is doubtful.
- Needle(s) are inserted, rotated or stimulated at different depths.
- Treatment is often given for about 30 minutes – optimum duration is unclear.

Acupuncture is used for numerous disorders. It is most effective for musculoskeletal rather than neuropathic pain. Side effects are infrequent. Despite potential for placebo effects, acupuncture provides powerful peripheral stimulation. Acupuncture carried out for long periods and at a stimulus intensity sufficient to cause pain raises the pain threshold and induces analgesia. Acupuncture-induced analgesia has been used to allow surgery to take place without general anaesthesia.

## Psychological Approaches

In chronic pain, it is the affective, behavioural and practical aspects that are crucial for the patient, rather than any fine print relating to perceived mechanisms. Whilst pain is anatomical and thus local, it has a major and general affective component. Structures such as the anterior cingulate, prefrontal cortex, amygdala and insula are implicated in encoding both pain and emotion. There is a tendency to assume that severity of perceived pain correlates with its intensity or seriousness – though neither can be measured, or conversely that chronic pain has some psychiatric cause. Really, any division between psychological and somatosensory aspects of pain is meaningless and reflects more upon the views/prejudice of the physician or others than upon reality.

Approaches to pain management can be divided into four aspects that require assessment:

- attention – the effect of pain on day-to-day life, as perceived by others and by the patient
- catastrophising – recognition and placing in perspective the severity of the problem, especially when the cause is neither malignant nor itself catastrophic
- avoidance – assessment of measures that help the patient avoid pain, and
- depression – recognition and enthusiastic treatment.

Psychologists who are members of the multi-disciplinary pain management team tend to use different approaches, and thus it is hard to compare different interventions. There is no doubt that CBT is effective. A considered psychiatric opinion is also valuable. However, it is distinctly unwise to attribute chronic pain to a psychiatric/psychological cause. Malingering and Munchausen's presenting as chronic pain are well recognised but rare. Chronic pain in a medicolegal context is multi-faceted and outside the scope of this chapter.

### The Placebo Phenomenon

The pain placebo phenomenon is evident – those who take an inert substance experience reduced pain. It is often thought that pain relief from sham treatment can have only a psychological basis, but there is some evidence that placebos have physiological effects:

- Placebo ultrasound after wisdom tooth extraction can reduce pain, swelling/trismus and reduce CRP levels.
- Naloxone can sometimes reverse placebo analgesia, suggesting that endogenous opioids are at work.
- Placebo analgesia is associated with altered cerebral blood flow, similar to that seen with opioids.
- Functional MRI suggests that placebo decreases activity in pain-subserving brain regions.
- Placebo effects occur following non-surgery – aborted or even faked surgery.
- Placebo effect is seen with non-painful disorders such as Parkinson's and depression.
- 'Nocebo' responses, when an inert treatment induces an adverse reaction are well recognised.

Ethical considerations: the consensus is that no one should receive a placebo without being informed about the possibility and consent secured.

## Diminished Sensitivity to Pain

In these rare conditions, stimuli that would normally be painful are not transmitted to the brain. This lack of pain input occurs in some hereditary small fibre neuropathies, notably HSAN type IV. Patients with this AR neuropathy develop painless injuries. They lack unmyelinated peripheral axons and sensory neurones in the DRG and elsewhere. Mechanisms relate to mutations in the TrkA gene that encodes the high-affinity receptor for NGF, crucial for nociceptive and sympathetic neurone development. Acquired causes include the occasional case of diabetes, tabes dorsalis and syringomyelia. Patients suffer painless injuries and develop Charcot joints and sometimes osteomyelitis.

### Congenital Insensitivity to Pain

In congenital insensitivity to pain (a.k.a. asymbolia for pain, congenital pure analgesia and congenital indifference to pain), patients have absent pain recognition from birth. They do not react to painful stimuli anywhere, but other sensory modalities and reflexes are normal. They sustain painless injuries. AD and AR families have been reported. In some damage to the insula perhaps leading to sensori-limbic disconnection has been reported. In others, the indifference to pain is caused by impaired function of the voltage-gated sodium channel gene *SCN9A*, encoding the $Na_v$ 1.7 sodium channel – a channelopathy-associated insensitivity to pain.

### Transient Indifference to Pain

In situations where severe pain might be expected, it may not be experienced at all, for several hours. Described in World War II, this is also seen rarely with civilian injuries. It was originally assumed that the absence of pain was a reaction to having survived, but these cases were noted to be distressed not elated. Moreover, analgesia was confined to the injury site – the soldier with a shattered leg would complain bitterly about venous cannulation. A postulated mechanism is transient cortical and spinal inhibition. Perhaps, comparable is the impaired pain perception during a parasomnia when an injury is sustained. Pain indifference occurs transiently with opiates, sometimes to an extraordinary degree – and also when drunk.

## Acknowledgement and Further Reading

I am most grateful to Paul Nandi for his contribution to *Neurology A Queen Square Textbook* Second Edition on which this chapter is based.

Nandi P. Pain. In *Neurology A Queen Square Textbook* 2nd edn. Clarke C, Howard R, Rossor M, Shorvon S, eds. Chichester: Wiley Blackwell, 2016. There are many useful references.

Also, please visit https://www.drcharlesclarke.com for free updated notes, potential links and other references. You will be asked to log in, in a secure fashion, with your name and institution.

# 24

# Autonomic Aspects of Neurology

## Anatomy and Neurotransmission

Autonomic pathways, the craniosacral parasympathetic and thoracolumbar outflows (Figure 24.1), are of importance to every organ. The system not only influences target organs but also operates centrally to control, for example blood pressure and core temperature. Neurotransmitters in each pathway influence ganglionic and post-ganglionic activity, which are summarised in Figure 24.2.

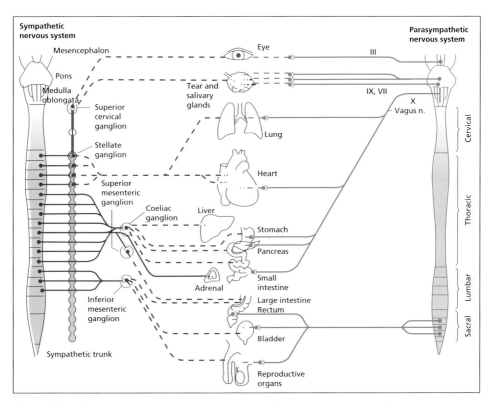

**Figure 24.1** Craniosacral parasympathetic and thoracolumbar sympathetic outflows.

*Neurology: A Clinical Handbook*, First Edition. Charles Clarke.
© 2022 John Wiley & Sons Ltd. Published 2022 by John Wiley & Sons Ltd.

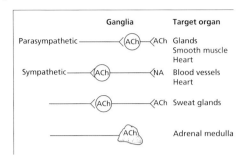

**Figure 24.2** Major neurotransmitters at autonomic ganglia..

I summarise here localised autonomic disorders, syncope, features of regional autonomic dysfunction and the main conditions seen in an adult general neurology clinic – autonomic failure with Parkinson's, multiple system atrophy (MSA) and pure autonomic failure (PAF). Rarities are also mentioned.

## Localised Autonomic Disorders

Localised disorders affect either an organ or a region. Some, such as Horner's and a Holmes–Adie pupil, will be familiar and are dealt with in other chapters.

- Crocodile tears, a.k.a. Bogorad syndrome, is the shedding of tears while eating or drinking in patients who have recovered from Bell's palsy – gustatory lacrimation. There is aberrant reinnervation of parasympathetic components of the facial nerve.
- Frey's syndrome is sweating while eating – gustatory sweating – and facial flushing caused by auriculotemporal nerve damage, typically after parotid surgery.
- Focal idiopathic hyperhidrosis most frequently affects the palms, axillae, soles or face. Sympathectomy is sometimes carried out for palmar and axillary sweating.

## Primary and Secondary Autonomic Disorders

Disorders are either primary or can be secondary to a disease – though the distinction is somewhat arbitrary. Intermittent autonomic dysfunction with recovery – for example, the familiar autonomic mediated syncope (AMS) and postural tachycardia syndrome (PoTS) – are generally manageable. Damage to the autonomic system secondary to neurological disease is typically irreversible and often untreatable. Classifications use different terminologies – for example, the term neurally mediated syncope is also used for AMS.

### Syncope

Syncope (fainting, autonomic mediated syncope, a.k.a. AMS) has many causes. In AMS, there is transient hypotension and bradycardia, without pre-existing orthostatic hypotension and often with a provoking factor. BP falls because of sympathetic withdrawal. Heart rate falls because of increased vagal activity. Effects are more likely when upright. There are typically no abnormalities between attacks. The history and recovery usually separate AMS from epilepsy. Recovery on lying flat usually is rapid. Tongue biting is exceptional. Rarely, a hypoxic convulsion can follow, especially if the subject is not laid flat, with urinary incontinence occasionally.

The three forms of relevance here are:

- Vasovagal syncope
- Carotid sinus hypersensitivity
- Situational syncope.

In vasovagal syncope, a.k.a. common faints, emotional syncope, provoking factors include fear, pain, sight of blood and medical procedures, especially needles. Nausea, palpitation and sweating occur in the pre-syncopal phase. In most, sitting or lying flat prevents syncope. Prolonged standing tends to provoke syncope. Diagnosis is usually evident.

Carotid sinus hypersensitivity is recognised as a cause of falls in the elderly, more in textbooks than in practice. There may be a history of syncope induced while shaving, head turning or buttoning a collar.

In situational syncope, a Valsalva manoeuvre and/or hyperventilation can provoke an attack. This occurs with weight lifters, trumpeters, with deliberate manoeuvres and following paroxysms of coughing. In micturition syncope, typical in males at night, hypotension follows the combination of vasodilatation caused by warmth and/or alcohol and straining during micturition – that induces a Valsalva – compounded by the release of the pressor stimulus arising from a distended bladder while upright. Swallowing-induced syncope can occur, if rarely, with glossopharyngeal neuralgia (Chapter 13).

## Orthostatic (Postural) Hypotension

Orthostatic hypotension is frequent and may point to an underlying disease. Definition: a BP fall of 20 mmHg systolic or 10 mmHg diastolic on rising from the supine, to sitting, standing or during a 60° tilt test. In neurogenic orthostatic hypotension, plasma noradrenaline levels do not rise when upright: they do so normally. Hypoperfusion, especially of organs above the heart such as the brain, causes malaise, nausea, dizziness and the visual disturbances that often precede syncope.

Hypotension can vary: syncope can occur instantly. Occasionally, a hypoxic seizure can follow cerebral hypoperfusion.

Many symptoms can occur:

- Coat-hanger pain (suboccipital and shoulders) develops when upright and is helped by lying flat.
- Exercising the arms when upright can reduce brain blood flow by a steal mechanism.
- Central chest pain can occur with normal coronary arteries – chest wall ischaemia.
- Oliguria, by day, when upright, follows reduced renal perfusion.
- Polyuria when supine occurs at night when BP is restored.
- Falls and unsteadiness can occur, without any other symptom of orthostatic hypotension.

Less defined complaints are weakness and fatigue. Prominent symptoms follow getting out of bed, on rising after a large meal, alcohol, sunbathing and on exercise. Many recognise the postural effect and sit down, lie flat, squat or assume curious postures. With time, some come to tolerate low cerebral perfusion. Orthostatic hypotension is often worsened by hypotensive treatment, by levodopa, insulin and sildenafil.

## Orthostatic Intolerance with Posturally Induced Tachycardia (PoTS)

Orthostatic intolerance without hypotension, but with a substantial rise in heart rate, is known as PoTS. This tends to affect women <50 years. Dizziness on postural change or modest exertion, pre-syncope or syncope may occur, without generalised autonomic features. Associations include joint hypermobility (Ehlers–Danlos III), chronic fatigue, mitral

**Table 24.1**  Autonomic investigations.

---

*Cardiovascular*

Heart rate responses: hyperventilation, standing, tilt tests, R–R interval, carotid sinus massage, Valsava, pressor stimuli and exercise testing

*Endocrine*

Plasma and urine catecholamine studies, renin and aldosterone

*Sudomotor*

Central thermoregulatory sweat test, sweat gland studies and sympathetic skin responses

*Gut*

Fluoroscopy, barium and endoscopy

*Renal, urinary tract and sexual function*

Urine constituents and urodynamic and penis studies

*Respiratory, eye and tears*

Laryngoscopy, sleep studies, pupil pharmacology and Schirmer's test

---

valve prolapse and hyperventilation. There is a range of opinion here about whether all the features have an organic basis, but the condition is well-recognised.

### Examination and Investigation

Physical examination with attention to autonomic features is essential. Postural BP is often omitted. In many syncope cases, frequently no tests are necessary. Tests carried out in autonomic laboratories are summarised in Table 24.1.

## Regional Autonomic Dysfunction

Regional features of evident dysfunction and some conditions in which they occur are summarised here. When BP falls, facial pallor with an ashen appearance can follow – common knowledge. With phaeochromocytoma, facial pallor can also sometimes occur during a hypertensive attack, usually with sweating.

- In Harlequin syndrome – damage to second and third thoracic root sympathetic fibres, sparing the first, from which oculomotor fibres leave – there is vasodilatation and anhidrosis on one side of the face with sparing of the pupil.
- Raynaud's can occur in both primary autonomic failure and multisystem atrophy.
- Raynaud's can also follow cold injury.
- *Livedo reticularis* can accompany sympathetic overactivity, as in phaeochromocytoma.
- Erythromelalgia (Chapter 23): limb discomfort and vascular changes.

### Sudomotor: Anhidrosis and Hyperhidrosis

Eccrine glands – temperature regulation – are innervated by sympathetic cholinergic fibres. Apocrine glands on palms and soles are influenced mainly by catecholamines.

- Anhidrosis is common in PAF.
- Anhidrosis can be isolated and congenital.
- Anhidrosis can be a component of a neuropathy, such as congenital insensitivity to pain with anhidrosis (HSAN type IV; Chapters 10 and 23).
- Anhidrosis, local or generalised, can occur with a Holmes–Adie pupil (Ross syndrome, Chapter 14).
- Hyperhidrosis can follow high cord lesions – sweating occurs over the face and neck.
- Parkinson's: facial and truncal hyperhidrosis can occur.
- Hyperhidrosis can occur intermittently in phaeochromocytoma and accompany hypertension/spasms in tetanus.

## Gut

- Reduced salivation with dry mouth, a.k.a. xerostomia, occurs in the rare pure cholinergic dysautonomia, sometimes with dysphagia.
- The smooth muscle of the lower two-thirds of the oesophagus is autonomically innervated. This is involved in Chagas' disease and in achalasia.
- In diabetes, gastric stasis can lead to distension and vomiting. Diarrhoea, especially at night, can be a feature of diabetic autonomic neuropathy.
- Constipation is common in primary autonomic failure.
- With PoTS and Ehlers–Danlos III, reflux, bloating and constipation can occur.

## Kidneys and Urinary Tract

Nocturnal polyuria is frequent in primary autonomic failure. There is BP elevation when supine, with redistribution of blood centrally with changes in renin, aldosterone and atrial natriuretic peptide levels. In MSA, there can be additional impairment of bladder and sphincter control. By day, low BP when upright can lead to oliguria.

Autonomic failure can cause urinary frequency, urgency, incontinence or retention. Loss of sacral parasympathetic function in the early phase of spinal cord injury causes an atonic bladder, with retention, whereas recovery of cord function causes a neurogenic bladder. Dyssynergia, with detrusor contraction but without sphincter relaxation, also occurs.

## Sexual Dysfunction

Erectile failure depends in part on the parasympathetic function. Ejaculation is a sympathetic function. To dissociate effects of increasing age, drugs, illness and depression from neurological causes of impotence is frequently impossible. Many drugs can have autonomic side effects and diminish sexual potency. The situation in females is less clear – male impotence dominates this field. See also Chapter 25.

## Respiratory

Involuntary inspiratory sighs, stridor and snoring of recent onset occur in MSA more frequently than in Parkinson's. Nocturnal apnoea, which occurs in the later stages of MSA, is caused by involvement of brainstem respiratory centres.

**Hypertension and Cardiac Changes**

High BP can sometimes occur:

- With high spinal cord lesions, paroxysmal hypertension can develop when an uninhibited increase in spinal sympathetic activity is caused by bladder contraction, large bowel irritation, pain or muscle spasms. This can cause a pounding headache, palpitation, bradycardia and sweating, with flushing over the face and neck. Limbs tend to be vasoconstricted and cold.
- In tetanus, hypertension can follow muscle spasms and/or tracheal suction in ventilated cases.
- In phaeochromocytoma, Guillain–Barré syndrome, acute intermittent porphyria and rarely with posterior fossa tumours, high blood pressure can occur, sometimes with bradycardia.
- Following subarachnoid haemorrhage, sustained hypertension can ensue, with or without vasospasm.
- In PAF, hypertension in the supine position can complicate orthostatic hypotension.
- Severe pain can cause severe hypertension as a transient phenomenon.
- Scombroid poisoning causes intense flushing, tachycardia and hypertension (Chapter 19).
- Essential hypertension perhaps the commonest form of autonomic dysfunction also deserves mention.

Severe bradycardia can sometimes occur:

- With ventilated high cervical cord injury cases with diaphragm paralysis. Intact vagi are sensitive to hypoxia: stimuli such as tracheal suction can induce bradycardia and even asystole. Similar responses occur in tetraplegic patients during anaesthesia.
- In neurally mediated syncope, with hypotension.

Other autonomic abnormalities:

- Cardiac denervation occurs following transplantation, typically permanently – and is often remarkably well tolerated at rest. However, the heart rate can only increase slowly via circulating catecholamines, and stroke volume can be insufficient in response to exercise.
- A fast pulse occurs in diabetes with a vagal neuropathy.
- Tachycardia occurs, by definition, in PoTS.
- Cardiac conduction disorders are common in Chagas' disease and in amyloidosis – sick sinus syndrome is typical.

# Parkinson's Disease, Multiple System Atrophy (MSA) and Pure Autonomic Failure (PAF)

These conditions have been mentioned above, and they are related by prominent autonomic features. In some reviews it may seem that each condition can be separated clinically. The reality is that it can be difficult to sort out a precise diagnosis, and equally, once an autonomic disturbance has caused a clinical problem, this can be difficult to treat.

In idiopathic Parkinson's disease, autonomic features can be present, particularly orthostatic hypotension, made worse by levodopa therapy. Idiopathic Parkinson's disease merges with PD with Autonomic Failure (PD + AF), where autonomic features become more prominent.

MSA is complicated by its three forms – parkinsonian multiple system atrophy (MSA-P), cerebellar multiple system atrophy (MSA-C) and mixed MSA – MSA-M. In MSA-P, there is some initial response to levodopa, but orthostatic hypotension can become a substantial problem. In MSA-C, ataxia can be difficult to separate from or perhaps be compounded by orthostatic hypotension.

Pure autonomic failure is a neurodegenerative disorder characterised by orthostatic hypotension, and once known as Bradbury–Eggleston syndrome from the 1925 description. Patients typically present in midlife with orthostatic hypotension and/or syncope. Autonomic failure can also cause bladder, bowel and thermoregulatory dysfunction. Pathologically, PAF is characterised by deposition of α-synuclein. Patients with PAF may progress into other synucleinopathies with CNS involvement.

## Rare Autonomic Disorders

The wider classification of these rare disorders is mentioned here. Table 24.2 can be used as a basis for further study.

**Table 24.2**   Classification of autonomic disorders.

| |
| --- |
| **Primary autonomic disorders** |
| *Acute/subacute dysautonomias* |
| Pure pandysautonomia and with neurological features |
| Pure cholinergic dysautonomia |
| *Chronic autonomic failure syndromes* |
| Pure autonomic failure |
| Multiple system atrophy (Shy–Drager syndrome) |
| Autonomic failure with Parkinson's |
| **Secondary autonomic disorders** |
| *Congenital/Genetic* |
| Nerve growth factor deficiency |
| Familial amyloid neuropathy (AD) |
| Familial dysautonomia – Riley–Day syndrome (AR) |
| Dopamine β-hydroxylase deficiency (AR) |
| *Metabolic diseases* |
| Diabetes mellitus and renal/hepatic failure |
| *Inflammatory and Infections* |
| Guillain–Barré, transverse myelitis, tetanus and HIV |
| *Cancer* |
| Posterior fossa, third and fourth ventricle, tumours and paraneoplastic syndromes |
| *Surgery and trauma* |
| Vagotomy and drainage procedures – 'dumping syndrome' and cervical/thoracic cord transection |
| *Drugs and toxins* |
| Direct neurotransmitter effects or via a neuropathy |

## Acknowledgements and Further Reading

I am most grateful to Christopher Mathias, Gordon Ingle and Valerie Iodice for their contribution to Neurology A Queen Square Textbook Second Edition on which this chapter was based.

Mathias C, Ingle G, Iodice V. Autonomic aspects of neurology. In *Neurology A Queen Square Textbook*, 2nd edn. Clarke C, Howard R, Rossor M, Shorvon S, eds. Chichester: John Wiley & Sons, 2016. There are numerous references.

Also, please visit https://www.drcharlesclarke.com for free updated notes, potential links and other references. You will be asked to log in, in a secure fashion, with your name and institution.

# 25

# Uro-Neurology and Sexual Dysfunction

The central neuroanatomy of micturition control is summarised in Figure 25.1.

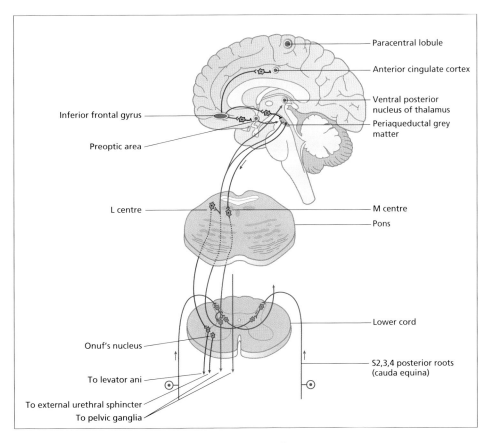

**Figure 25.1**   Central neuroanatomy of micturition control.

*Neurology: A Clinical Handbook*, First Edition. Charles Clarke.

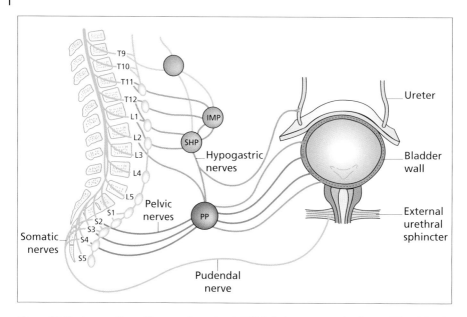

**Figure 25.2**  Innervation of lower urinary tract. IMP, inferior mesenteric plexus; PP, pelvic plexus; SHP, superior hypogastric plexus.

## Lower Urinary Tract: Neurological Control

The nerve supply of the bladder is shown in Figure 25.2. The bladder and urethra have two functions: storage and periodic elimination of urine that require synergistic activity between smooth and striated muscles. The lower urinary tract differs from other visceral organs: micturition is under voluntary control and also depends on learned behaviours. This reflects the role that the CNS has in controlling it but also renders the lower urinary tract susceptible whenever there is CNS disease. Many other autonomic systems are regulated involuntarily and are maintained even after damage to their innervation.

The lower urinary tract has two main modes of operation, with a phasic regulator:

- Storage: the bladder is in this phase much of the time. Micturition is once every 3–4 hours, except during sleep. The bladder capacity is 400–600 mL.
- Voiding: switching to void mode is initiated in part by conscious decision, by the state of bladder fullness, assessment of social appropriateness and sensory inputs, such as sudden exposure to cold.

During the storage phase, the tension within the bladder outlet is raised to maintain continence, mediated through sympathetic and pudendal nerve activation of the internal and external urethral sphincters. Inhibition of the parasympathetic outflow prevents detrusor contraction. Throughout the storage phase, our perception of bladder fullness enables us to plan the next appropriate place to void, before reaching that uncomfortable position – being desperate to micturate. To effect proper storage and voiding, connections between cortex, pons, cord and peripheral innervation must remain intact:

- Voluntary control of micturition originates in the cortex
- Switching to void mode takes place in the brainstem
- Impulses pass to the sacral cord S2–S3
- Neurones of the lower urinary tract are activated.

The periaqueductal grey matter (PAG) is a crucial relay centre. PAG has connections with the thalamus, insula, cingulate and prefrontal cortices and serves as a conduit for afferent activity from the pelvic organs, to inform the pontine micturition centre about bladder fullness.

The prefrontal cortex, the seat of cognitive and appropriate social behaviour, is activated on bladder filling – the social control of bladder function.

With the decision to void, fMRI activation appears in the prefrontal cortex, insula, hypothalamus, PAG and the pontine micturition centre. The pontine micturition centre is no longer inhibited. Sphincter–detrusor activation reverses. There is relaxation of both urethral sphincter and pelvic floor muscles and parasympathetic contraction of the detrusor. Thus, micturition takes place, sometimes with relief.

## Bladder Dysfunction and Neurological Disease

Many lesions cause bladder dysfunction – the character depends on the level of the lesion. This is complicated by the effects of ageing, the male prostate, a female tendency to stress incontinence and by the fact that written descriptions of the effects of lesions at different levels vary. In some cases, disorders of the urethral outlet are present – potentially correctable conditions. In the elderly, there is also evidence of detrusor and local axonal degeneration. If one adds to these the fact that individual patients react in different ways and that therapies are limited, the management of bladder dysfunction needs to be very much tailor-made.

### Frontal Disease and Stroke

When a lesion is above the level of the pons, inhibitory control of the pontine micturition centre is lost. This causes involuntary spontaneous contractions of the detrusor muscle, a.k.a. detrusor overactivity. Early frontal pathology causes frequency of micturition and urge incontinence, but the patient is socially aware. When frontal lobe disease progresses, loss of social inhibition increases. The patient may become unconcerned. Either incontinence or socially inappropriate voiding follows. To complicate matters, urinary retention occasionally occurs with cortical disease.

Following a stroke, detrusor overactivity is common and the usual cause of long-term incontinence. At a general level, incontinence at 7 days following a stroke is an indicator of both poor independence later on and thus lower survival. Haemorrhagic stroke cases tend to have initial urinary retention.

## Parkinson's Disease

Nocturia is common. There is reduced capacity and detrusor overactivity, usually with incomplete emptying, a common enough situation – and obviously, prostatic outflow obstruction is common in males with PD anyway.

One hypothesis to explain bladder symptoms in PD is that dopaminergic neurone degeneration cause loss of tonically D1-mediated inhibition of the pontine micturition centre. Effects of levodopa vary: levodopa exacerbates detrusor overactivity during bladder filling, but also improves bladder emptying, through increased detrusor contractility, so that post-micturition residual volumes diminish.

## Multiple System Atrophy

Bladder control can fail early, before postural hypotension. There are several explanations:

- Selective atrophy in the pons.
- Atrophy of axons of the intermediolateral cell column that carry autonomic innervation to sacral region.
- Degeneration in Onuf's nucleus.

The effects in MSA are detrusor overactivity, incomplete emptying, an open bladder neck in men and sphincter weakness, all compounding to produce early and severe incontinence. Bladder dysfunction may change during the course of MSA: a reduction in detrusor overactivity and increase in post-micturition residual volume.

## Spinal Cord Disease

Following acute spinal cord injury (SCI), the bladder becomes acontractile during the stage of spinal shock. Over several weeks, reflex detrusor contractions develop. C fibres, formerly quiescent, have emerged as the main neural drivers to activate a new spinal reflex that causes detrusor overactivity. The cord lesion that has enabled the emergence of the new reflex also causes UMN signs in the lower limbs: urge incontinence is particularly likely to affect patients with spastic paraparesis.

In addition, in SCI, because there is disconnection from the pontine micturition centre, control of synergy between sphincter and detrusor fails: the sphincter tends to contract when the detrusor is contracting, a.k.a. detrusor–sphincter dyssynergia (DSD).

This, together with poor neural drive on the detrusor muscle during attempts to void, produces incomplete bladder emptying. Incomplete bladder emptying can in turn exacerbate the symptoms caused by detrusor overactivity, but these difficulties may not be evident. Following SCI, detrusor overactivity and DSD can cause ureteric reflux and hydronephrosis. Renal failure was once a common cause of death following SCI. These patients need to remain under joint care with a urologist. The situation is summarised in Table 25.1.

**Table 25.1**  Cord lesions and the bladder.

| Dysfunction | Symptoms |
| --- | --- |
| Detrusor overactivity: involuntary detrusor contractions at low filling volumes | Urgency, frequency |
| | Urge incontinence |
| Detrusor–sphincter dyssynergia (DSD) | Interrupted stream, incomplete bladder emptying |
| Detrusor underactivity | Poor stream, incomplete bladder emptying |
| Loss of central connections | Impaired initiation of voiding voluntarily, inability to suppress urgency |

## MS and Peripheral Lesions

MS affects the cord, from the uro-neurological perspective in ways similar to those of SCI, but with increasing disability and brain lesions, the patient's needs may be different. Bladder symptoms become especially difficult as mobility deteriorates. The common problem is detrusor overactivity. Patients also have difficulty with voiding, hesitancy, an interrupted stream and incomplete emptying – commonly based on the observation that having passed urine, the patient can and needs to do so again within 5–10 minutes.

Pelvic nerve injuries: nerves and nerve roots can be damaged by surgery, such as resection of rectal cancer, prostatectomy and hysterectomy, or trauma. Incontinence following radical prostatectomy or hysterectomy can also be caused by damage to the parasympathetic innervation of the detrusor.

# Urinary Retention

Retention, typically a male problem with prostatism, also occurs in neurological disease. Examination may reveal:

- Sensory loss in sacral dermatomes – saddle area – perineal and perianal sensory loss
- Weak voluntary contraction of the anal sphincter
- Absent anal and bulbocavernosus reflexes
- Lower limb areflexia.

Innervation of the lower bowel and genitalia is shared through S2, 3 and 4. Patients in retention because of a *cauda equina* lesion, such as a central disc – a neurosurgical emergency – frequently have saddle sensory loss and bowel and sexual dysfunction.

## Urinary Retention in Women: Fowler's Syndrome

Unexplained urinary retention in women was once thought to have a psychogenic cause. In 1985, an EMG abnormality of the striated urethral sphincter was described. It was thought that this impaired urethral relaxation caused obstructed voiding, incomplete bladder emptying and/or retention. Some cases have polycystic ovaries. Fowler's syndrome is characterised by painless retention and a bladder capacity in excess of 1 L. Many Fowler's cases have had an incident that triggered the onset, such as surgery, a urinary infection or childbirth. It has been postulated that a hormonally sensitive channelopathy of the striated urethral sphincter causes this involuntary continuous contraction. However, the mechanism for retention has become unclear. In many cases, a chronic pain syndrome is also present. It has even been suggested that both Fowler's and other cases of retention are the result of cord and/or neuronal intoxication by enkephalins.

Painless isolated unexplained retention in men not associated with prostatism, constipation or sexual dysfunction is most uncommon. Investigation fails to reveal an abnormality. It is speculated that such retention is caused by some abnormality of intrinsic afferent innervation, thought to be part of the bladder stretch-sensing apparatus.

## Management

The bladder has a small repertoire. Incontinence and retention are the product of many pathologies. Treatments are limited.

### Storage Dysfunction: Simple Measures

Before any tests and drugs, simple measures help:

- Fluid intake control – around 1–2 L/24 hours.
- Caffeine reduction – or a change of product may be helpful.
- Alcohol is a bladder stimulant and affects individuals in different ways. Alcohol interferes with sleep in many, especially after the age of 50.
- Bladder retraining – void by the clock. 'Hold on' – voluntarily.
- Pelvic floor exercises can also help.
- Perineal hygiene and clean clothes focus attention and are socially appropriate.

### Investigations

Initial assessment consists of routine tests, renal function, outflow obstruction investigations and imaging, if required. Urodynamic testing and sphincter EMG are carried out in some cases.

### Other Measures and Drugs

The two initial interventions for detrusor overactivity and incomplete emptying are shown in Figure 25.3.

If these measures are insufficient, detrusor injection with botulinum toxin is considered. Botox is injected into multiple sites within the detrusor. This helps storage symptoms – reducing frequency, urgency, nocturia and incontinence. Benefits last for up to a year. Retention is a potential issue. Patients must be shown how to perform clean intermittent self-catheterisation (CISC).

Antimuscarinics, such as oxybutynin, are the first line drugs for the overactive bladder. They block parasympathetic effects on M2/M3 receptors of the detrusor, though their actions may be more complex.

Desmopressin, an arginine vasopressin analogue, reduces urine production temporarily by promoting water reabsorption in the kidney. It is useful for frequency or nocturia in MS and also helpful for the nocturnal polyuria in PD. However, in the over 60s, it should be used with caution: oedema, hyponatraemia and congestive failure need to be considered.

***Neuromodulation*** Tibial nerve stimulation is effective in some with an overactive bladder.

Sacral neuromodulation is also used to treat detrusor overactivity and urgency incontinence and in Fowler's syndrome. The procedure consists of introduction of an electrode into the sacral extradural space, testing stimulation and if appropriate, a second stage – a permanent subcutaneous stimulator. Stimulation is continued at a level that is sub-sensory.

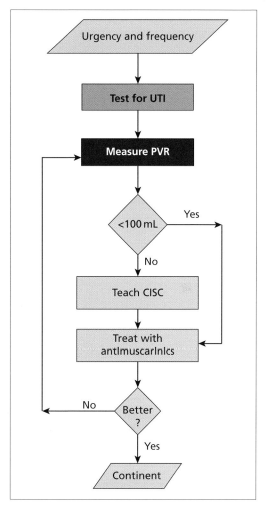

**Figure 25.3** Algorithm for incontinence. CISC, clean intermittent self-catheterisation; PVR, post-void residual.

## Voiding Dysfunction

Prior to prescribing an antimuscarinic, it is important to measure the post-void residual (PVR) volume, particularly if symptoms suggest incomplete voiding. PVR can be measured by catheterisation or with a hand-held ultrasound bladder scanner. The importance of recognising incomplete emptying is that any residual volume can trigger volume-determined reflex detrusor contractions, exacerbating the situation. If a patient with symptoms has a PVR >100 mL, CISC is advocated.

## Clean Intermittent Self-Catheterisation

A specialist nurse is usually the best person to instruct how to carry out CISC. Women may require a mirror to locate the urethral orifice, but once learnt, even blind or partially sighted patients become proficient. Frequency of CISC will best be determined by the patient, but initially they should perform this 3–4 times/day. Symptomless bacteriuria is common with CISC and is not an indication for antibiotics. A suprapubic vibrating stimulus also helps some to improve bladder emptying.

## Sexual Function

Sexual function depends on nervous system integrity at all levels: higher centres determine cognitive and emotional aspects of sexual drive, hormonal levels drive libido via the hypothalamus, and the ability to effect a sexual response depends on spinal autonomic reflexes. Malfunction of some aspect of this system is therefore common in neurological disease and of course without any disease at all.

Widespread brain responses on sexual arousal are well shown by fMRI. There is barely a cerebral structure that is not involved in some way. Activation of the prefrontal cortex, anterior cingulate, occipitotemporal cortex, thalamus, amygdala, hypothalamus, insula and claustrum is seen, many long known to be important in sexual activity. On fMRI:

- Penile stimulation by a partner shows activation on the right side of the insula, the somatosensory cortex – and deactivation of the amygdala and hypothalamus.
- Male ejaculation and female orgasm show prominent fMRI activity in the dopamine-rich mesodiencephalic junction–ventral tegmentum, an area activated in the rush of heroin and cocaine.

Two pathways subserve the male erectile response: a psychogenic pathway via the thoracolumbar sympathetic outflow (T12–L2) and a sacral spinal reflex pathway, whereby genital stimulation results in a short-lived erection. In neurological health these two responses fuse to produce an erection adequate for intercourse. Comparable pathways mediate vaginal lubrication and hyperaemia, the analogous female sexual responses.

Penile erection follows increased blood flow into the corpus cavernosum, a response mediated by the efferent parasympathetic pathway originating in the cord (S2–S4) via the pelvic nerves. The preganglionic neurotransmitter here is acetylcholine. Post-ganglionic nerve fibres that terminate either on vascular smooth muscle of the corporeal arterioles or non-vascular smooth muscle of trabecular tissue, surrounding the corporeal lacunae, release nitric oxide (NO).

Vaginal arousal is associated with increased blood flow, erection of cavernous tissue in the clitoris and the outer vagina. Erectile responses of these tissues are NO dependent. Nerve fibres containing vasoactive intestinal polypeptide (VIP), calcitonin gene-related peptide (CGRP) and substance P have also been described in the clitoris. Vaginal lubrication, also NO mediated, that increases markedly with arousal, is dependent both on intact innervation and by oestrogen levels and thus affected by drugs such as letrozole that depress the latter.

Detumescence after orgasm in both genders is mediated by noradrenaline in the sympathetic system. In the absence of stimulation, the sympathetic maintains both penile flaccidity and the vagina in its unaroused state.

Orgasm and ejaculation:

- Orgasm involves contraction of pelvic floor muscles via the perineal branches of the pudendal nerves.
- Ejaculation involves forceful emission of semen into the posterior urethra and closure of the bladder neck. In neurological disease, either can be affected.
- Female orgasm also involves contractions of the pelvic floor muscles and vaginal muscles.
- Immediate cerebral components of orgasm are prominently vascular – there is brief hypertension in both genders.

## Sexual Dysfunction and Neurological Disease

Sexual dysfunction is significant and frequently underestimated.

### Traumatic Brain Injury and Stroke

Sexual dysfunction, usually with reduced sexual desire, is common following TBI, particularly if there has been substantial cognitive damage. However, damage to prefrontal areas can result either in erotic apathy or inappropriate disinhibition. Similar problems can follow encephalitis. Partner dissatisfaction has an important role. Hypothalamic and pituitary damage following TBI is recognised but generally overstated.

### Epilepsy

Temporal lobe epilepsy can have sexual manifestations. Sexual auras can occur in complex partial seizures and genital automatisms. Occasionally hypersexuality occurs in TLE, but the usual story is failure of arousal – probably, the result of temporolimbic involvement, rather than the consequence of the diagnosis, psychosocial factors or antiepileptic drugs.

### Parkinson's and Multi-System Atrophy

Sexual dysfunction in PD is unresolved. One survey of PD patients and their partners revealed dissatisfaction – typically in male PD cases who complained of erectile dysfunction and premature ejaculation. Another study compared men with PD against those with arthritis and found similar sexual dysfunction in both. Age, disease severity and depression, testosterone levels and enthusiasm of the patient and/or partner are the major determinants of sexual dysfunction in PD, as in other situations. Sexually compulsive behaviour – very damaging – can develop in PD with impulse control disorder (Chapters 7 and 21).

Dopaminergic mechanisms are involved both in libido and penile erection. The medial preoptic area of the hypothalamus regulates sexual drive: stimulation of D2 dopaminergic receptors increases sexual activity. In 2001, the proerectile effect of apomorphine was recommended as a treatment for erectile dysfunction. Other drugs, such as sildenafil, are now preferred. Deep brain subthalamic nucleus stimulation may help sexual well-being in men but not women. In MSA, erectile dysfunction can be an early symptom, initially intermittent.

## Spinal Cord Injury, MS and other Spinal Lesions

Early SCI studies showed that the level and completeness of a lesion determined the extent of preserved erectile and ejaculatory capacity in paraplegic men. These observations led in part to the concept of both spinal reflex and psychogenic pathways for erection. Following a complete cervical lesion, psychogenic erections were lost, but spontaneous reflex erections remained intact. In low lesions, particularly if the *cauda equina* was involved, there was erectile dysfunction. The thoracolumbar sympathetic outflow originates between T12 and L2. Psychogenic erectile responses are mediated through this pathway. Occasionally, men with low lumbar cord lesions but intact sacral roots retain psychogenically driven erectile responses. In women with SCI, many aspects of genital neurology are affected. Women have little genital sensation, poor vaginal lubrication and have difficulty in reaching orgasm.

### Multiple Sclerosis

Cord plaques in men with MS can cause initially partial erectile dysfunction with pre-served nocturnal and morning erections. Typically, this worsens. Sildenafil is used widely by men with MS. Some are helped; others continue to have difficulty. Yohimbine can be tried. One recourse is to use a vibrating sex aid, if this acceptable. Women with MS report sexual dysfunction less frequently, but the problem is common, increasing with disability.

### Sympathetic Thoracolumbar Outflow T10–L2 Lesions

Thoracolumbar sympathetic pathways emerge at T10–L2 and then course through the ret-roperitoneal space to the aortic bifurcation to enter the pelvic plexuses. Sympathetic fibres are injured during retroperitoneal lymph node dissection. Loss of sympathetic innervation causes disorders of ejaculation with either failure of emission or retrograde ejaculation, though ability to experience orgasm can be retained.

### Conus, Cauda Equina and Other Lesions

The *cauda equina* contains the sacral parasympathetic outflow and both somatic efferent and afferent fibres. A lesion results in sensory loss and a parasympathetic defect. Both men and women complain of loss of perineal sensory and of erotic genital sensation – for which there is no effective treatment. Diabetic neuropathy is a common cause of male ED, and in females decreased vaginal lubrication and capacity for orgasm.

## Sexual Dysfunction: Management

Many factors, quite obviously, influence sexual function in neurological disease. Measures such as pelvic floor exercises, electrical stimulation and cognitive therapy, which can improve the neurologically intact, have not been found to be generally effective. Treatment is distinctly limited. However, there is no doubt that discussion of this topic can be helpful, if this is desired by the patient and/or their partner. Health workers should be aware that the needs and aspirations of one partner may differ from the other and that anyone con-ducting an interview is likely to know little of the true sexual history of either party.

***Type 5 Phosphodiesterase Inhibitors*** In the 1990s, in men with neurogenic erectile dysfunction, corporeal injections of papaverine and alprostadil were used, until sildenafil citrate, the type 5 phosphodiesterase inhibitor (PDE-5), appeared in 1998. Normal erectile function is dependent on the smooth-muscle relaxing effects of NO mediated by the cyclic nucleotide pathway. Down-regulation of this pathway is central to erectile dysfunction. Hence, selective inhibition of PDE-5, which catalyses degradation of cyclic guanosine monophosphate, promotes erectile responses. The efficacy of sildenafil transformed the situation and also opened discussion. Vardenafil, which has high *in vitro* potency, and tadalafil enable couples to have sex with less planning. Female sexual dysfunction is much less helped: this does not mean it is not a problem.

## Acknowledgememts, References and Further Reading

I am most grateful to Jalesh Panicker for his contribution to *Neurology A Queen Square Textbook* Second Edition on which this chapter is based and to Clare Fowler who was the Lead Author of the chapter in the First Edition.

The late Professor MJ Turlough Fitzgerald, Professor of Anatomy, National University of Ireland, Galway provided Figure 25.1 from Fitzgerald MJT, Gruener G, Mtui E. *Clinical Neuroananatomy and Neuroscience* 6th Edition. Elsevier 2012. Figure 25.2: courtesy of www.deckerpublishing.com, with permission. Professor Clare Fowler CBE provided Figure 25.3.

Fitzgerald MJT, Gruener G, Mtui E. *Clinical Neuroananatomy and Neuroscience*, 6th edn. Philadelphia, PA: Elsevier, 2012.

Fowler CJ, Panicker JN, Drake M, Harris C, Harrison SCW, Kirby M, *et al*. A UK census on the management of the bladder in multiple sclerosis. *J Neurol Neurosurg Psychiatry* 2009; **80**: 470–477.

Panicker J. Uro-neurology. In *Neurology A Queen Square Textbook*, 2nd edn. Clarke C, Howard R, Rossor M, Shorvon S, eds. Chichester: John Wiley & Sons, 2016. There are numerous references.

Also, please visit https://www.drcharlesclarke.com for free updated notes, potential links and other references. You will be asked to log in, in a secure fashion, with your name and institution.

# 26

# Systemic Conditions and Neurology

This chapter is an overview of the neurology of general medicine and pregnancy. Conditions include vascular disease, endocrine conditions, diabetes and electrolyte disturbances, hepatic and uraemic encephalopathy and blood disorders. Vitamin deficiencies are mentioned in Chapter 19.

## Cardiac and Aortic Disease

Relevant vascular anatomy is outlined here. Stroke and TIA – the main effects of embolism from the heart and/or great vessels – are covered in Chapter 6. Aortic disease and/or surgery can lead to damage to the brain, cord and peripheral nervous system. The great vessels of the aortic arch that supply the brain, brainstem and cord are illustrated in Figures 26.1 and 26.2.

### Cerebral Ischaemia and Aortic Disease

Aortic atheroma, aortitis or aneurysm can cause cerebral ischaemia, typically via an embolic stroke. Steal syndromes can also follow innominate or subclavian disease, proximal to a vertebral artery origin. Steal describes a theft of blood, meaning reverse flow, usually in a left vertebral artery with exercise of that arm, that increases limb blood flow. Subclavian steal syndrome implies posterior circulation ischaemia, *i.e.* vertigo, visual disturbances and ataxia. Most steals are asymptomatic.

### Spinal Cord Ischaemia and Aortic Disease

A thoracic anterior spinal artery syndrome is typical – abrupt loss of spinothalamic sensation and paralysis below the lesion and loss of sphincter control but some preserved dorsal column function. Radicular thoracic pain is often severe. Cervical cord infarction is uncommon – the cervical cord has a more robust blood supply than lower regions.

Infarction can follow aortic disease or surgery, but no cause is found in most. Atheroma and thromboembolism in the anterior spinal artery itself are rare.

Aortic atheroscleroma, aortitis, dissection, aneurysms or coarctation can also cause cord ischaemia – pathology generally involves the suprarenal aorta.

*Neurology: A Clinical Handbook*, First Edition. Charles Clarke.
© 2022 John Wiley & Sons Ltd. Published 2022 by John Wiley & Sons Ltd.

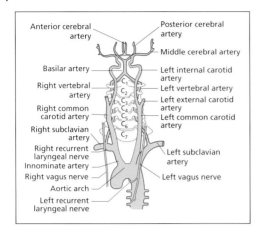

**Figure 26.1** Arteries arising from the aorta.

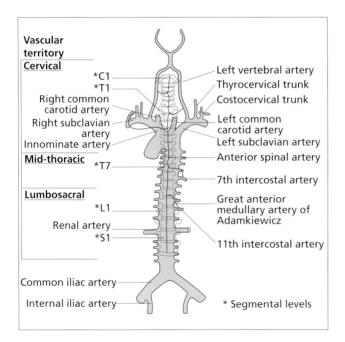

**Figure 26.2** Arterial supply: spinal cord.

Spinal infarction is usually evident clinically (paraparesis/paraplegia, Chapter 16). MRI shows cord signal abnormalities. Cardiac/aortic surgery with clamping of the aorta, and aortic angiography, can also cause an anterior spinal artery syndrome.

Dissection of the thoracic aorta causes searing interscapular pain, shock and asymmetric arm pulses. Dissection can cause ischaemia of the midthoracic cord. Syphilitic aortitis is now rare – this typically affected the thoracic aorta, with cerebral embolism. In the abdominal aorta, aneurysmal dilatation is usually atheromatous.

Takayasu's disease, the rare large vessel vasculitis, causes aortitis, typically in females below the age of 30. There is a pre-pulseless phase with fever, weight loss, arthralgia, myalgia, night sweats and chest pain. The pulseless phase follows, with aortic arch vessel occlusion, aortic regurgitation, aneurysm formation and hypertension. Stroke/TIA can occur.

**Table 26.1** Causes of cardiac embolism.

---

*Rhythm disturbances*

Atrial fibrillation/flutter, sick sinus syndrome

*Cardiomyopathy*

Congenital, alcohol, cocaine, amyloid, sarcoid, ischaemic heart disease

*Valve disease*

Endocarditis, rheumatic heart disease, mitral valve prolapse, prosthetic valves

*Other cardiac lesions*

Atrial myxoma, ventricular aneurysm, patent foramen ovale, ventricular akinesia following infarction

---

### Cardiac Surgery: Neurological Complications

Early sequelae of bypass grafting (CABG) include stroke, delirium, seizures and encephalopathy. Mechanisms include microemboli and hypoperfusion during surgery and atrial fibrillation. Embolism is the most common mechanism of post-operative stroke. Pre-existing cerebrovascular diseases, especially carotid stenosis, are risk factors. If carotid stenosis is greater than 70% or bilateral, surgical intervention is considered. Other complications include cognitive abnormalities – executive, memory, attention and processing speed. Most improve over months, but not all.

### Cardiac Embolism

Cardiac embolism accounts for about a quarter of ischaemic strokes (Table 26.1). About 80% of these emboli enter the anterior cerebral vessels. Cardioembolism to the posterior circulation is less common, but certain stroke syndromes are characteristic:

- Top of the basilar syndrome – stupor/coma, visual field loss, limb sensory or motor symptoms
- Unilateral posterior cerebral artery occlusion causing hemianopia.

## Endocrine Disease

### Thyroid Disorders

Thyroid disease can affect the CNS, peripheral nerves and muscle, via high or low levels of T4 and/or T3 and/or immune-mediated damage.

#### Hyperthyroidism

Hyperthyroidism is frequently autoimmune (Graves' disease), but other causes are thyroiditis, multi-nodular goitre or, quite exceptionally, a pituitary tumour. A myopathy is present in almost all with hyperthyroidism, sometimes symptomless. Onset is subacute, with weak proximal limb muscles – difficulty ascending stairs or rising from a chair. Muscle pain is common. Proximal wasting involves shoulder and pelvic girdles, with limb hyperreflexia but normal tone. Bulbar weakness can be prominent occasionally.

Hyperthyroidism can be associated with hypokalaemic periodic paralysis, seen mainly in SE Asia (Chapter 10).

Creatine kinase is normal. EMG: polyphasic motor potentials and/or decrement in CMAP on repetitive stimulation.

Hyperthyroidism can occasionally cause an upper motor neurone syndrome, with leg spasticity, weakness and extensor plantars and mimic cord compression. A mixed UMN and LMN picture can resemble amyotrophic lateral sclerosis.

The typical fine tremor is common. Myoclonus and chorea occur and, oddly, even parkinsonism.

Polyneuropathy is rare, but a flaccid paraparesis can occur, a.k.a. Basedow's paraplegia.

Thyroid eye disease is a common feature of Graves' disease – lid retraction, inflammation of orbital soft tissues – redness and swelling of lids and conjunctivae, proptosis and extraocular ophthalmoplegia. Both eyes are affected, sometimes asymmetrically.

Hyperthyroid encephalopathy is rare but can occur in untreated cases, after radioiodine, during intercurrent illness or following surgery. Signs: florid thyrotoxicosis, confusion, agitation, fever and seizures, a.k.a. thyroid storm.

About one-fifth of myasthenia gravis cases have a thyroid disorder, mostly hyperthyroidism.

### Hypothyroidism

Hypothyroidism is easily curable. Encephalopathy with lethargy and slow cognition develops. When severe, myxoedema coma can follow, with hypothermia, usually following sepsis or trauma. Neuropsychiatric features can also develop – psychosis with hallucinations, a.k.a. myxoedema madness. Hypothyroidism should be excluded in any dementia.

Muscle weakness is common. Mild limb weakness with depressed or slow-relaxing reflexes – once seen never forgotten (a.k.a. pseudomyotonia). Percussion can cause slow muscle rippling. Some pain is typical.

Cerebellar ataxia occurs, if rarely, in hypothyroidism. Hypothyroidism also causes carpal tunnel syndrome. Check thyroid function in any suspected case. Treatment avoids surgery. A mild polyneuropathy sometimes develops.

***Hashimoto's Encephalopathy*** Hashimoto's encephalopathy, a.k.a. steroid-responsive encephalopathy associated with autoimmune thyroiditis (SREAT), describes a subacute, sometimes relapsing encephalopathy, responding to steroids and associated with antithyroid antibodies. The encephalopathy is not explained by thyroid hormone levels, which can be normal.

## Diabetes Mellitus

Diabetes can cause many effects on the nervous system – hyperglycaemia, hypoglycaemia and diabetic neuropathies.

### Acute Metabolic Disturbances

Diabetic ketoacidosis occurs because of insufficient insulin levels in type 1 diabetes, usually because of insulin omission or undertreatment and/or intercurrent illness. Drowsiness occurs but not usually coma. Rarely, cerebral oedema follows over-rapid correction of hyperosmolality, especially in children.

Hyper-osmolar non-ketotic coma (HONK) occurs mainly in type 2 diabetes with high glucose and high sodium levels and thus high osmolality. Seizures can occur.

Hypoglycaemia can follow excess of oral hypoglycaemics or insulin. With a low blood sugar, there is often a warning, such as sweating, trembling, tingling hands and palpitation. Features of hypoglycaemia include confusion, dysarthria, altered behaviour and agitation, seizures and focal signs that can mimic a TIA or stroke. Coma follows. If hypoglycaemic coma remains unrecognised, brain injury can ensue.

### Diabetic Neuropathies

Distal sensorimotor neuropathy is found commonly with long-standing diabetes. Others include (Chapter 10) autonomic neuropathy, acute painful neuropathy, cranial neuropathy – especially III nerve, painful proximal neuropathy a.k.a. diabetic amyotrophy and thoracoabdominal neuropathy.

## Other Endocrine Disorders

Pituitary tumours are covered in Chapter 21. Pituitary apoplexy (Sheehan's syndrome) is mentioned in the section on pregnancy.

## Adrenal Disorders

### Cushing's

Cushing's disease means pituitary ACTH hypersecretion and thus high plasma cortisol, from a pituitary adenoma. Cushing's syndrome follows steroid therapy or primary hyper-adrenalism – ACTH is low. Disease and syndrome are typically indistinguishable – obesity, hypertension, hirsutism, striae, acne, menstrual irregularity, immunosuppression, myopathy and psychosis.

### Addison's

Adrenal insufficiency in the past was sometimes caused by adrenal TB. Autoimmunity is now the common cause. Features are faintness, episodes of unexplained stupor or coma, weight loss, apathy, vomiting and skin/mucous membrane pigmentation. Addison's can be life threatening during intercurrent illness. A rare cause is adrenoleukodystrophy, with brain and spinal cord involvement (Chapter 19). Secondary adrenal failure is due to ACTH deficiency – iatrogenic or from pituitary failure.

### Phaeochromocytoma

This catecholamine secreting tumour of the adrenal medulla, a cause of hypertension, can sometimes be extramedullary (paraganglioma) and/or multiple. Other features: palpitation, headaches, weight loss, accelerated hypertension and rarely intracranial haemorrhage.

# Electrolyte Disturbances

Electrolyte abnormalities range from being symptomless to causing disturbances in both central and peripheral nervous systems. Severity is greatest when an abnormality has developed rapidly. The CNS effects of electrolyte imbalance are related to fluid shifts/brain volume changes, with secondary neurotransmitter changes.

### Potassium, Calcium and Magnesium

Hyperkalaemia and hypokalaemia are features of periodic paralyses (Chapter 10), and whatever the cause, the main neurological effect of low – or sometimes high – potassium is weakness.

Calcium abnormalities do sometimes present to a neurologist. Tetany is the prominent feature of hypocalcaemia – tingling or numbness (perioral and in hands/feet), cramps and carpopedal spasm, laryngospasm, seizures or generalised tonic contractions. Other features include fatigue, irritability and anxiety, but even with severe hypocalcaemia some have no neuromuscular symptoms. Occasionally chorea is a presenting feature of chronic hypocalcaemia. Key causes are hypoparathyroidism, pseudohypoparathyroidism and vitamin D deficiency. Chronic hypocalcaemia can lead to basal ganglia calcification.

Isolated low magnesium is uncommon. Features overlap with the associated hypocalcaemia. Hypomagnesaemia can occur in eclampsia.

## Blood Disorders

### Anaemias

A low haemoglobin, usually below 8 g/dL, can cause fatigue, dizziness, impaired concentration, syncope, irritability and headache. Occasionally, severe anaemia (<6 g/dL, typically) can cause TIAs, usually with stenosis in an extra- or intracranial artery. Iron deficiency anaemia has been questioned as a rare cause of intracranial hypertension. Iron deficiency is also associated with restless leg syndrome (Chapters 6 and 20, and the section on pregnancy). Retinal haemorrhages occur with severe anaemias, especially with $B_{12}$ deficiency.

Vitamin $B_{12}$ deficiency, the prominent cause of megaloblastic anaemia, and its neurology are covered in Chapters 16 and 19. Before $B_{12}$ was discovered – finally, in1948 – pernicious anaemia and its sequelae such as subacute combined degeneration of the cord (SACD) could be fatal, though there were treatments with liver extracts.

Nitrous oxide exposure and low serum copper are rare causes of a syndrome resembling SACD.

Sickle cell disease causes neurological problems. Intravascular sickling of erythrocytes produces a large vessel arteriopathy, small vessel occlusion and coagulopathy. Stroke in sickle cell disease is common. Sickling is exacerbated by low oxygen saturation and/or intercurrent illness. Small vessels occlusion causes subcortical infarction, often symptomless. Large intracranial vessels can develop intimal proliferation to produce stenosis and thromboembolism.

Following large artery stroke, there can be distal collateral formation, a.k.a. secondary Moyamoya. Haemorrhage can occur, notably subarachnoid. Many have imaging evidence of cerebrovascular disease. Treatments include partial-exchange transfusion, hydroxyurea and bone marrow transplantation.

Thalassaemia is a rare cause of neurological problems. Haematopoiesis outside the marrow occurs in lymphoid tissue, spleen, liver and bone. Myelopathy can occur.

## Leukaemias

Neurological problems are caused by tissue infiltration, haemorrhage with low platelets, hyperviscosity or infection.

Meningeal leukaemia is most commonly associated with acute lymphocytic leukaemia – a subacute meningitis with headache, drowsiness, neck stiffness, cranial neuropathy and papilloedema. CSF contains leukaemic cells and high protein. Impaired CSF resorption can lead to hydrocephalus. Solid leukaemic deposits may occur in any part of the CNS. Peripheral nerve involvement can occur – for example, an apparent Bell's palsy.

## Plasma Cell Dyscrasias

Plasma cell dyscrasias include myelomas, Waldenstrom's macroglobulinaemia, monoclonal gammopathy of undetermined significance (MGUS), plasmacytoma and plasma cell leukaemia.

Multiple myeloma affects bones and cause pain, fractures and sometimes cord, *cauda equina*, root compression or cranial neuropathies. Polyneuropathy can occur – by a paraneoplastic mechanism, amyloid deposition or direct nerve infiltration.

Waldenstrom's macroglobulinaemia is secondary to lymphoplasmacytoid lymphoma, causing hyperviscosity with an IgM gammopathy. A progressive sensorimotor neuropathy results from IgM antibody binding and/or lymphocytic infiltration in about a quarter. Hyperviscosity can cause stroke.

The rare Bing–Neel syndrome describes CNS infiltration by neoplastic lymphoplasmacytoid cells in brain parenchyma, meninges and/or CSF to cause seizures, hearing loss and cognitive impairment.

MGUS is a benign condition, but some develop a malignant plasma cell dyscrasia, with a chronic demyelinating polyneuropathy.

## Lymphomas

Hodgkin's and non-Hodgkin's lymphomas can affect the nervous system. Usually, patients have evidence of lymphoma elsewhere. Cord and meningeal infiltration occur. The *cauda equina* and lumbosacral roots and/or the hemispheres, cerebellum and brainstem can be infiltrated. Paraneoplastic syndromes include polyneuropathy, necrotising myelopathy, leukoencephalopathy and polymyositis.

Primary CNS lymphoma: see Chapter 21.

### Langerhans Cell Histiocytosis

Langerhans cell histiocytosis is a rare disorder. Histiocytes derived from skin and mucosa produce osteolytic lesions, in bone – especially skull, in multiple organs and within the CNS. Cases present with local bony pain/swelling, seizures and/or cranial nerve palsies.

Related, absolute rarities:

- Erdheim–Chester disease – a multisystem, infiltrative and histiocytic disorder that can affect the CNS.
- Rosai–Dorfman disease – histiocytosis with massive lymphadenopathy involving mediastinum, axilla, groin, head and neck.

### Polycythaemia and Thrombocythaemia

Polycythaemia is either primary (*polycythaemia vera*) or secondary to another condition such as chronic hypoxia, for example Monge's disease (Chapter 19).

Symptoms: ill-defined – poor concentration, mild headaches, tinnitus, paresthesiae or acute vascular events, permanent or transient. Chorea occurs with polycythaemia related to a mutation in the erythropoietin receptor gene, *JAK2*. *Polycythaemia vera* can transform into leukaemias, or myelofibrosis.

Thrombocythaemia (platelets >800 000/mm$^3$) is associated with CNS thrombosis and haemorrhage and also occurs with leukaemia or myelodysplasia. Thrombosis can occur in arteries, veins or venous sinuses. Sagittal sinus thrombosis, mimicking idiopathic intracranial hypertension, can occur.

### Thrombotic Thrombocytopenic Purpura and Bleeding Disorders

Thrombotic thrombocytopenic purpura (TTP), a rarity of early adult life, is characterised by occlusion of small vessels – recurrent microangiopathic haemolysis with platelet microthrombi, familial or acquired. Endothelial cells secrete abnormally large von Willebrand factor multimers that are not degraded because of lack of the cleavage enzyme ADAMTS-13. Features: fevers, hepatic and renal disease with a low platelet count and encephalopathy – the presenting feature in many cases often provoked by an intercurrent illness. Ischaemic stroke and cerebral haemorrhage also occur. Fragmented red cells, elevated LDH, bilirubin and reticulocyte count also point toward TTP.

Haemophilia, disseminated intravascular coagulation and von Willebrand's disease are also rare causes of intracerebral haemorrhage.

### Coagulation Disorders

The antiphospholipid antibody syndrome, usually characterised by venous thromboses, is also a rare cause of arterial cerebrovascular events, sometimes with rashes, migraine and recurrent miscarriage. Thrombophilias including protein C and S deficiency, antithrombin III deficiency, factor V Leiden and the *MTHFR* mutation are associated with cerebral venous thrombosis (Chapters 6 and 19).

Anticoagulants, especially when improperly monitored, are prominent causes of cerebral and spinal haemorrhage.

### Primary Immunodeficiency

Inherited immune defects affect humoral immunity, cell-mediated immunity, phagocytic and/or complement function.

Combined immunodeficiency is caused by mutations of the genes coding for both T and B cell functions: a severe form causes early death from infection. Incomplete forms present in late childhood with recurrent or chronic respiratory infections, chronic viral disease, opportunistic infection, chronic lymphoma or the onset of autoimmune disease. T-cell disorders include *ataxia telangiectasia*, Wiskott–Aldrich syndrome and X-linked lymphoproliferative disease.

Common variable immunodeficiency (CVID) is characterised by impaired B-cell differentiation with defective immunoglobulin production. Features are chronic infections and susceptibility to lymphoma. CVID is a collection of hypogammaglobulinaemia syndromes associated with multiple genetic defects.

## Hepatic Encephalopathy

Toxins responsible for hepatic encephalopathy include ammonia, aromatic amino acids, mercaptans, short-chain fatty acids and endogenous benzodiazepines. The speed of onset of encephalopathy parallels that of the hepatic failure – from a matter of hours to slow progression over months. Hepatic foetor is the sickly sweet odour detectable in some. Delirium typically fluctuates; a flapping tremor of the hands (asterixis) occurs. Untreated delirium progresses to stupor, coma and death.

## Renal Disease

Kidneys and the nervous system are affected by vasculitides, connective tissue diseases, genetic disorders such as Fabry disease, Wilson's, von Hippel–Lindau (VHL) disease, infections and plasma cell dyscrasias.

### Uraemic Encephalopathy

With rapidly increasing uraemia, clouding of consciousness progresses to confusion and coma. A coarse irregular tremor with asterixis and a stimulus-sensitive multi-focal myoclonus with seizures can develop. Agitation with hallucinations sometimes supervenes before uraemic coma and respiratory arrest. Uraemic encephalopathy is generally reversible with treatment.

### Dialysis Encephalopathy

Dialysis encephalopathy (dialysis dementia) is the rare but potentially fatal condition that previously complicated chronic dialysis. This was caused by the aluminium in gels and dialysates. Purified dialysate has led to its disappearance. Long-term haemodialysis can also rarely lead to Wernicke's encephalopathy and sensorimotor axonal polyneuropathy.

### Dialysis Disequilibrium Syndrome

Changing osmotic gradients between plasma and brain during rapid dialysis causes nausea, visual blurring and headache – and later confusion, clouding of consciousness, seizures and tremor. Symptoms are usually mild and can be helped by slow flow rates during dialysis.

### Neuropathy Associated with Renal Disease

Uraemic neuropathy is a distal axonal degeneration with secondary myelin loss in chronic renal failure, usually reversible with treatment.

## Malabsorption

Malabsorption is the result of gluten sensitivity and many other conditions affecting the small bowel.

*Coeliac Disease*   Many neurological syndromes can occur with coeliac cases – epilepsy, myoclonus, cerebellar atrophy and ataxia, multifocal leukoencephalopathy, dementia and peripheral neuropathies, both axonal and demyelinating. Immunological mechanisms or trace vitamin deficiencies may underlie these associations. Neurological features can occur in the absence of overt coeliac disease, to be considered in cryptogenic ataxias and neuropathies (Chapter 17).

*Inflammatory Bowel Disease*   Both ulcerative colitis and Crohn's are associated, if rarely, with thromboembolic complications such as cerebral venous thrombosis and cord ischaemia. Scattered white matter lesions are seen on brain MRI more frequently than in controls. Inflammatory bowel disease is also associated with polyneuropathies and occasionally with dermatomyositis.

## Neurology and Transplantation

Many transplants now proceed without incident. Neurological problems relate to organ failure, immunosuppression/infection, allograft rejection, drugs and/or the surgical procedures.

Infections: the probability of infection depends on the degree of immunosuppression, exposure to pathogens and the time since transplantation. Opportunistic infections are covered in Chapter 9.

Seizures and encephalopathy: sepsis, drugs – ciclosporin and OKT3.

Stroke: underlying atheroma, bypass, air embolism, endocarditis and fungi.

Drugs: ciclosporin – tremor, headache and rarely posterior reversible leukoencephalopathy syndrome (PRES). OKT3, the murine E monoclonal – aseptic meningitis and encephalopathy. Tacrolimus – tremor.

Malignancy: intracerebral B-cell lymphoma and possibly *glioblastoma multiforme*. Previous EBV infection may be relevant.

Mononeuropathies and critical illness neuromyopathy: anaesthesia, surgery and ITU.

### Some Specific Complications

Kidney: cord ischaemia. The iliac artery is diverted for graft revascularisation – a particular hazard when there is an anomalous blood supply to the cord from the internal iliac rather than an intercostal artery.

Liver: encephalopathy. Previous liver damage, drugs, hypoxic–ischaemic injury and sepsis. Coagulopathy: haemorrhage.

Heart and lung: hypoxic-ischaemic brain injury.

Bone marrow: acute GvHD: within first 100 days – primarily affects skin, liver and gut. Chronic GvHD: >80 days. Vasculitis – scleroderma-like skin involvement, bronchiolitis, Sjögren's, myasthenia gravis, neuropathy and polymyositis – sometimes years later.

## Systemic Vasculitides and Related Disorders

Neurological sequelae are common, but apart from giant cell arteritis (GCA) and isolated cerebral angiitis (ICA), it is unusual for patients to present with solely neurological problems.

Cases divide into broad groups:

- Neurological problems develop because of increased disease activity.
- A specific nervous system complication develops that needs investigation, medical or surgical treatment – e.g. an entrapment neuropathy or cord compression in rheumatoid arthritis (RA).
- A problem may be iatrogenic – steroid myopathy, PRES with immunomodulation.
- A separate, often common condition – ischaemic stroke in SLE with hypertension and diabetes.

Vasculititides are classified by:

- predominant size and type of vessel
- granulomas
- antineutrophil cytoplasmic antibodies (ANCA). ANCA-positive vasculitides are granulomatosis with polyangiitis (GPA), microscopic polyangiitis (MPA) and eosinophilic granulomatosis with polyangiitis (EGPA), a.k.a. Churg–Strauss.

### Pathological Mechanisms

The final common pathway is ischaemic damage to neural tissue, usually permanent, typically with a necrotising arteritis and a transmural leucocyte infiltrate – a mixture of polymorphs, lymphocytes and eosinophils. Proportions, subtypes and behaviour of these cells vary, both within and across different vasculitides. Granulomas form in GPA and GCA.

Cell populations also vary with the lesion's age – neutrophils acutely, intimal proliferation and fibrosis later. All conspire to reduce blood flow. With an individual nerve, arteritis affects pre-capillary arteries. In the CNS, vessel calibre associates with disease type, but overlap is common.

Secondary thrombotic events can lead to distal embolism. However in some, damage follows thrombosis of arteries, capillaries or veins (see SLE).

### Polyarteritis Nodosa (PAN) and Microscopic Polyangiitis (MPA)

Polyarteritis nodosa (PAN), the prototype necrotising vasculitis, affects medium-sized arteries; microaneurysms form. A third with PAN are HbsAg-positive, but ANCA-negative.

A progressive painful mononeuritis multiplex occurs in about 50%. Encephalopathy, seizures, stroke, aseptic meningitis, ischaemic myelopathy and cranial nerves palsies can also develop.

MPA is related to PAN but ANCA-positive. A perinuclear (pANCA) pattern is associated with the myeloperoxidase antigen, and cytoplasmic (cANCA) pattern with the neutrophil enzyme proteinase 3. Both occur in MPA. RA and SLE can also be ANCA-positive. The neurology of MPA is similar to PAN.

### Granulomatosis with Polyangiitis (GPA)

There are respiratory tract granulomas – typically nasal mucosa, inner ear, lung and a necrotising glomerulonephritis. Skin and joint symptoms also occur. cANCA is usually present.

About one-third develop lesions in the nervous system:

- polyneuropathy/mononeuritis multiplex
- cranial neuropathy, +/− hearing loss
- ophthalmoplegia
- stroke
- seizures
- cerebritis.

### Giant Cell Arteritis (GCA)

GCA (temporal arteritis) is the commonest vasculitis, affecting those over 50 years almost exclusively, M>F. Typically, extracranial branches of the aorta are involved, rarely with intracranial involvement, probably because intracranial vessels lack the internal elastic lamina that is the focus of the inflammatory response.

Headache, unilateral with scalp tenderness, is the commonest complaint, but can be absent. Other symptoms include jaw claudication, and weight loss, malaise, fever and myalgia which are present in at least one-third. There is overlap with *polymyalgia rheumatica* (Chapter 10).

Blindness is the commonest serious sequel, with monocular, bilateral or rarely homonymous visual loss (Chapter 14). Monocular visual loss is caused by arteritis of the posterior ciliary arteries, leading to optic nerve head infarction. Sequential ischaemic optic neuropathies or even bilateral occipital infarction can follow. Strokes in MCA territory also occur, rarely.

Sometimes, an inflamed artery is cord-like and pulseless, such as a superficial temporal artery, a facial artery as it runs under the mandible and/or an occipital artery.

The ESR and the CRP are almost always raised. Anaemia is present in many, with leucocytosis and raised transaminases in one-third. Temporal artery biopsy is essential, if practicable, but often treatment must start without this confirmation – and skip lesions occur, so a normal biopsy does not absolutely rule out GCA. GCA should be treated with high dose steroids, though there is incomplete protection from ischaemic events.

### Isolated Cerebral Angiitis (ICA)

ICA, a.k.a. primary cerebral vasculitis, is rare. There are neither clues from other inflamed organs nor specific tests. There are three main patterns:

- an encephalopathy with headache, confusion and coma
- isolated or multiple intracranial mass lesions and/or of focal CNS signs, raised ICP
- MS-like, with a relapsing–remitting course, optic nerve involvement, sometimes with stroke-like episodes and seizures.

Brain MRI is abnormal in ICA but not pathognomonic. Brain (with meningeal) biopsy leads to a diagnosis in most. However, many biopsies for presumed ICA show an alternative pathology. Infection, lymphoma and MS are high on this list. Treatment: steroids and immunosuppression. Outcome: variable.

## Rheumatoid Arthritis (RA)

RA is the multi-system disorder usually presenting with a symmetrical distal polyarthropathy. Entrapment neuropathies are common. Cord or brainstem syndromes are secondary to erosion of the atlantoaxial, odontoid and other vertebrae and/or *pannus*. The cervical spine is most frequently affected, but extradural *pannus* can cause compression at any location, including *cauda equina* (Chapter 16). Aseptic rheumatoid meningitis also occurs, exceptionally.

## SLE and Mixed Connective Tissue Disease (MCTD)

Lupus is also a multi-system disorder. Antinuclear antibodies (ANAs) are often present but with a high false positive rate; more specific antibodies – double-stranded and single-stranded DNA – occur. CNS complications develop in about half, now labelled neuropsychiatric lupus (NPSLE). Strokes, seizures, frank psychosis, neuropathies, myopathy, and a relapsing MS-like condition certainly occur, but it is sometimes difficult to sort out the genuine complications of this serious disease.

Antiphospholipid antibodies tend to be associated with stroke in NPSLE. Anticardiolipin antibodies are more common in NPSLE than in pure SLE.

Mixed connective tissue disease (MCTD) is the rare disorder with features seen in SLE, scleroderma, polymyositis and RA. Some are positive for the U1-RNP antibody – associated with pulmonary hypertension, a serious complication.

## Antiphospholipid Syndrome

Antiphospholipid syndrome (APS) is characterised by thrombosis – venous, arterial or microvascular – with a heterogeneous group of antiphospholipid antibodies (aPL). Positive aPL implies one or more of these antibodies:

- lupus anticoagulant (LA) – prolongs *in vitro* phospholipid-dependent clotting assays
- anticardiolipin antibodies (aCL)
- anti-$\beta$2 glycoprotein-1 ($\beta$2-GPI) antibodies.

These antibodies also occur in other autoimmune disorders – SLE, RA, systemic sclerosis, Behçet's and Sjögren's; in lymphoproliferative disorders and some infections.

SLE: about one-third have aPL; of these, less than half will develop APS. aPL probably accounts for <10% of all cases of acute venous lower limb thromboembolism (VTE).

Many neurological syndromes have been described with aPL: an MS-like syndrome, migraine, cognitive impairment, epilepsy, psychiatric disorders and visual disturbances.

Catastrophic antiphospholipid syndrome (CAPS) is exceedingly rare but life threatening – sudden extensive microvascular thrombosis leading to multi-organ failure.

## Sjögren's Syndrome (SS)

In Sjögren's syndrome (SS), there is lymphocytic infiltrates and destruction of epithelial exocrine glands. The main symptoms are dry eyes (*keratoconjunctivitis sicca*) and dry mouth (*xerostomia*). Several types of neuropathy occur. The most common (c. 50%) is of an asymmetrical, segmental or multi-focal sensory distal neuropathy progressing to involve the trunk or face. A large proportion have a sensory ataxia, severe in some, with high signal in the cord posterior columns on T2W MRI. Neuropathic pain is sometimes prominent. Progression tends to be over years. Mononeuritis multiplex is less common.

Neuropathology indicates that the sensory–ataxic pattern is caused by a ganglioneuronitis – lymphocytic infiltration of dorsal root ganglia.

Cranial neuropathies in SS tend to be either a sensory neuropathy of the trigeminal nerve(s) without motor features or a cranial polyneuropathy. Hearing loss (VIII) may develop suddenly.

Autonomic features are frequently associated with SS: Holmes–Adie pupils, sweating and orthostatic hypotension are the commonest. A pure autonomic neuropathy also occurs. Many older patients diagnosed with SS turn out to have had a chronic neuropathy for years.

MS-like features can occur, with an optic neuropathy and cutaneous vasculitis. CNS involvement can be in many forms: meningoencephalitis, stroke-like episodes, intracerebral or subarachnoid haemorrhage, internuclear ophthalmoplegia, nystagmus, movement disorders, focal/generalised seizures and organic affective disorders. Cord involvement: an acute transverse myelitis or slow progression. MRI T2W changes can be indistinguishable from MS.

## Other Cerebral Arteriopathies

### CADASIL

CADASIL (cerebral AD arteriopathy with subcortical infarcts and leukoencephalopathy) is a disease of small vessels caused by mutations in the *notch 3* gene on chromosome 19q13. *Notch 3* is a gene coding for a transmembrane protein involved in intracellular signalling. Headaches and recurrent subcortical ischaemic strokes begin in mid-adult life. There is cognitive impairment, incoordination and progression to pseudobulbar palsy and subcortical dementia (Chapter 5). Prognosis: poor.

### CARASIL

CARASIL (cerebral AR arteriopathy with subcortical infarcts and leukoencephalopathy) is a rare small vessel disorder, affecting mainly Japanese. CARASIL is caused by mutations in the *HTRA1* gene encoding HtrA serine peptidase/protease 1. Progressive cognitive impairment and recurrent ischaemic subcortical strokes are typical. Other features include premature alopecia and low back pain, with disc herniation and/or *spondylosis deformans*.

### Fabry's Disease

Fabry's disease, the X-linked lysosomal storage disease, is mentioned in Chapters 6 and 19.

## Susac's Syndrome

Susac's is a rare microangiopathy, with a triad of encephalopathy, sensorineural hearing loss and retinal artery branch occlusion, seen largely in women. Prodromal headache can last for months before cognitive and psychiatric features, sometimes with seizures and myoclonus. Hearing loss is often acute and bilateral, suggesting infarction from occlusion of cochlear arteries. Fundoscopy: multiple branch retinal artery occlusions and a macular cherry red spot. MRI: multiple small high signal white matter lesions on T2W. Brain biopsy: microinfarcts with arteriolar occlusion. Treatment: uncertain – steroids, immunosuppression.

## Sneddon's Syndrome

Sneddon's syndrome is another rare disorder – recurrent strokes in young patients, often with a migraine history. There is *livedo reticularis* (a violaceous and net-like rash on limbs and trunk). Antiphospholipid antibodies and antiendothelial cell and antiprothrombin antibodies are sometimes found. Pathology: arteriopathy of small- and medium-sized vessels.

## Degos' Disease

Degos' disease is a multi-system small vessel occlusive arteriopathy. Ischaemic and haemorrhagic stroke can occur.

## Hereditary Angiopathy with Neuropathy, Aneurysms and Cramps (HANAC)

Mutation in the *COL4A1* gene that encodes type IV collagen alpha 1 chain, a crucial component of basement membranes, causes hereditary angiopathy with neuropathy, aneurysms and cramps. There is a diffuse leukoencephalopathy with intracranial aneurysms, cramps, polyneuropathy, retinal tortuosity, haemorrhage and optic nerve disease.

## Reversible Cerebral Vasoconstriction Syndrome (RCVS) and Posterior Reversible Encephalopathy Syndrome (PRES)

These serious conditions, possibly identical are mentioned in Chapter 6.

# Sarcoidosis

Sarcoidosis, the multi-system granulomatous disorder of unknown cause, affects the nervous system in some 5%. Its hallmarks are non-caseating epithelioid cell granulomas and fibrosis.

## Clinical Features

Sarcoid affects the lungs alone in 90% – this varies from asymptomatic bilateral hilar lymphadenopathy to severe interstitial lung disease. Other organs involved are the liver, heart, lymph nodes, skin, endocrine system and muscles.

Neurosarcoidosis (NS) carries a worse prognosis than pulmonary disease. The heart and eyes (Chapter 14) may be involved. In some with NS, the presenting features are neurological; in others, neurology develops later, but usually within 2 years. Chronic NS can cause cranial nerve palsies, aseptic meningitis, parenchymatous brain and cord lesions, hydrocephalus, encephalopathy, neuropathy and myopathy.

### Cranial Neuropathy

About half NS patients present with facial palsy, unilateral or bilateral. Optic neuropathy develops in over one-third and is often subacute. There may be anterior uveitis, disc swelling, optic atrophy and/or granulomatous infiltration of the optic nerve. Oculomotor palsies and bulbar weakness can occur. Deafness (VIII) can also follow.

### Peripheral Neuromuscular Sarcoid

This develops in about one-fifth of sarcoid cases. An isolated mononeuropathy or a mononeuritis multiplex occurs, with granulomatous vasculitis and/or compression from granulomas. Polyneuropathy develops. Muscle involvement is common, and often symptomless, but there can be acute or chronic myopathy with inflammation and occasionally palpable nodules.

### Meningeal and Parenchymatous NS

An aseptic meningitis can develop or occasionally a meningeal mass lesion. Parenchymal lesions are unusual. Pituitary and hypothalamic involvement can occur. At the base of the brain, infiltration can lead to hydrocephalus. CSF diversion procedures tend to fail. A chronic or relapsing sarcoid encephalopathy and, rarely, cerebral venous thrombosis can occur.

### Diagnosis and Prognosis

Diagnosis can be difficult. MRI – hyperintense lesions on T2W – is non-specific. CSF findings are also non-specific – a pleocytosis of up to 100 cells/mm$^3$, with elevated protein, usually <2 g/dL. Sometimes CSF glucose is low, and oligoclonal bands present. Muscle biopsy can be helpful: non-caseating granulomas are found in about a quarter. Biopsy of brain lesions and meninges is also sometimes helpful: non-caseating granulomatous changes are diagnostic. Generally, established NS is a serious disease. One third of neurosarcoid cases have progressive disease despite immunosuppression.

## Behçet's Syndrome

Behçet's is a multi-system disease – recurrent oral ulceration and two of the following: recurrent genital ulcers, skin lesions, ocular lesions and a positive pathergy test. Neurological features occur in <10% and fall into two patterns:

- Parenchymal CNS lesions, either relapsing-remittng or progressive, commonly affecting the brainstem.
- Cerebral venous sinus thrombosis (CVST).

## Pathergy Test

The forearm is pricked with a fine sterile needle. With a positive pathergy test, a small red bump at the site develops 1–2 days later – a largely lymphocytic reaction. Behçet's cases from the Mediterranean coastal region tend to have positive tests, around 50% from the Middle East and Japan but fewer from northern Europe. A positive test is thus not diagnostic.

### Treatment

Steroids and immunosuppressants are used.

# IgG4-Related Disease and CLIPPERS

IgG4-related disease is a fibroinflammation with tumour-like dense infiltrates rich in IgG4-positive plasma cells. Elevated serum IgG4 is found in most. Lesions can develop in most organs: pancreatitis and salivary gland disease are common. Neurology: lesions in the pituitary and meningeal masses. Some respond to steroids and immunosuppression.

Chronic lymphocytic inflammation with pontine perivascular enhancement responsive to steroids (CLIPPERS) is a rare inflammatory condition. MRI: nodular enhancement mainly in the pons and cerebellum with perivascular and parenchymal CD3+ T-cell infiltrate. Patients present with local brainstem signs, cranial nerve lesions, pyramidal signs and ataxia, without systemic involvement.

# Neurocutaneous Syndromes

Neurocutaneous syndromes (a.k.a. phakomatoses) are multi-system disorders with characteristic CNS and skin manifestations. The skin lesions are important pointers towards potential neurological complications.

## Neurofibromatosis Types 1 and 2

These are also mentioned in Chapter 21.

## Xeroderma Pigmentosum (XP)

Xeroderma pigmentosum (XP) is an uncommon AR disorder caused by mutations in nucleotide repair genes. There is severe solar sensitivity leading to basal and squamous cell carcinoma and melanomas beginning in early childhood. Ocular abnormalities include keratitis, corneal opacification, iritis and melanoma of the choroid. Many with XP have progressive cognitive and mobility problems.

## Tuberous Sclerosis (TS)

Tuberous sclerosis (TS) is characterised by multiple hamartomatous lesions which affect many organs – brain, skin, eye, kidney, heart and lung.

### Von Hippel–Lindau Disease (VHL)

VHL is an AD condition caused by a germline mutation in the *VHL* gene. Two forms are recognised depending on the risk of developing pheochromocytoma. Neurological involvement is characterised by the development of haemangioblastoma, particularly affecting the cerebellum, brainstem or cord, often at a young age.

### Ataxia Telangiectasia

*Ataxia telangiectasia* (Chapter 17) is an autosomal recessive ataxia caused by a gene mutation at 11q 22.3. Features: progressive cerebellar ataxia, conjunctival and skin telangiectasia, oculomotor apraxia and deficiencies of both cellular and humoral immunity with particular impairment of IgA and IgG. These cases can be wheelchair bound by the age of 12. Other features: recurrent infections, bronchiectasis, pulmonary fibrosis, lymphomas, acute leukaemia and diabetes mellitus.

### Sturge–Weber Syndrome

SW is characterised by a facial capillary malformation (port wine stain) and an associated capillary–venous malformation affecting the brain and the eye. Sturge–Weber syndrome can lead to seizures, associated with cortical malformations including polymicrogyria and cortical dysplasia; intellectual impairment; behavioural problems and focal signs caused by stroke-like episodes. Hydrocephalus can occur.

## Neurological Aspects of Pregnancy

### Epilepsy and Pregnancy

Fertility rates are low in women with treated epilepsy. Reasons include

- low rates of marriage/partnership and stigmatisation.
- avoidance of pregnancy – risk of epilepsy in offspring and teratogenic potential of drugs.
- one third of menstrual cycles in TLE cases are anovulatory (8% in controls).

Epilepsy is the commonest neurological condition that needs to be managed in an obstetric unit. The majority of such pregnancies proceed without incident.

#### Reducing Risks to Mother and Child

Ideally, drugs should be reviewed before conception is contemplated. It is important to establish whether antiepileptic drugs are needed at all. With tonic–clonic seizures, it is usual to continue therapy. However, some women with partial seizures elect to withdraw therapy. Conversely, others who are seizure free will choose to continue therapy because of the risks of seizure recurrence.

The small teratogenic risk of antiepileptic drugs needs to be discussed. In some, and because of this, it is even reasonable to withdraw therapy for the first half or whole of pregnancy – the teratogenic risks are greater in the first trimester, but the physical effects of seizures are greater in the later stages of pregnancy. These matters need to be assessed, and the decisions recorded.

### Teratogenicity and Antiepileptic Drugs

Many antiepileptic drugs are teratogenic, as is well known. However, some data are uncertain, and additional factors include:

- poor diet and poverty that increase the risk both of epilepsy and of malformations.
- seizures themselves may cause malformations – a small effect.

Of the drugs commonly used, carbamazepine, lamotrigine and levetiracetam probably carry a lower risk than valproate, barbiturates, phenytoin or topiramate.

*Major Malformations and Antiepileptic drugs*   The commoner malformations associated with antiepileptic drugs (phenytoin, phenobarbital, primidone, benzodiazepines, valproate, carbamazepine and topiramate) are cleft palate/lip, cardiac and neural tube defects, hypospadias and renal and skeletal abnormalities. Polytherapy carries higher risks than monotherapy.

Phenytoin as monotherapy has a relatively low incidence of major defects, though there is minute risk of neuroblastoma.

With spina bifida, the background population risk is 0.2–0.5%. Valproate is associated with a 1–2% risk, and carbamazepine a 0.5–1% risk.

*Other Abnormalities and Neurodevelopmental Delay*   In addition to major malformations, dysmorphic changes occur, a.k.a. foetal syndromes. The foetal phenytoin syndrome was the first described. However, most features are minor and overlap with normal variation.

Primidone, phenobarbital, carbamazepine and valproate syndromes have been described, and there are questions of developmental delay – a contentious field, confounded by opinion rather than firm evidence, and by litigation.

The effects of newer antiepileptic drugs have not been established. This does not imply safety. Major malformations were not noticed until the older drugs had been in use for decades, and negative results from mammals are not reliable indicators in *homo sapiens*.

### Antiepileptic Drugs During Pregnancy

If informed decision is to continue therapy, monotherapy is preferable. A few with severe epilepsy will need drug combinations. Drug levels should be monitored. In most, monotherapy with carbamazepine, lamotrigine or levetiracetam will be possible. Difficulties arise when seizures are best controlled by valproate, such as in idiopathic generalised epilepsy. Replacement of valproate with levetiracetam or another drug is sometimes recommended – usually a matter for specialist opinion.

Dosage increases of lamotrigine (and less so with carbamazepine, phenytoin and phenobarbital) may be needed: antiepileptic drug levels can fall in the second half of pregnancy. With lamotrigine, levels can drop rapidly – weekly blood levels are needed.

### Foetal Malformations: Screening

Over 90% of neural tube defects can be detected prenatally – such as, cleft palate, major cardiac and renal defects. It should be made clear that not all malformations are detectable even with sophisticated technology – ultrasound imaging, α-fetoprotein levels and amniocentesis. Therapeutic termination of pregnancy may be advised, on occasion, if this is acceptable.

*Folic Acid*   Folic acid supplementation is strongly recommended for all women who may become pregnant. The foetus of a mother with epilepsy is at a greater-than-expected risk of a neural tube defect, particularly if the mother is taking valproate. Folic acid has some protective effect.

### Pregnancy, Labour and Delivery

Epilepsy increases the risks of many pregnancy complications. Perinatal mortality is twice that of the general population. About 2% with active epilepsy have seizures during delivery. The foetal heart rate can slow dramatically with a maternal seizure. Obstetricians tend to recommend caesarean section. Home birth should not usually be contemplated.

Although epilepsy from other neurological disorders can be worsened, such as MS, AVMs and meningiomas, pregnancy has a little effect on seizure frequency in the majority.

Occasionally, presumably because of hormonal influence, some experience seizures exclusively during pregnancy (gestational epilepsy). Symptomatic epilepsy can present in pregnancy for various reasons – for example, the size of a meningioma can increase and thus cause epilepsy.

During labour, antiepileptic drugs must be continued. Any history of status is usually an indication for caesarean section. There is maternal and infant mortality with severe seizures during delivery. Maternal hypoxia with a seizure can be profound because of foetal oxygen demands.

### Eclampsia and Pre-Eclampsia

Many new-onset seizures after 20 weeks are the result of eclampsia. Pre-eclampsia causes hypertension, proteinuria, oedema and clotting changes. Some 5%, if untreated, progress to eclampsia. Eclamptic encephalopathy causes seizures, confusion, stupor, focal signs and cerebral haemorrhage. *Status epilepticus* can follow. The incidence in Europe is about 1/2000 pregnancies.

Magnesium sulphate has long been used to treat seizures in eclampsia and is superior to phenytoin and/or diazepam. The mechanism is unclear; magnesium may influence NMDA receptors or free radicals, prostacyclins or reverse intense eclamptic cerebral vasospasm.

In the latter stages of pregnancy, a convulsion can damage the placenta and/or the foetus, especially if the mother falls, but generally a single short-lived seizure is well tolerated. However, *status epilepticus* during pregnancy or delivery is hazardous, with a high infant and maternal mortality. Partial seizures have no known effects on a foetus.

HELLP is a serious if unusual complication, allied to eclampsia, described in 1982: haemolysis (H), elevated liver enzymes (EL) and low platelets (LP).

*Vitamin K and Antiepileptic Drugs*   Enzyme-inducing antiepileptic drugs can induce deficiency of infantile vitamin-K-dependent clotting factors (factors II, VII, IX and X) and protein C and S, predisposing to infantile haemorrhage. The newborn should receive vitamin K at birth and at 28 days. It is sometimes recommended that the mother take oral vitamin K in the last trimester. Fresh frozen plasma may be needed, if clotting factors fall greatly, or if there is neonatal bleeding – a matter for specialist advice.

***Post-Partum Period***   There is tendency for a slight increase in seizures within 6 weeks of delivery. Clobazam 10 mg for a few days after delivery is sometimes given. Drug levels should be monitored: with high maternal levels, an infant may be drowsy.

***Breastfeeding***   Concentrations of most antiepileptics in breast milk are <30% than in plasma, and the amount ingested by the baby is insignificant. However, lamotrigine, levetiracetam and phenobarbital require precautions. Phenobarbital can be a problem: in neonates, its half-life is long and the free fraction higher than in adults; neonatal levels can even exceed maternal levels.

***Maternal Epilepsy and an Infant***   A mother at a high risk of seizures should not be left alone with a small child, and sensible precautions should be taken – often easier to recommend than to follow. Post-partum seizures pose greater risks to infants than to the foetuses.

### Cerebral Ischaemia, Haemorrhage and Emboli

In pregnancy, there is a small increased risk of both ischaemic and haemorrhagic stroke. Ischaemic (arterial) stroke is most frequently in the middle cerebral artery territory. Occlusion of cortical veins or venous sinuses can also occur (Chapter 6). Both tend to occur towards the end of pregnancy or post-partum. With a cortical or venous sinus, thrombosis, headache and seizures can be prominent.

Cerebral haemorrhage can be caused by a pre-existing aneurysm or AVM. Pre-eclampsia and eclampsia are mentioned earlier.

Other rare causes of cerebrovascular events are cerebral angiitis and Moyamoya disease, Takayasu's arteritis, cardiac emboli, sickle cell disease, antiphospholipid antibody syndrome, deficiencies in antithrombin, proteases C and S, factor V Leiden and PRES/RCVS.

Amniotic fluid embolism causes encephalopathy, seizures and cardiovascular collapse during or immediately after labour and can lead to maternal and foetal death.

Air embolism: air enters the myometrium during delivery and then the venous circulation.

TTP is a rarity, usually of the second or third trimester: acute thrombocytopenia, microangiopathic haemolytic anaemia, fever and renal dysfunction. Neurology: headache, seizures and focal signs. PRES/RCVS (Chapter 6) may develop.

## Pregnancy and Other Neurological Conditions

### Pituitary Disorders

Pregnancy causes the pituitary to enlarge. Sheehan's syndrome is the rarity of maternal pituitary infarction +/−haemorrhage, following postpartum haemorrhage and hypotension, and/or the vascular demands of the pituitary exceeding its blood supply. This causes shock, +/− coma and acute pituitary insufficiency, a.k.a. pituitary apoplexy.

Lymphocytic hypophysitis, another rarity possibly autoimmune is usually self-limiting.

### Headache

The most common headache is tension-type headache. Migraine improves in many, presumably because of hormonal changes. If migraines require treatment, propranolol can be used; paracetamol is the safest analgesic. Triptans are not recommended. Ergotamine, seldom used today, is contraindicated. New onset headaches should be investigated and not ascribed to pregnancy.

### Neuromuscular Disorders

- Restless leg syndrome can occur during the third trimester. High-dose folic acid may help.
- Pregnancy has an unpredictable effect on myasthenia gravis.
- Bell's palsy is possibly more common in pregnancy and the puerperium than at other times.
- Carpal tunnel syndrome is common in the third trimester and typically resolves after delivery.
- *Meralgia paraesthetica* can occur late in pregnancy because of compression of the lateral cutaneous nerve of the thigh. It tends to improve following delivery.
- Gestational polyneuropathy – a rarity – follows nutritional deficiency from general malnourishment and/or *hyperemesis gravidarum*. Hyperemesis can exceptionally cause Wernicke's encephalopathy.
- A lumbosacral plexus neuropathy is usually caused by compression by the descending foetal head, by extrinsic neural compression (e.g. stirrup supports) or from ischaemia because of prolonged nerve stretching of the nerves during labour.
- A femoral neuropathy can also develop – quadriceps weakness with sparing of adduction.
- Peroneal nerve compression with typical foot drop can occur.
- Obturator neuropathy causes medial knee pain and adductor weakness.
- Sciatic nerve: compression can occur in the lithotomy position as the hip is flexed or by the foetal head near the sciatic notch.

Most peripheral nerve lesions improve and recover completely.

### Multiple Sclerosis

Unless there is severe disability, MS has no known effects on fertility, pregnancy, delivery, congenital malformations or perinatal death rates. Pregnancy affects neither relapse frequency nor disease progression.

### Chorea Gravidarum

*Chorea gravidarum* (CG) refers to chorea in pregnancy. It is uncommon and typically begins in the first trimester. About one-third have had rheumatic fever or previous Sydenham's chorea. CG probably follows reactivation of basal ganglia damage. CG can also be secondary to other causes of chorea such as lupus and Huntington's. In a mild case, the patient may be unaware of the involuntary movements. Symptoms generally resolve.

### Tumours

CNS malignancies develop no more commonly in pregnancy than at other times, but meningiomas present more often than expected, usually during late pregnancy – a presumed effect of oestrogen level changes. Gliomas and AVMs occasionally enlarge aggressively during pregnancy. Choriocarcinoma (Chapter 21), a malignancy seen in pregnancy, often metastasises to the brain. Pituitary adenomas are slightly more common in pregnancy; large tumours can cause visual failure.

### Idiopathic Intracranial Hypertension

Idiopathic intracranial hypertension can occur. Weight control is essential. A short course of corticosteroids is sometimes given and/or other measures (Chapter 14). Acetazolamide is best avoided – its teratogenicity is unknown.

### Regional Obstetric Anaesthesia

Systemic toxicity can cause hypotension, pruritus, nausea and vomiting.

Upward progression of the level of anaesthesia usually follows injection of anaesthesic intrathecally rather than into epidural space. A serious reaction can develop with hypotension. Hypoperfusion of the brainstem can cause respiratory depression. Dyspnoea can follow intercostal muscle, diaphragm and bulbar weakness.

Pneumocephalus: air is introduced intrathecally. This causes a severe headache.

Spinal epidural haematoma is a rarity but can occur with anticoagulants or coagulation disorders. Haematoma compresses nerve roots and/or the cord – a surgical emergency.

Post-spinal headache can follow dural puncture with CSF leakage.

Infection – epidural abscess and/or meningitis can follow epidural puncture. Pregnancy may predispose, if marginally, to most infections.

## Acknowledgements, References and Further Reading

I am most grateful to David Werring, Robin Howard and Simon Shorvon for their contribution to *Neurology A Queen Square Textbook* Second Edition on which this chapter is based.

Figures 26.1 and 26.2 are from Aminoff MJ, ed. *Neurology and General Medicine.* New York: Churchill Livingstone, 1992.With permission of Elsevier.

Aminoff MJ, Josephson SA. *Aminoff's Neurology and General Medicine*, 6th edn. Amsterdam: Academic Press, 2021.

Werring D, Howard R, Shorvon S. Systemic conditions and neurology. In *Neurology A Queen Square Textbook*, 2nd edn. Clarke C, Howard R, Rossor M, Shorvon S, eds. Chichester: John Wiley & Sons, 2016. There are numerous references.

Also, please visit https://www.drcharlesclarke.com for free updated notes, potential links and other references. You will be asked to log in, in a secure fashion, with your name and institution.

# Index

*Neurology: A Clinical Handbook*, First Edition. Charles Clarke.
© 2022 John Wiley & Sons Ltd. Published 2022 by John Wiley & Sons Ltd.